Introductory Linguistics for Speech and Language Therapy Practice

Jan McAllister
Senior Lecturer, University of East Anglia

Jim Miller
Emeritus Professor, University of Edinburgh

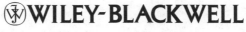

WILEY-BLACKWELL

A John Wiley & Sons, Ltd., Publication

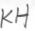

Contents

1 Introduction

This book is a practical introduction to the aspects of linguistics that generalist speech and language therapists (SLTs) need to understand in order to be able to use the published tools that are available for analysing clients' language abilities. Linguistics is the study of the organising principles of language. It is concerned with language in general, not with specific languages, although from a practical point of view we may wish to apply the principles to a particular language (here, English).

If you are reading this book you are probably interested in Speech and Language Therapy. Perhaps you are studying on a degree course leading to registration as an SLT – if so, one would certainly <u>hope</u> that you are interested in Speech and Language Therapy! Or perhaps you are considering enrolling on such a degree, or are a qualified SLT already but want to brush up on your language analysis skills. Whatever your interest, read on!

1.0 Why do speech and language therapy students need to study linguistics?

We said in the previous section that this book was about linguistics, but some students seem to wonder why, when they have enrolled on a degree in Speech and Language Therapy, they need to spend time studying linguistics, which is, after all, a separate academic discipline which can be studied to degree level in its own right. A short answer to this question is that professional bodies say that students need this knowledge. The Royal College of Speech and Language Therapists (RCSLT), which is the professional body that provides leadership and sets professional standards for SLTs in the United Kingdom, produces curriculum guidelines that specify the knowledge bases that speech and language therapists must acquire before registration, and one academic discipline that they stipulate is general linguistics. This is in addition to the related subjects of phonetics, psycholinguistics, sociolinguistics, bilingualism and language development.

The RCSLT curriculum guidelines are drawing attention to the fact that linguistics is one of the key underpinning disciplines of Speech and Language Therapy, alongside

Introductory Linguistics for Speech and Language Therapy Practice, First Edition. Jan McAllister and Jim Miller.
© 2013 John Wiley & Sons, Ltd. Published 2013 by John Wiley & Sons, Ltd.

subjects like anatomy and physiology, psychology and sociology. A newly qualified speech and language therapist who had not mastered these different disciplines to the required level would struggle to carry out their role.[1] Understanding the structure and function of language systems is as fundamental to the job of an SLT as understanding the structure of the human body is to the job of a doctor. It would be strange, not to say worrying, to be treated by a doctor who did not know about the structure or function of the human body, and it would be just as strange and worrying to be treated by an SLT who did not know about the structure and function of language.

1.1   Why do speech and language therapy students need this book?

Learning linguistics in the context of a Speech and Language Therapy degree presents various challenges. Like most students entering higher education today, those studying Speech and Language Therapy typically arrive with little prior knowledge of linguistics or even basic grammar. Many 'introductory' texts assume that students already have an accurate understanding of, for example, part-of-speech labels, but for many, this is not the case. Also, though a practical understanding of linguistics is fundamental to Speech and Language Therapy practice, it competes for space in the curriculum with the other knowledge bases that students need to acquire during their degree (life sciences, clinical skills, etc.). Given that they must acquire quite sophisticated linguistic knowledge in a very limited time, students need to focus on just those aspects of linguistics that they will need to master in order to be able to carry out their clinical work, rather than equally interesting but less relevant topics that are covered in many introductory linguistics texts, such as language evolution, historical linguistics or non-human communication.

There are some texts that omit these peripheral subjects and just focus specifically on the core areas of linguistics. These are typically written for students on linguistics degree courses or people with an interest in linguistics *per se*, rather than as one of several disciplines underpinning their main focus of study. As such, they usually provide more detail than is strictly necessary for an introductory text for SLTs, often illustrating them with examples from a wide range of languages. This is not to say that the material covered in these texts is not interesting and important in its own right; this approach is appropriate where the aim is to provide a wide-ranging and in-depth understanding of the subject.

But the needs of students on Speech and Language Therapy courses are different. A comparison of core linguistics texts with assessments and other clinical resources that are routinely used by SLTs shows that the latter focus on only a subset of

---

[1]Admittedly, the remit of specialist SLT posts may involve tightly focused areas that do not require linguistic analysis skills. Specialisms in dysphagia or motor speech disorders are two areas that spring to mind. But SLTs who occupy such posts generally only do so after working for some time as a generalist, using the wider spectrum of SLT skills.

the structures and concepts covered in the former. Most of these resources also focus on the English language; whilst we acknowledge that many SLTs work in multicultural and multilinguistic settings, the one language that students on UK speech and language therapy courses absolutely must be able to describe is English. Given the limited amount of time that students of speech and language therapy have to devote to the linguistics strand of their degree, they need a text that will focus tightly on the core structures that are examined in the most commonly used clinical resources, and for students graduating in the United Kingdom, the language that they most need to know about is English.

1.2   Aims of this book, and what this book will *not* aim to do

The aim of the book will therefore be to provide the student with a practical introduction to those core linguistic concepts that are most often the subject of clinical resources and to illustrate these concepts with examples from English. As an introductory text with this applied aim, it will avoid reference to formal linguistic models and engagement with current controversies in the field of linguistics. By introducing the concepts and terminology of traditional linguistic description alongside those employed within speech and language therapy (where these differ), it will enable students to explore the subject in more detail using more advanced texts.

The book will focus on the core areas of (to use traditional linguistic terminology) morphology, syntax, semantics, discourse and pragmatics. It will not attempt to cover phonology, which is traditionally considered part of 'speech' rather than 'language' by SLTs.[2] Similarly, we will not attempt to provide in-depth coverage of any psycholinguistic or sociolinguistic concepts, although we will refer to concepts from these fields where necessary to elucidate relevant material. It is beyond the scope of the book to analyse languages other than English, and such topics can be dealt with more effectively in more specialised texts.

The focus of this book is the techniques of core linguistics that are needed to carry out analysis of disordered language, rather than the products of such analysis. The latter is the province of clinical linguistics, and the interested reader is referred to the further reading list at the end of this chapter. This decision has motivated the choice of language data that we analyse in this book. For example, occasionally in exercises we have used picture materials to generate extended pieces of language for analysis. For the reasons just stated, we have deliberately not attempted to reproduce the kinds of disordered samples that SLT clients would be likely to produce in response

---

[2]Phonology is a linguistic system just as much as morphology, syntax and the other topics that we will cover. We note that in the RCSLT Curriculum Guidelines published in 2010, phonology is listed under General Linguistics, and that it is an area assessed in the CELF-4; but, for example, phonology is grouped with 'articulation' rather than 'language' in the RCSLT Clinical Guidelines (Section 5.3). It is not possible to cover phonology without first providing at least an outline account of phonetics; so inclusion of phonology would increase the size of the text considerably. So although phonology is certainly part of theoretical linguistics, we decided, in the interests of keeping the text to a manageable size, to exclude this topic.

to such materials. Instead, we have chosen to illustrate the concepts that we are trying to impart by using examples from non-disordered language, reasoning that this is appropriate for an introductory linguistics text. Once readers have acquired these concepts, they are in a position to understand texts that focus on disordered samples.

Many of the examples that we have used are modelled on those found in clinical resources. We have avoided directly quoting the resources themselves because of copyright restrictions. It should be borne in mind that the specific examples used in the clinical resources have been validated using normative data; our examples, though they imitate the structure of these resources, have not been normed in this way.

Linguistics is a huge subject area, and as we noted earlier, introductory texts cover a great deal that is not directly relevant to speech and language therapy. In choosing which topics to cover in this text, we have been guided by the concepts that are addressed in speech and language therapy resources. Where we judged it necessary, we have explored additional topics that are not directly addressed in clinical resources, to provide relevant background to those topics that are addressed, or to set them in a wider context.

We recognise that there is a great deal more to communication than we will aim to cover in this text. Particularly when language is disrupted, non-verbal means of communication such as gesture are potentially extremely important, both to the client, and from a professional point of view, to the SLT. But we are concerned here with language, not communication. Communication is a means of conveying meaning (social, emotional, transactional, informational, etc.) between individuals. Language is one form of communication, albeit a highly intricate form that is characterised by a large number of complex rules.

This book will not attempt to impart any clinical knowledge at all. In particular, it will not try to teach students how to administer, score or interpret specific assessments or use therapy materials. For this, students must use the guidance of their clinical educators and the manuals that are provided with clinical resources.

1.3   Some preliminaries

We will continue this chapter by noting a few fundamental assumptions that should be stated explicitly before we begin.

A first observation concerns the notion of 'standard English'. Our main focus here is core linguistics, and we are using data modelled on the material that will be encountered in the widely available clinical resources that SLTs use. In these resources, target items are almost always framed in terms of a notional 'standard English' – the variety of English that is considered not to contain particular dialectal variants. It is obviously of great importance that students of Speech and Language Therapy should acquire theoretical concepts and practical knowledge and skills relevant to language variation, and indeed sociolinguistics, whose province these concepts are, is a curriculum requirement for Speech and Language Therapy courses. It is not, however, the topic of this book. The core linguistic concepts that we wish to elucidate here can perfectly well be illustrated using standard English, and that is what we will do. But readers should not conclude that this is the whole story.

Clinically, it is important to distinguish between the **processing** (mental operations) involved in **receptive** language (**comprehension**) and **expressive** language (**production**). Although students need to understand the psycholinguistic frameworks that differentiate these activities, the descriptive linguistic frameworks that are relevant are common to them both. Similarly, we are mainly focusing on aspects of language that are common to both the spoken and written forms.

We should also draw the distinction between **competence**, the body of abstract knowledge that a speaker has about the way that language works, and **performance**, the way that a piece of language is produced on a particular occasion, when it is subject to competing processing demands, limitation of resources such as working memory and so on. Our goal here is to provide a background to enable the reader to understand the model of competence that is encapsulated in the resources that SLTs use.

1.3.1   Levels of description in language

Having set out the scope of this book, we now turn to a preliminary discussion of the way that a subject as broad as language can be split into manageable components.

1.3.1.1   Three aspects of language

We suggested earlier that language, as one form of communication, was a means of conveying meaning. In fact, it is useful to distinguish at least three aspects of language of which meaning is just one. Let us start by cutting the linguistic cake three ways. We can think of language as involving **meaning, form** and **function** (alternatively, **meaning, form** and **use**).

Many words in English have more than one **meaning**. This ambiguity is the source of many children's jokes: *Why wouldn't the elephant travel by train? – Because his trunk wouldn't fit in the luggage rack*; *Why do you always stand on a chair when you sing? – So that I can reach the high notes.*

The **form** dimension involves what words or sentences look or sound like. If the form of a word is disrupted, it may be mispronounced or misspelt. Sentence form may be disrupted by words being used in the wrong order. Think of the way that the Star Wars character Yoda speaks: he consistently produces utterances that violate the standard form of English, saying things like *Take you to him I will*, or *Help you I can*. His meaning is clear, but there is no denying that his form is non-standard.

A speaker may select words with the meaning that they want to convey and pronounce all the words correctly and in the right order, with nothing omitted, and yet the utterance may still be put to an inappropriate **use** or may be interpreted by the listener as having a **function** other than the one that the speaker intends. Misuse of function often occurs in comedy. In the US sitcom 'The Big Bang Theory', one of the characters, Sheldon, is very brainy but struggles with many social conventions including the interpretation of sarcasm. On one occasion he irritates his neighbour, Penny, in several ways including claiming that she snores. 'You might want to see an otolaryngologist', says Sheldon, then realising that she does not know what that word means, adds '. . . a throat doctor'. Penny replies, 'What kind of doctor removes shoes from asses?', to which Sheldon helpfully responds 'Depending on the depth, that's either a proctologist or a general surgeon'. There is no problem here with the meanings of the individual words, or with the form of the words or the sentences. Instead, Sheldon interprets Penny's utterance as a request for information, rather than recognising its intended function, namely a threat. One could argue that this example is about the 'meaning' of Penny's utterance, but it is not 'meaning' in the same sense as was being used earlier with the children's joke examples, where the alternative meanings of *trunk* or *high* could be found in a dictionary. In the Sheldon/Penny example, there is no dictionary where we can look up the appropriate interpretation of Penny's utterance – it is all down to the context in which the utterance occurs and Sheldon's failure to recognise the absurdity of having a doctor whose role is to remove shoes from asses.

These are light-hearted examples, but the three-way distinction between meaning, form and function has a serious point in the context of speech and language therapy, because each of these dimensions can be separately affected in clients with language problems. An example of a clinical problem with meaning might occur when a client is unable to select a word with the intended meaning but selects a meaning-related word instead, such as saying *son* for *daughter*. Clients present with various types of problem with form, from difficulties with articulating speech sounds to omission of words or parts of words (e.g. saying *I go now* instead of *I am going now*) or putting words in the wrong order (e.g. *What you are doing?* instead of *What are you doing?*). A client may correctly interpret the form and word-by-word meaning of *Who do you think you're looking at?* but not realise that it functions as a threat.

Exercise 1.1

Discuss these examples in terms of meaning, form and function/use:

Stan: I've got free tickets for the new James Bond movie – would you like to
    come?
Archie: Is the Pope a Catholic?

The former President of the United States, George W. Bush, was often satirised for errors that he made when speaking in public. On one occasion he complained about 'rumours on the Internets'.

Someone intends to say 'Atlas carried the world on his shoulders' but says instead 'Atlas carried the world on his elbows'.

1.3.1.2   A more detailed characterisation of language

The meaning/form/function characterisation of language is useful, but it is not fine-grained enough for all purposes. Linguists identify a larger number of dimensions to language and these dimensions are also recognised in the literature and clinical resources that SLTs use, though the labels that are used sometimes vary. The following are the main elements of the language system as they are conceptualised in this approach:

- **Phonetics**: the physical characteristics of the sounds that are used in language.
- **Phonology**: the sound system of the language.
- **Prosody**: This refers to the sound level of language, and it is related to both phonetics and phonology, but it refers to aspects such as intonation, the 'melody' of spoken language, and stress pattern. For example, the word *trusty* meaning 'able to be trusted' is stressed on the first syllable, while *trustee* meaning 'official of a trust' is stressed on the second syllable but is pronounced in exactly the same way in other respects.
- **Lexicon**: The store of words that the person knows. For each word that a person knows, specifications of the meaning, pronunciation, spelling and grammatical properties are stored in the lexicon.
- **Morphology**: This level of representation is concerned with the internal structure of words. The basic units of morphology are called **morphemes**. Our knowledge of the morphology of English tells us that the word *clinical* consists of two morphemes, *clinic* and *-al*, and that these two elements must occur in this order; it also tells us that the word *clinical* is related to the words *clinic* and *clinician*. It also allows us to work out the meanings of new words that we have not encountered before, that are made up of morphemes that we already know. For example, the term *Bushisms* was coined to refer to the speech errors produced by George W. Bush, making use of three existing morphemes combined in a way that allowed people who had never seen the word before to work out what it meant.
- **Syntax**: This level is concerned with the way that words are combined to produce phrases (e.g. *a whale*), phrases are combined to produce clauses (e.g. *a whale is a mammal*) and clauses are combined to produce sentences (e.g. *A shark is a fish but a whale is a mammal*). It tells us that *The nurses are going on strike* is a permissible sentence of English but that randomly ordering the words to say *Nurses the on going are strike* is not. It also tells us when the use of particular form of a word is dictated by features of another word in the sentence, so that we can recognise that **The nurse are going on strike* contains an error (and how to fix it). Note that in the previous example we have adopted the convention of indicating an unacceptable form by placing an asterisk before it.
- **Semantics**: This system is concerned with the meaning of individual words, phrases and sentences. Our knowledge of semantics tells us, among other things, that *walk*, *skip* and *run* are words related in meaning, that *big* and *small* have opposite meanings, and that *Eric is taller than Iain* cannot be true at the same time as *Iain is taller than Eric*, if *Iain* and *Eric* refer to the same entities in both sentences.

- **Discourse**: This term is used in various disciplines that focus on language, but here it is used to explain the way that longer sequences of sentences, such as paragraphs, are structured. For example, in paragraphs it is unusual to continue to refer to individuals by their full name after they have first been mentioned; in subsequent sentences we might use *he* or *she*. In SLT, the term **narrative** is often used when we are concerned with longer sequences of sentences.
- **Pragmatics**: This label is given to a wide range of phenomena that relate to language in use. It includes language function as discussed in the previous section, and this aspect of pragmatics explains the way that we use language to make jokes, be sarcastic, pay a compliment, apologise and so on. It is also concerned with the rules of conversation.

In addition, we could identify **orthography**, the spelling system of the written language. Though many of the aspects of language that we will consider in this book are common to its spoken and written forms, there are some instances where the two differ, and we will identify these as we go along.

Exercise 1.2

Use the terms that we have just introduced to comment on the following examples:

An advertisement of a Mazda car (with a picture of a car parked on the driveway leading to a large mansion): 'The perfect car for a long drive'.

George W. Bush, who was mentioned earlier, claimed soon after his election that 'They misunderestimated me'.

Two more Bushisms: 'Rarely is the question asked "is our children learning?" '; 'The literacy level of our children are appalling'.

Judy is sitting in the living room huddled in front of the fire when Howard walks in and sits down, leaving the door wide open. Judy says 'Were you born in a barn?' Howard gets up and closes the door.

1.4   How this book is organised

Each chapter will provide an introduction to a specific area of linguistic description that is relevant to the work of a generalist SLT. Chapter 2 will consider the issues relevant to evaluating processing of words and non-words. Chapters 3 and 4 look at semantics, at the word and sentence levels, respectively. Chapter 5 takes a preliminary look at parts of speech. Chapter 6 considers some relevant aspects of morphology (word structure). Chapters 7 to 10 are concerned with syntax (sentence structure). Chapters 11 to 13 are concerned with pragmatics (language in use). Chapters 14 to 16 look at the issues relevant to analyses of discourse or narratives – extended pieces of language.

1.5   Exercises

The text of each chapter is interspersed with practical exercises to help readers to consolidate their learning. At the end of each chapter is a set of exercises that draw on clinical resources (assessments and therapy packages) that readers may be able to access. We also constantly refer to such resources during chapters to show readers that the concepts that we are presenting are relevant to clinical practice. Because many resources have long and complicated names, clinicians tend to refer to them by abbreviations, and where such abbreviations are widely used, we have employed them in the chapter as well. In case students are unfamiliar with them, at the start of each of the following chapters we have listed in full the names of all the resources that we will reference in that chapter, along with abbreviations where appropriate. Full details of the resources that we have referenced are in Appendix B.

Exercises using clinical assessments

1.3. The Children's Communication Checklist (CCC-2) is a parent-completed screening instrument that is used to help the clinician to identify areas that need further investigation. Have a look at the following items in the response booklet: 12, 15, 19, 36, 43, 54, 55. Which of the areas listed below do they address (a single item may address more than one)?
   - Lexicon
   - Morphology
   - Syntax
   - Semantics
   - Pragmatics

1.4. For each of the areas identified in your answer to the previous question, identify an assessment that explores that area in more detail.

Further reading

Introductory text for psycholinguistic topics that will not be covered in detail in this book: Fernandez and Cairns (2011).

To get a feel for the field of Clinical Linguistics, consult the journal *Clinical Linguistics* or the textbook of the same name by Cummings (2008).

2   Words and Non-words

2.0   Introduction

Most native speakers of English, if asked 'what are the basic units of language?', would probably say 'words'. Certainly individual words can be used to great communicative effect. Think of the first utterances of small children, which always consist of single words – 'More!', 'No!' or 'Juice!'; despite being so rudimentary, they communicate their message in a very direct way.

In this chapter we will explore the factors that are relevant to the clinical evaluation of a client's knowledge of words. Although we suggested in the previous chapter that we would be focusing on clinically relevant aspects of linguistics and in general ignoring other related topics that are often covered in introductory linguistics texts,

Introductory Linguistics for Speech and Language Therapy Practice, First Edition. Jan McAllister and Jim Miller.
© 2013 John Wiley & Sons, Ltd. Published 2013 by John Wiley & Sons, Ltd.

the factors that are relevant to a discussion of the word knowledge are just as much the province of psycholinguistics, and we will touch on some relevant background to this subject to clarify our discussion. In the interests of brevity, it will not be possible to explore the psycholinguistic background in any detail, but more comprehensive references are signposted at the end of the chapter.

We will also explore some of the kinds of resources that use words and word-like items – non-words. These kinds of materials are sometimes used as measures of language development, because a child's ability to repeat such items is a useful index of language difficulties. Because some of the same linguistic and psycholinguistic principles apply to both kinds of resource (those that target vocabulary knowledge and those that target repetition as an index of language development) it is appropriate to explore them together in this chapter.

An important aspect of our knowledge of words is our understanding of their meanings. Models of word processing take meaning into account alongside other factors that will be considered in this chapter, but within linguistics as well as psycholinguistics a distinction is drawn between meaning and other factors. Since we will be considering word meanings in the next chapter, this aspect of word knowledge will not be considered in detail in this chapter. Here, we will focus on other factors that are relevant to the processing (production/expression and reception/comprehension) of words, and that sometimes motivate the selection of items in clinical resources.

2.1   Why do SLTs need this knowledge?

Suppose that you have a client with aphasia who has word finding difficulties. Perhaps they can produce certain words but struggle to produce others. Are there principles that can help you to predict what kinds of words are likely to be easier to produce and which will be more difficult? Or consider a 4-year-old girl with language delay; given her age, what words might you expect her to know?

The programme overview of the Vocabulary Enrichment Intervention Programme summarises the importance of this aspect of the language system for children and adolescents. During the school years, children are exposed to tens of thousands of new words. Vocabulary abilities are key to the development of literacy and other language skills. A rich vocabulary improves access to the school curriculum and promotes academic achievement. Children's vocabulary knowledge is one of the best predictors of the likelihood of escaping the adverse impact of social deprivation early in life. Difficulties with vocabulary are among the most significant problems for children with speech, language and communication needs. Fortunately, this is an area that responds well to direct intervention.

There are many clinical resources that have been designed for assessing vocabulary knowledge and carrying out relevant interventions. If you can identify the principles that typically motivate the design of these resources, it will enhance your understanding of them. The resources cover several hundred lexical items in total, which may seem like a respectable quantity. But this is probably only a small fraction of the number of words that a typical mature native speaker knows. Clinicians will frequently need to supplement intervention materials with items that they generate themselves, and they need to be aware of the relevant considerations when doing so. Finally, although standardised, norm-referenced resources are generally used for assessment, to some extent materials for intervention may need to be devised or adapted to suit a particular client. For example, a person with aphasia whose hobby is gardening may want to access one set of vocabulary items; another person whose hobby is photography may want to access another. But when designing such customised sets of vocabulary, it is as well to bear in mind the factors that we introduce here.

Also, as noted earlier, poor ability to repeat words and non-words is considered by many researchers to be a useful index of language difficulty. Some assessments focus on this ability, and in order to use and interpret these resources correctly, clinicians need to understand the linguistic and psycholinguistic principles that underpin them.

2.2   Learning objectives

After reading this chapter and doing the exercises listed at the end, you should be able to:

* Explain the difference between lexemes and word-forms;
* Describe some tasks that clinicians commonly use to investigate clients' ability to use words;
* Outline some of the lexical characteristics that are relevant when creating materials for use in such tasks;
* List some resources that can help you to create such materials;
* Explain why non-words are often used in clinical resources;
* Identify items in clinical resources that exemplify the concepts covered in the chapter.

2.3   Words, word-forms and lexemes

The remarks that we made in the introduction assume a common understanding of what we mean when we refer to a *word*. For example, if we asked how many words are in the sentence

The Big Bad Wolf ate two of the pigs but the third pig got away.

most readers would say that there are 15. This reflects the fact that speakers' informal definition of *word* includes the knowledge that, in continuous text, words are the elements that are separated by spaces (though in spoken language we do not typically pause between words).

Suppose, however, that we are trying to make a list of the words that a child knows based on a recording of their interaction during play, and the utterance above was one of the ones that we recorded. In this context would we want to count *pig* and *pigs* as two different words? It depends on exactly what theoretical or clinical question we were trying to answer, but if what we really wanted to know about was the number of items in the child's vocabulary, we would probably not count them as different words. We would want to treat the list of words that the child knew as a sort of dictionary or lexicon; indeed, we refer to this list of the words that a person knows as the **mental lexicon**. Just as, in a real dictionary, we would not expect separate entries for *pig* and *pigs*, we would not count them as separate 'words' in this second sense either.

To clarify the distinction between these different senses of *word*, linguists use different terms to refer to them. A word in the 'dictionary entry' sense is termed a **lexeme**; the *lex-* part indicates 'word' (as it does in the word *lexicon*) while the *-eme* part is found in many linguistic labels (e.g. *phoneme, morpheme*) and indicates a unit of analysis. For the example we are discussing, linguists would say that there are at least two different **grammatical word-forms** (*pig* and *pigs*) and both associated with the same **lexeme**, PIG. Notice that by convention the grammatical word-forms are written in italics and the lexeme in capitals. Though SLTs would not necessarily use these terms, it is useful to be aware of the distinction, partly because it will deepen your own understanding of the concepts around word knowledge, but also for purposes of further reading in this book and elsewhere. We will, however, continue to use the term *word* unless it is useful to make more precise distinctions. In the first part of this chapter, we are mainly concerned with the lexemes that individuals know, rather than the word-forms, although we will need to refer to this distinction again later.

We have already introduced the concept of the mental lexicon, the store of words that an individual knows. It is worth saying a little more about what the mental lexicon contains. Most of the entries in the mental lexicon relate to what we would conventionally call a single word. But the mental lexicon may contain other kinds of unit as well. Occasionally phrases or even whole sentences may be stored, in cases where the group of words has a unitary, idiosyncratic meaning such as occurs in **idioms** like *under the weather* or fixed word combinations like *cold call*. The meaning of forms like this must be stored because if they were analysed by our normal phrase- and sentence-processing mechanisms, an incorrect interpretation would result. The fact that such forms are stored as unitary entities is also clear from the fact that we cannot alter them; for example, a native speaker of English would not say that someone was *beneath the weather* or *below the weather*, even though *beneath* and *below* mean roughly the same as *under*. Therefore idioms or other fixed word combinations are stored in their entirety. But usually we do not store the meanings of phrases and sentences; we work out the meaning of each one afresh when we encounter it, as we discussed in Chapter 1 and will explore in detail in later chapters.

2.4   Testing word processing and related abilities

As we noted in Chapter 1, in this book we are not attempting to explain how to conduct clinical assessments or carry out interventions; our goal is to help you to understand the linguistic structures and concepts that are addressed in these clinical resources. Nonetheless, it is useful to refer to the kinds of tasks that are used clinically, to make the subsequent discussion in this chapter less abstract. We do not attempt here to give a comprehensive picture of the range of tasks that clinicians use, but if you look at the resources that we cite in this and other chapters, you will gain an overview of them.

Some of the most commonly used methods for assessing a client's ability to produce and recognise words involve pictures (or sometimes video, particularly if the words of interest refer to actions rather than objects). To assess expressive abilities, **naming** (or **confrontation naming**) tasks are used; here the client is shown a series of pictures like the ones shown in Figure 2.1, and is asked to name each one. Examples of this kind of expressive test are the Renfrew Word Finding Vocabulary Test and the Expressive Vocabulary subtest of the CELF-4. Alternatively, a person may be asked to read aloud a printed word. This is also sometimes referred to as (word) naming.

To test receptive abilities, **picture selection** is often used; here, a set of pictures is presented simultaneously and the task is to choose one in response to an instruction.

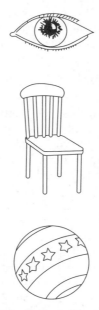

Figure 2.1   Confrontation naming. Adapted from Snodgrass and Vanderwart (1980). © American Psychological Association.

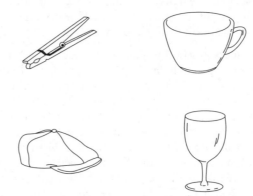

Figure 2.2 Picture selection. Adapted from Snodgrass and Vanderwart (1980). © American Psychological Association.

The clinician says (or writes, or signs) the **target** word, and the client's task is to select it (e.g. point to it) while ignoring the other items (the **distractors**). In the set of pictures in Figure 2.2, if the picture of the cup was the target, the distractors would be the glass, the cap and the peg. The PPVT and the BPVS are examples of this kind of test.

A third kind of task that is used is **repetition**. Such tasks may involve words, non-words, sentences or other sequences, though we are particularly interested in the first two kinds of item in this chapter. As was noted earlier, the ability to perform such repetition accurately is a good index of language development and processing ability. Examples of clinical instruments that use repetition are the ERB and the CAT.

2.5 Principles of selection of items in clinical resources

Only a few of the resources that clinicians use to work on lexical knowledge give an explicit account of the factors that motivated their choice of word items. Here, we will consider the sorts of factors that are relevant.

For picture- or video-based tasks, an obvious requirement is that it should be possible to illustrate the target word in some way. It is much easier to provide a picture that will reliably elicit the response *car*, for example, than, say, *fact* or *way*. Some words, for example *the* or *for*, are probably impossible to illustrate.

Another factor that could be relevant is how early in life a word is typically learned. This is obviously the case for paediatric assessments that require young children to produce a spoken response. It would be unreasonable to expect most 2-year-olds to know the word *system*, for example. A related issue is how early the sounds in the word are acquired, or how easy it is for a young child to produce a particular sequence of sounds, such as the consonant sequence at the start of the word *straw*. A proper understanding of these factors requires a knowledge of phonology, which is beyond the scope of this book, but see further reading at the end of this chapter.

A further factor that seems to be implicit in item selection in many resources is familiarity; it seems obvious that a client will not be able to produce or understand a word that is unfamiliar to them. Unfortunately for anyone who aims to produce an assessment that can be used by a wide range of people, familiarity is a very individual characteristic. For example, a child who takes part in cooking activities at home might know the names of kitchen implements such as *colander* or *spatula* that are unfamiliar to some other children of the same age. A word that is very familiar to a lawyer, such as *tort*, may be unfamiliar to the average person. Nonetheless, as mature speakers we feel that we have an intuitive knowledge about what words are likely to be familiar to the majority of other speakers (though this knowledge is inevitably coloured by our own lexical experience). So writers of assessments often seem to make a guess at which items are likely to be familiar to their target user group.

Occasionally, assessment manuals provide explicit information about the factors that were involved in the choice of the items used. Examples of assessments that do so are the ERB, a paediatric assessment which includes a test of word and non-word repetition, and the VAN[1] which focuses on word-finding ability. It would be instructive to read the manuals for these assessments, since they discuss several characteristics that have been controlled in their design and which are known to influence lexical processing. Some of the factors that they have taken into account are outlined below. When generating your own intervention materials, it is appropriate to bear these factors in mind.

Imageability: This characteristic is related to the idea that was mentioned earlier that it should be possible to illustrate the objects, actions, etc., that are referred to by words used in tests. Imageability is, however, a broader, meaning-based concept that refers to the extent to which an entity can be perceived by the senses. For example, the word *pineapple* is highly imageable because it can be perceived by nearly all of the senses – it has a distinctive visual appearance, taste and smell, and it can be touched. Other words are far less imageable; it is much more difficult to pinpoint sensory experiences that we might associate with a word like *obedience* or *honesty*, for example. Though some clinical resources, such as the RDLS or the Western Aphasia Battery, provide real objects as part of the package, in practice, because of the tendency to use picture-based tasks in published SLT resources, it is nearly always the visual aspect of items' imageability that is relevant, but presumably there is nothing to stop clinicians from designing their own smell- or taste-based materials! Identifying words that can readily be represented pictorially

---

[1] As noted at the start of the chapter, VAN stands for Verbs and Nouns Test. If you do not yet feel sure what a verb or a noun is, do not worry; this distinction, which is explored in detail in Chapter 5, is not crucial to our discussions here.

is not necessarily a straightforward task, as anyone who has played the game Pictionary can testify.

Imageability has been shown to be an important factor when the task involves the processing of written or spoken words. For example, people with aphasia find it easier to access words with high imageability in various tasks, and the RCSLT clinical guidelines recommend controlling for this factor when selecting materials.

Information about imageability has been collected by researchers in various studies in which the participants have been asked to rate particular words for this characteristic. Some references to published papers that report imageability ratings are given at the end of this chapter. Some information about imageability can be found online in publicly available resources such as the MRC Psycholinguistic Database, which can be found at http://websites.psychology.uwa.edu.au/school/MRCDatabase/uwa_mrc.htm. This has amalgamated the ratings for words from several studies, and provides ratings ranging from 100 for low imageability to 700 for high imageability. For example, to get the database to propose a list of highly imageable words, go to the first set of tick-boxes (under 'Select the database fields to be displayed in the output') and tick 'Word' and 'Imageability rating'; then scroll down to 'Optionally set upper and/or lower limits for selected word properties' and type a minimum imageability rating, say 500, and a maximum rating, say 700; finally, scroll down to the bottom of the page, and click 'GO'. This returns a few hundred words, such as *crown* and *beach*, with imageability scores in this range. For a particular word, if the database has a score for it, you can discover what that score is by removing the upper and lower limits (i.e. 600 and 700 in the example just given) and under 'simple letter match' type in the word or set of words that you are interested in, one per line; then press 'GO'. A limitation of this resource is that for imageability it only has information for a subset of words, but the database can be used to investigate other factors for which there is more extensive information. If you invest a little time to get to grips with the way that the database works, you will find that you can use it to identify words with various combinations of the characteristics discussed in this chapter. Another resource that contains information about imageability and other characteristics is the Bristol Norms which can be accessed at http://language.psy.bris.ac.uk/bristol_norms.html

Familiarity: As noted above, familiarity is a rather individual characteristic of words: a word that is familiar to you may be unfamiliar to someone with a different cultural background, experience, age, etc. Nonetheless, if we ask large numbers of people to rate the familiarity of words, we can average these ratings and come up with a rough index of how familiar a word is likely to be. Like imageability, familiarity is a factor for which rating scores have been collected by researchers, and these scores can be accessed via some publicly available resources such as the MRC Psycholinguistic Database and the Bristol Norms as previously mentioned. For example, in the Bristol Norms, *clement* and *wigwam* receive low familiarity scores, while *dinner* and *goodbye* receive high scores.

<u>Word frequency</u>: We have pointed out more than once that familiarity is a very individual characteristic, but that an intuitive estimate of this factor does seem to have been a criterion in the selection of items for several tests. A more objectively measurable characteristic that relates to (but is not the same as) familiarity is word frequency. Word frequency can be defined as the number of times that a word appears in a particular sample of language. For example, in the nursery rhyme 'Hey Diddle Diddle' (here it is in case you don't know it!):

Hey diddle diddle,
The cat and the fiddle,
The cow jumped over the moon,
The little dog laughed to see such fun,
And the dish ran away with the spoon.

the word *the* occurs seven times, but the word *spoon* only occurs once, so *spoon* has a lower frequency than *the* in this context. A useful distinction to make is between **types** and **tokens**. To calculate word frequency, we need to count up the number of tokens that occur in a particular piece of text; there are seven tokens of *the* in the rhyme 'Hey Diddle Diddle', and one token of *spoon*. The term type refers to distinct words. In this rhyme, 22 different word types, that is 22 different words, occur (*hey, diddle, the, cat, and, fiddle, cow, jumped, over, moon, little, dog, laughed, to, see, such, fun, dish, ran, away, with, spoon*). There are 30 words in total in the rhyme, so some word types are represented by more than one token (specifically, *diddle, the* and *and*). Of course, a word frequency count based on such a tiny sample would not be of any use, but as we will see below, it is possible to access word frequency information that is based on very large samples indeed.

We will say more about resources for getting word frequency in a moment, but first we will continue with our discussion of types and tokens. **Type–token ratio** (or **TTR**) is a measure that is sometimes calculated to work out how diverse a person's vocabulary is. TTR is calculated by dividing the number of types in a text by the total number of tokens, so for 'Hey Diddle Diddle' the TTR is 22/30, or 0.73, or 73% (though it is desirable to use many more than 30 tokens for an accurate result). A person with a diverse vocabulary will have a higher TTR than a person with a very restricted vocabulary. Suppose that a person produced a short description of a picture consisting of 25 tokens, but used only 5 different word types: here, TTR = 5/25 = 0.20 = 20%. Suppose that another person gave a 40-word description, but they used 16 different word types: TTR = 16/40 = 0.40 = 40%. So even though the descriptions were of different lengths, we can tell that the second person's vocabulary is twice as diverse as the first person's. Again, in a real study we would aim to use much larger language samples; although this example illustrates the concept, such small samples would not yield valid conclusions.

When word frequency is investigated in psycholinguistic and clinical studies, it is customary to use very large bodies of text containing many different language samples to determine the score for a particular word. Here, 'text' is used to refer to a set of samples of language of any type, spoken, written or signed. The group of samples that is used for a word frequency count, the 'body of texts' that the numbers are based on, is called a **corpus**.

Psycholinguists and clinicians have found word frequency to be an important predictor of the speed and accuracy with which a word can be processed. Healthy adults and people with various kinds of acquired language problem can generally process high-frequency words more easily than low-frequency words.

There are many online resources that provide information about word frequency, although not all of them are freely accessible. One useful word frequency resource, which has the advantage of being publicly available (at least in a rudimentary form), is the British National Corpus (BNC), which can be seen at http://www.natcorp.ox.ac.uk/. The BNC consists of a body of text (corpus) of around 100 million words; the individual texts in the corpus were drawn from a large range of sources, gathered in the late twentieth century. The written texts include extracts from regional and national newspapers, specialist periodicals and journals for a range of ages and interests, academic books and popular fiction, published and unpublished letters and memoranda, and school and university essays. The spoken texts, which represent about 10% of the total word count, consist of orthographic transcriptions of unscripted informal conversations (recorded by volunteers selected from different age, region and social classes in a demographically balanced way) and spoken language collected in different contexts, ranging from formal business or government meetings to radio shows and phone-ins. If you go to the BNC link above and type the word *the* into the box labelled 'Look up', you will find that this word occurs 6,055,159 times in the 100 million or so words of the corpus, or about 60,000 times per million words. *Spoon* occurred only 797 times in the BNC, or fewer than 8 times per million words.[2]

The MRC Psycholinguistic Database, which was mentioned in the discussion of imageability, is another publicly available resource that can be used to quantify frequency, although its corpus of texts is much smaller (about one million words) and older (it was collated in the 1960s). However, the MRC Psycholinguistic Database does have the advantage that you can input a combination of factors such as the ones covered in this chapter and get it to suggest sets of words which will yield a word list with particular characteristics.

Another very useful, publicly available tool for getting an idea of word frequency is the Google Ngram Viewer, which you can find at http://books.google.com/ngrams (or google it!). 'Ngram' refers to letter combinations, or it might be more accurate to say character combinations. The corpus in this case is derived from over 5.2 million books published between 1500 and 2008, which between them cover about 500 billion words in American English, British English, French, German,

---

[2]In the publicly available version of the BNC, requesting a frequency count for *pig* will give you the number of instances where the three-letter word *pig* appears in the corpus, plus the number of instances of *pig's*; it would not include the number of instances of *pigs*. In psycholinguistic studies of frequency effects, for many words it is relevant to take into account all the different grammatical word-forms associated with a lexeme (e.g. add together scores for *pig*, *pigs*, *pig's*). See Further Reading.

Spanish, Russian, or Chinese. Only words that have appeared in more than 40 of the books are listed in the publicly available database. You can select specific language samples, e.g. British English, and you can restrict your search to particular time windows. You can search for individual words, and see when historically they began to be used by more than a handful of people. You can also input phrases, or sequences that contain non-alphabetic characters like *B&B*. You can compare two or more sequences by typing them with a comma between them. The Google Ngram Viewer does not deliver a numerical result, but provides a graph instead, which can be more useful than a number for some purposes.

Exercise 2.1

Use the Google Ngram Viewer at the previously given link to compare the usage of the terms *cell phone* and *mobile phone* in British English between 1980 and 2008.

Length: Length can be measured in terms of phonemes, syllables or letters. There is some evidence that shorter words are processed more easily than longer words. On the whole, shorter words tend to be of higher frequency than longer words.

Word length is one of the easier lexical characteristics to compute for yourself, though you can also use the MRC Psycholinguistic Database to suggest words of particular length in terms of phonemes, syllables or letters, perhaps in combination with particular frequency ranges.

Exercise 2.2

Use the MRC Psycholinguistic Database to identify a set of five words that are one or two syllables long and have a frequency of less than 10 per million. What are the frequencies of these words in the British National Corpus?

Neighbourhood density: Another characteristic that has been shown to affect lexical processing is called neighbourhood density, which is a measure of how similar a particular word is to other words in the lexicon. For example, thinking for the moment about the spellings of words, we could define neighbourhood density in terms of the number of words that could be produced by changing, adding or deleting a single letter. These other words form the neighbourhood of the target word, and so a word which is similar (according to this definition) to many other words is said to come from a dense neighbourhood, while a word that has few similar neighbours come from a sparse neighbourhood. The word *cat*, for example, comes from a relatively dense neighbourhood; many words can be created by changing, adding or deleting a single letter, including *sat*, *cot*, *can*, *at* and *coat*. Other words, such as *emu*, result in fewer words when we try changing, adding or deleting a single letter; *emu* belongs to a relatively sparse neighbourhood. The same approach is applied to defining neighbourhood in phonemic terms.

Many recent studies have investigated the impact of lexical neighbourhood on language processing and acquisition. Healthy adults, adults with aphasia, typically developing children and children with specific language impairment all respond differently to words from dense and sparse neighbourhoods.

Neighbourhood density is another characteristic that you can compute for yourself relatively easily, but again there are resources that can help. An online tool that is publicly available and that can be used to investigate neighbourhood density is provided by Washington University at http://128.252.27.56/Neighborhood/Home.asp. It allows you to generate orthographic neighbours (based on the word's spelling) or phonological neighbours (based on the pronunciation). Although the phonological representations are drawn from US English rather than British English, and the resource uses its own phonetic transcription system rather than that of the International Phonetic Association, the resource provides a useful means of checking your own results.

Exercise 2.3

Use the Washington University resource at http://128.252.27.56/Neighborhood/Home.asp to determine the average number of orthographic neighbours of the words in the list that you constructed in your previous answer.

Age of Acquisition: The age at which a word is typically acquired is obviously relevant to investigating developmental difficulties with lexical processing. It would be foolish to use words in an intervention with a pre-schooler that are not typically acquired until one's teens. However, age of acquisition has more subtle psycholinguistic effects on lexical processing. For example, words that are acquired early in life are more likely than later-acquired words to be preserved in aphasia; it may be that words that are acquired early are integrated into the developing lexical network in a way that makes them more resistant to loss. Though age of acquisition is logically distinct from word frequency, there is a reasonably strong correlation between the two, and it has been argued that many published effects that are attributed to word frequency are in fact more likely to be due to age of acquisition.

Some studies of age of acquisition effects have used subjective, retrospective information from adults, usually university undergraduates; that is, participants were given a list of words and asked to rate them to indicate the age at which they thought they had acquired them. Information about this kind of subjective judgement about some words is available in the MRC Psycholinguistic Database that was mentioned previously. A more objective approach is taken in another publicly available resource, the MacArthur Bates Communicative Development Inventories (or CDI; see http://www.sci.sdsu.edu/lexical/select.php) which focuses on word acquisition during the early years. A CDI typically takes the form of a questionnaire completed by parents, who are asked to indicate which words from a list their child already uses or understands. When results for children of various ages are combined, it is possible to work out the percentage of children who can be expected to have acquired a given word at a particular age, and to use this to identify which words are acquired early and which are acquired later. The MacArthur Bates CDI has information about 350 words in the expressive and receptive vocabularies of children between 8 and 30 months of age. Though the MacArthur Bates CDI concerns children acquiring US English, results for British English are broadly similar, and this CDI has the advantage of being publicly available.

Though it may appear that the subjective estimates of age of acquisition would be unreliable, in fact there is reasonable correlation between them and the more objective measures, so you may decide to use either or both depending on the client group with which you are working.

Exercise 2.4

Construct a set of items that, according to the MacArthur Bates Communicative Development Inventory, should be in the expressive vocabularies of 50% or more of 30-month-olds. Choose items that you can draw, so that you could make this into a resource for working on productive vocabulary.

Spelling-sound regularity: In tasks involving reading, a further factor to consider is spelling-sound regularity. The concept of regularity crops up at various levels of linguistic description. An item is **regular** if it follows the same pattern or rule as the majority of similar items; otherwise it is **irregular** (an **exception**). For example, the words *beak, leak, teak, weak, tweak, creak* and *freak* all rhyme with each other; these words demonstrate the regular spelling-sound correspondence for the letter sequence e-a-k. The word *break* does not obey this rule; it is irregular. Spelling regularity is one of the features that the PALPA manipulates as a means of determining the source of reading difficulties in clients with aphasia.

2.6   Words and non-words

Clinical resources often include **non-words**, which, as the name suggests, are strings of sounds or letters that do not constitute actual words of English. In fact, it would be more accurate to say that the resources include **pseudo-words**: strings of sounds or letters that happen not to constitute actual words of English, but that obey the structural rules of the language so that they could in theory be (or become) real words. For example, *frex* is a pseudo-word because, although it is not a real word of English, it conforms to the rules that govern the spelling (orthography) and sound structure (phonology) of the language; but *frxe* is an orthographically and phonologically illegal non-word because it violates these rules.

One reason for employing pseudo-words in clinical resources is to avoid the meaning-related effects that might occur if real words were used. An example of such an effect is imageability, which was discussed earlier. In the PALPA, pseudo-words are used when the clinician wants to determine whether a person with aphasia is having word-finding difficulties because of damage to the meaning representations of words or for some other reason. The PALPA builds on research in cognitive neuropsychology that has been going on for many decades. This approach has more recently been extended to analysing children's abilities, where it is particularly associated with the frameworks for speech and language therapy described by Stackhouse and Wells in the 1990s. There are now several resources that specifically target non-word processing abilities in children, such as the CNRep, which uses only non-words, and the ERB, in which children are asked to repeat both words and non-words. Various studies have shown that the ability to repeat words and non-words correlates with measures of receptive and productive vocabulary and other indices of language ability.

Pseudo-words can vary in terms of word length and neighbourhood density, but not in terms of the other factors covered in this chapter. Imageability, word frequency and age of acquisition can, by definition, only be characteristics of real words. With regard to spelling-sound regularity, this is what determines the target pronunciation of pseudo-words in reading-aloud tasks: for example, we would expect the pseudo-word *foad* to be pronounced in such a way as to rhyme with *load, road*, etc., not *broad*.

You can easily construct your own pseudo-words for use in the clinical situation; for example, you could take a list of real words and re-arrange the letters or sounds, which is the approach taken in the ERB. Alternatively, you could use one of the many freely available online resources for generating non-words and pseudo-words, such as the ARC database at http://www.maccs.mq.edu.au/~nwdb/

Exercise 2.5

Invent two one-syllable pseudo-words: one should be from a sparse orthographic neighbourhood and one should be from a dense orthographic neighbourhood.

Chapter summary

- Clinical resources that investigate clients' knowledge and processing of words often use pictures in tasks such as confrontation naming and picture selection.
- Repetition of words and non-words (or pseudo-words) is considered to be a useful index of language development and language processing ability.
- The design of such resources often implicitly or explicitly takes into account psycholinguistic and linguistic factors including imageability, familiarity, word frequency, length, age of acquisition and neighbourhood density.
- Various online resources exist that can help you to create your own intervention materials taking these factors into account.
- Some questions that clinicians need to ask are best addressed via tasks involving pseudo-words.

Exercises using clinical resources

2.6. The BPVS divides items into sets. Compare the average length of items in the first and last sets in terms of (a) letters and (b) syllables. How many of the words in each set can you find in the MRC Psycholinguistic database?

2.7. Consider the first five items in the Renfrew Word Finding Vocabulary Test, all of which are also items in the MacArthur Bates Communicative Development Inventories. Judging from the CDI data, which of these items is least likely to be in the productive vocabulary of an 18-month-old?

2.8. Look at the manual for the ERB. Which of the factors discussed in this chapter are used to group responses in the Preschool Repetition (PSRep) subtest of this assessment?

2.9. Look at the manual for the VAN. What factors were able to be matched across nouns and verbs? Were there any factors that could not be matched?

2.10. Look at the five non-words in the CAT, Section 14, 'Repetition of Non-words'. Which item is from the most dense orthographic neighbourhood?

2.11. Look at Section 8 of the PALPA (Non-word repetition). Which of the factors discussed in this section have been used to group the scores?

2.12. What is the average word frequency of items 1–8 of the items on the Boston Naming Test (Standard Form)? What is the average frequency of items 53–60? Use the British National Corpus to get frequency scores.

2.13. Which of the factors that are covered in this chapter are manipulated in subtest 20 of the CAT?

Further reading

The introductory sections of the Vocabulary Enrichment Intervention Programme provide a good introduction to this clinical area.

For further information about the psycholinguistic background to this area, see introductory texts such as Harley (2008). The main focus of this text is processing by adults.

The psycholinguistic approach is also adopted with children. One of the best-known frameworks among SLTs was proposed by Stackhouse and Wells (1997).

The manuals of the ERB and the VAN give useful and concise introductions to some psycholinguistic factors that are relevant in this area.

For a more linguistics-oriented discussion of vocabulary, see Bauer (1998).

The British National Corpus is explored by Leech, Rayson and Wilson (2001).

3 Word Meaning

> **Clinical resources that will be referenced in this chapter:**
>
> ACE – Assessment of Comprehension and Expression 6–11
> Boehm Test of Basic Concepts
> Bracken Basic Concept Scale
> Bracken Concept Development Program
> CELF-4, CELF-Preschool – Clinical Evaluation of Language Fundamentals
> LIST – Listening Skills Test
> MCLA – Measure of Cognitive-Linguistic Abilities
> PALPA – Psycholinguistic Assessment of Language Processing in Aphasia
> Pyramids and Palm Trees
> Semantic Links
> TOAL-4 – Test of Adolescent and Adult Language
> TOWK – Test of Work Knowledge
> Understanding Ambiguity
> Vocabulary Enrichment Intervention Programme
> Western Aphasia Battery

3.0 Introduction

Speech and language therapists frequently help clients to improve their ability to process meaning in both expression/production and reception/comprehension of language. The term **semantics** is used by clinicians and linguists when discussing meaning. In this chapter and the next we consider the aspect of semantics that relates to the inherent meanings of linguistic expressions such as words and sentences. For example, we can look at the sentence *A week consists of seven days* and judge that it is true. Our judgement would be based on our knowledge of the meanings of the individual words and our knowledge of the grammatical rules of English. There are various ways that we might interpret what we mean by 'meaning'. For example, we might say that the 'meaning' of the question *Do you know what time it is?*, when spoken as a casual enquiry to a passer-by, has a rather different meaning

Introductory Linguistics for Speech and Language Therapy Practice, First Edition. Jan McAllister and Jim Miller.
© 2013 John Wiley & Sons, Ltd. Published 2013 by John Wiley & Sons, Ltd.

from that of the same utterance spoken to a caller who has rung up at 3 am. This contextual aspect of meaning, which has more to do with function than with form, will be covered in later chapters. In many clinical resources, words and sentences are presented out of any social or interpersonal context, and it is the meaning that we are able to derive from such linguistic expressions that we are concerned with in this chapter and in the next one.

In this chapter, we will focus on semantic frameworks for describing the meanings of items, such as words, whose meanings we store in the mental lexicon; this aspect of meaning is called **lexical semantics**. Larger linguistic units such as sentences are not usually stored in the mental lexicon; instead, we compute the meanings of these larger units as and when we encounter them. We will have more to say about this aspect of meaning in Chapter 4 and in subsequent chapters.

3.1   Why do SLTs need this knowledge?

The RCSLT clinical guidelines make many references to meaning and semantics. Learning about meaning is a critical part of typical language development. Many children in language support services have word-finding difficulties, that is, problems producing a word with the appropriate meaning, resulting in either a complete failure to produce the required word or a semantic error – the production of a word that is similar in meaning but different from the target. People with aphasia often have similar kinds of word-finding difficulties.

Models of word processing, such as the one presented in the PALPA, generally assume that the same semantic system is used for producing and understanding words; so clinicians need to consider semantics when tackling receptive as well as expressive problems. In such cases, RCSLT recommends that therapy should aim to strengthen and improve access to word meanings by enhancing the links between word forms (e.g. *chalk*) and word meanings (e.g. 'substance used for writing on a blackboard'). The resources that clinicians use to work on word-level meaning use frameworks developed in linguistics, and SLT students need to understand these frameworks in order to use the resources effectively.

3.2   Learning objectives

After reading this chapter and doing the exercises listed at the end, you should be able to:

- Describe some tasks that clinicians commonly use to assess semantic abilities;
- Explain the difference between two types of 'meaning' – reference and sense;
- Define and/or give examples of the following:
  - semantic features
  - semantic fields
  - hyponymy
  - synonymy
  - oppositions.

3.3   Reference and sense

The meaning of words is fundamental to linguistic communication. During the first year of life, typically developing children go through a developmental stage called babbling where they produce meaningless sequences of sounds such as 'doo', often repetitively. We can say that they are meaningless because the child does not use them consistently in association with any particular object, context, action, etc. A while later, the parents are overjoyed when the child reaches for her cup of juice and says 'doo' – she has produced her first word! Yet her utterance is identical in form to a sound sequence that was produced during the babbling phase and bears only a slight resemblance to the word as an adult would produce it. The difference is that now the child produces the syllable as part of a consistent sound–meaning relationship – always saying 'doo' to refer to or request juice, for example. It is only once this sound–meaning pairing is in place that we can say that the child is producing words. In technical terms, a child's use of a particular sound sequence can only be considered a word if it is consistently associated with a particular **referent** – that is, the particular entity (object, person, concept, etc.) that the sound sequence refers to. The term '**reference**' is of course not confined to the relationship between spoken language and entities – written or signed forms also have referents.[1]

The LIST explicitly uses the term 'referent' in the title of its sub-test 'Referent Identification', but the concept is implicit in many clinical resources. If you look at the 'Message' column in this sub-test you will see that we often need to use expressions consisting of several words when we want to identify a referent. The technical term for linguistic expressions that are used to identify referents is **referring expression**. The set of potential referents for a referring expression is called a **category** – a set of entities of the same kind. The category denoted by *orange juice* consists of all the entities that a speaker would consider to be orange juice. Equally, a category may consist of a single individual: *the winner of the gold medal in the Men's Keirin finals in the 2012 Olympics* refers to a single individual. Of course, more than one referring expression can be used to denote a referent: an alternative way of referring to the referent of *the winner of the gold medal in the Men's Keirin finals in the 2012 Olympics* is *Chris Hoy*.

Picture selection tasks such as those mentioned in the previous chapter may be used to investigate this 'reference' aspect of word meaning. An example of this kind of task is shown in Figure 2.2. The clinician might ask the client to point to the *cup*. Notice that there are several distractor pictures as well as the target picture. One picture represents an object with a similar meaning to *cup* (*glass*, another drinking receptacle), another depicts an object whose name sounds similar to *cup* (*cap*) and a final distractor has neither a sound nor a meaning relationship (*peg*).

---

[1] A related concept is **denotation**. Denotation is part of the dictionary meanings of lexical items; APPLE **denotes** the set of entities to which that lexical item can be applied. Reference is the act of using an expression to direct the addressee's attention to an entity or a set of entities: *the apple in the blue bowl*, *the apple you bought yesterday* and *the apple you want to eat* may be used to refer to three different apples or to one and the same apple. *Apples* is used to refer to all the members of the set of entities that count as apples. We will consider this point again in Chapter 11.

An alternative interpretation of 'meaning' relates to a more abstract representation that is stored in the mental lexicon, which linguists call **sense**. This abstract representation of meaning is also sometimes called a **concept**, although the term is often used more loosely in speech and language therapy. For example, the 'sense' meaning of *orange juice* is something like 'liquid produced by squeezing the round, reddish-yellow, sweet or bitter, edible citrus fruit'. So sense is the aspect of meaning involving the properties of a given entity.

The 'sense' aspect of word meaning is also explored in clinical resources; see, for example, the 'Word Definitions' sub-test of CELF-4 (ages 9–16), which involves tasks such as 'Define the word *butter* as in *Would you like butter on your toast?*' Another task that may use the 'sense' aspect of meaning is **semantic cueing**, in which the client is given a definition of a word and is asked to retrieve it – for example, 'a sweet substance produced by bees' to elicit the target *honey*.

3.4   Lexical semantics

As we noted in the introduction to this chapter, lexical semantics refers to the frameworks that are used to represent meanings of items stored in the mental lexicon. For the most part these are words, but as we explained in Chapter 2, sometimes we store the meanings of word sequences in the lexicon if misinterpretation would otherwise result. For example, in the Multiple Meanings in the Context section of the clinical resource Understanding Ambiguity, some of the items are single words, but many are multi-word idioms like *barking up the wrong tree* or *dropping like flies* which (depending on context) usually have to be interpreted as a unitary concept because word-by-word processing will yield the wrong meaning. However, we will confine ourselves to a discussion of the meanings of individual words here.

3.4.1   Lexemes, categories and concepts

In Chapter 2, we introduced the notion of a lexeme – a word in the 'dictionary entry' sense, such as PIG, as distinct from grammatical word forms such as *pig* and *pigs*. In the previous section, we drew a distinction between category, the set of referents that are denoted by a particular referring expression and concept or sense, the abstract representation of meaning of a lexeme that is stored in the mental lexicon. The relationship between a lexeme's form (e.g. pronunciation, spelling) and these different aspects of meaning is sometimes shown as a triangle like the one in Figure 3.1.

The line between the linguistic form and the set of referents is dashed because this relationship is indirect: a person can only identify a set of referents on the basis of a lexeme's form if they can first access the stored concept. The relationship is also arbitrary: there is nothing inherent in the lexeme's form that indicates what set of referents should be accessed; so there is no visual clue in the letter sequence d-o-g that would point the reader towards the set of referents that are canine

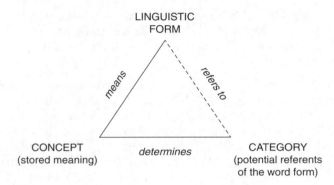

Figure 3.1   The semiotic triangle.

creatures. A few forms have a less arbitrary sound–meaning relationship: these are **onomatopoeic** forms, in which the meaning of the word is supposedly suggested or evoked by its sound, for example, *zip, hiccup, clank, cuckoo, zoom* or *purr*. But **onomatopoeia** is the exception rather than the rule. Onomatopoeic forms also have a more arbitrary meaning–sound relationship than is often suggested: the sound of a balloon bursting is the supposedly onomatopoeic word *pop* in English, but it is *pan* in Japanese and *thaa* in Hindi.

3.4.2   Decomposition of word meaning

It is beyond the scope of this book to explore in detail the many different semantic theories that have been proposed to explain word meaning, but a fundamental notion in most of them is **decomposition**: the idea that word meanings are complex entities that can be analysed into more basic meaning components. For example, an analysis of the word *princess* would identify components related to being royal and of a particular rank, as well as being female. Most of the components that would be identified are shared with the semantically related word *prince*, with the obvious exception of the component relating to gender.

The concept of decomposition in lexical semantics is analogous to that of factorisation in mathematics, in which a composite number, such as 30, is represented as a set of prime numbers which, when combined using multiplication, result in the number ($2 \times 3 \times 5$). In fact, some semantic theories seek to define a set of **semantic primes** or **semantic primitives**, basic semantic concepts whose meaning cannot be further analysed. Examples of semantic primes that have been proposed are 'do', 'move', 'people', 'not' and 'because'. These are seen as being **universal**, that is, part of the general knowledge that humans have about language, rather than being specific to a particular language.

SLT resources that are concerned with word meaning sometimes draw implicitly on the notion of decomposition and the related concept of **componential analysis**, which seeks to identify fundamental meaning components or **semantic features** that capture the similarities and differences between related words. For example, the words *woman, girl, man* and *boy* form a semantically related set. They are all terms that are used to refer to human beings, so Human would be an appropriate semantic feature to identify.

We could identify at least two other features that characterise the meanings of the words: two (*woman, man*) refer to Adult entities while the other two do not; and two (*woman, girl*) refer to Female entities while the other two do not. Semantic theorists who have taken this approach seek to identify a set of semantic features that are general, in that they apply to a wide range of words rather than just a small *ad hoc* set, and universal, in that they embody meaning distinctions that are represented in all languages of the world. They also seek to formulate rules that specify the way that these elements are combined to form lexemes. In practice, no one has ever managed to carry out a comprehensive analysis of this sort. Nonetheless, the approach is still widely used.

A popular method of componential analysis involves the use of **binary** semantic features. A binary feature is one that has two (and only two) potential values, usually represented with the symbols + and −. The concept was originally developed to describe the simpler systems that are encountered in other areas of linguistics such as phonology and morphology, which deal with a more restricted set of items, but it has been applied to semantics as well. To continue the example of *woman, girl, man* and *boy* from the previous paragraph, we can evaluate each word against the three semantic features that we identified, and assign each one a plus or a minus symbol to indicate whether or not it possesses the feature in question. All four words referred to Human entities, so they would all be assigned a + symbol for this feature. *Woman* and *girl* would be given + for Female and *man* and *boy* would be given −. *Woman* and *man* would receive + for Adult and *girl* and *boy* would receive −. We might represent the features in a matrix as shown in Table 3.1.

If the only entities that we were interested in describing were *woman, girl, man* and *boy*, the feature human would be **redundant** – it would not provide us with any useful information for discriminating between entities; we will, however, retain it for present purposes. Notice that each column has a unique combination of + and − symbols: for example, *woman* is characterised as [+Human +Female +Adult], while boy is [+Human −Female −Adult]. This analysis suggests that *girl* and *man* have a closer semantic relationship to *woman* than *boy* does, because they share more semantic features. Clients' understanding of the relative closeness of semantic relationships is exploited in the Semantic Links resource.

Table 3.1 Binary semantic example

	Woman	Girl	Man	Boy
Human	+	+	+	+
Female	+	+	−	−
Adult	+	−	+	−

Exercise 3.1

Extend Table 3.1 [woman girl man boy] to incorporate the words *mare, stallion, colt* and *filly*.

Many assessments require implicit or explicit manipulation of semantic features. A further example is sub-test 3 'Spoken Analogies' in the Test of Adolescent Language (TOAL-4), in which clients have to respond to items similar to the following: 'Eye is to see as ear is to ___'.

3.4.3   Basic concepts

Think for a moment about the process of looking up a word in a dictionary. Any word that has an entry in the dictionary is defined in terms of other words, which ought to lead to an unsatisfactory degree of circularity. For example, in the online Cambridge dictionary at http://dictionary.cambridge.org/, *man* is defined as 'an adult male human being' but *human being* is defined as 'a man, woman or child'. This circularity is not restricted to this particular dictionary but is a property of dictionaries in general. Some dictionaries actually list explicitly the words that they are not going to attempt to define. To this extent, dictionaries would be fundamentally flawed if their typical users were individuals who had no knowledge of human language at all. Fortunately, users of dictionaries are able to make sense of dictionary entries because they are <u>not</u> complete linguistic novices; even the most inexperienced user of a dictionary already has access to the meanings of a small set of basic vocabulary items, such as *person*. Dictionary writers do provide definitions for words like *person,* but in fact, they write dictionary entries for other words with the assumption that meaning of words like *person* will be understood. The notion of semantic primitives that was mentioned in the previous section captures a similar concept.

SLT resources also appeal to the idea of a basic set of items whose meaning is usually assumed to be a part of the knowledge base of even quite young children with typically developing language abilities. These basic concepts were first researched in detail in the latter part of the twentieth century. Educational psychologists and researchers writing about language testing in the 1970s and 1980s remarked that preschool and primary school clients would often perform poorly in standardised assessments that were available at that time because they did not understand the test instructions, which were ironically often more complex than the test items themselves. This was because many of the paediatric resources available at that time were just scaled-down versions of resources that had originally been developed for adults, with little attempt to adapt to the needs of their younger target group. For example, a child who does not understand the concept of 'opposite' will not be able to respond correctly when asked to supply 'the opposite of *big*'. Classroom teachers also generally assumed that their pupils would understand basic concepts such as 'opposite' that they used in their lesson activities, but children with language difficulties might well fail to comprehend them. Such observations led to research into the emergence of basic concepts in children, which ultimately resulted in the development of resources such as the Boehm Test of Basic Concepts and the Bracken Basic Concept Scale. These resources cover the concepts that young children should be able to understand by the time they are engaged in the early years of formal education.

Resources like the Boehm Test of Basic Concepts, the Bracken Basic Concept Scale and the Bracken Concept Development Program focus on assessing school readiness and bringing children to the required level. To do so they target concepts that are clearly fundamental in, and specific to, a child's early formal education, such as letters, numbers and shapes. They also include more general concepts: colours (e.g. *red, violet, black*), size/comparison (e.g. *big, small, long, short, similar, different*), direction/position (e.g. *under, over, right, left*), emotions and physical states (e.g. *happy, excited, tired, sick*), gender (e.g. *boy, girl, male, female*), family relationships (e.g. *mother, father, sister, brother*), characteristics of materials (e.g. *wet, shiny, rough, smooth*), time (e.g. *morning, day, night, week, month, year*), sequence (e.g. *first, second, once, twice, before, after*), speed (*fast, slow*), relative age (*old, young, new*) and quantity (e.g. *whole, part, more, less, most, least, half*). Other resources that are not so focused on school readiness, such as the CELF-Preschool, also investigate children's grasp of basic concepts.

Another fundamental semantic feature that is relevant to linguistic analysis is **animacy**. This has to do with whether an entity is **animate** (humans and other animals) or **inanimate** (everything else – objects, abstract concepts, etc.). This distinction is relevant to the way that we can describe the semantics of sentences.

3.4.4   Semantic fields

Imagine the following scenario: A man with aphasia performs well on a naming task, except for the following words: *pineapple, pear, grape, banana*. The client's problems with lexical processing are not random; they seem to involve the names of fruits. Though this is a very contrived example, it is not unusual for people with aphasia to have problems with groups of words with similar meanings like this. The words in the group share a common semantic property. Linguists refer to such a group of words as a **semantic field** (sometimes also called a **semantic domain, word field** or **lexical field**). Semantic fields are essentially the set of lexemes that are used to talk about a particular phenomenon. The 'fruit' example is an instance of a particular kind of semantic relationship that will be explored in Section 3.4.5.

Kinship terms (terms such as *son* or *cousin* that are used to refer to members of one's family) provide an interesting example of a semantic field that is often discussed in linguistic texts. Although all languages have kinship terms, they may differ with respect to the relationships that are grouped together under a single term. For example, where we have separate words in English for *niece, nephew, granddaughter* and *grandson*, Italian has one word, *nipote*, while Serbian has three

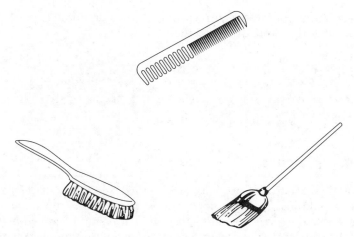

Figure 3.2   Items similar to those used in the Pyramids and Palm Trees resource. Adapted from Snodgrass and Vanderwart (1980). © American Psychological Association.

words corresponding to the English word *aunt* (*tetka* refers to the sister of one's mother or father, *ujna* to the wife of one's mother's brother and *strina* to the wife of one's father's brother). In fact, there are many gaps in this semantic field in English, compared with other languages; for example, there is no single word in English to describe the relationship between one's mother and one's mother-in-law, but in Yiddish there is (*mekhuteneste*). Other, more loosely defined semantic fields could be represented by the words that are associated with cooking, such as *pan, knife, spatula, ingredient, recipe, oven* and *hob* or words associated with hairdressing, such as *scissors, spray, drier, shampoo, cut* and *style*.

Words that belong to the same semantic field are **semantic associates** of each other. The notion of semantic associates is exploited in the Pyramids and Palm Trees resource, which is often used to evaluate the semantic processing abilities of people with aphasia. The items in the assessment are presented in triads (sets of three), with one item at the top and two below it, as in Figure 3.2. The items may be represented in pictorial or print form. The client is asked to choose which of the two lower items is more closely associated with the one at the top. A similar format is used in the Semantic Decisions sub-test of the ACE, although in this resource there are four options to choose from.

A television quiz show called 'Only Connect' draws on the notions of semantic fields and semantic associates. In one activity in the show, players are presented with 16 words or phrases that are drawn from 4 different semantic fields and they have to sort the words appropriately; the correct solution has 4 words in each semantic field. The complicating factor is that the words may belong to more than one semantic field. For example, the following word list might be presented: *brush, canvas, close-up, cut, drier, easel, fade, knife, paint, palette, pan, recipe, scissors, shampoo, spatula, temperature*. Notice that several words in this list are also mentioned earlier in this section, but in the correct solution they do not necessarily belong to the semantic fields that were discussed there.[2]

Exercise 3.2

Construct a set of 16 words that could be used in the 'Only Connect' game described in this section.

3.4.5   Sense relations

The influential psychiatrist Carl Jung (1875–1961) pointed out that 'The word "happiness" would lose its meaning if it were not balanced by sadness'. Admittedly, he was probably interested in the psychological states denoted by the words rather than their semantics, but an important aspect of our knowledge of a word's meaning concerns its relationship to other words – that is, its **meaning relations** or **sense relations**. To some extent the concepts of semantic fields and semantic associates that were discussed in the previous section rely on sense relations, but when this term is used by linguists, they are usually referring to some particular types of relationship, such as synonymy, opposition and hyponymy. The meaning of these three terms is explained and elaborated in the following sections. Clinical assessments and other resources frequently include items that are based on these sense relations.

Hyponymy. This meaning relation is concerned with the membership of sets. *Dog, ostrich, trout* and *boa constrictor* are all members (or **hyponyms**) of the set 'animals'; conversely, 'animals' is called the **superordinate, hypernym** or **hyperonym**, of the set. *Blue, purple, beige* and *violet* are hyponyms of the set 'colours'; the hypernym of *Pikachu, Popeye, Marge Simpson* and *Danger Mouse* is 'cartoon characters'. Referring back to an earlier example in the previous section, *pineapple, pear, grape* and *banana* are all hyponyms of the hypernym 'fruit'. So a hypernym is a broad, superordinate label that applies to many members of a set, while the members themselves are the hyponyms. We could also use the term **co-hyponym** when referring to more than one member of a set – we could say, for example, that *pear* and *grape* are co-hyponyms within the superordinate category 'fruit'. It should be obvious that the notion of hyponymy is related to the concept of semantic fields that we have already encountered, although a semantic field usually involves a more loosely defined relationship than hyponymy.

Hyponymy is a hierarchical relationship, and it may consist of a number of levels. For example, *dog* is a hyponym of *animal*, but it is also the hypernym of *poodle, alsatian, chihuahua, terrier, beagle* and so on. In some linguistic theories, a sub-category like *dog* which has hyponyms of its own is not considered to be

---

[2]Here is the solution: *temperature, recipe, spatula* and *knife* are all words associated with cooking; *palette, paint, easel* and *canvas* are all associated with painting; *cut, fade, pan* and *close-up* are all associated with film photography; and *brush, shampoo, scissors* and *drier* are terms from hairdressing.

a hyponym of the overarching hypernym (e.g. *animal*). Different authors in linguistics also adopt subtly different interpretations of the concept of hyponymy, depending on whether it is a relation between lexical items or meanings (senses). But clinical resources that include tasks involving hyponymy do not typically draw these distinctions.

Clients' access to hyponymy is very regularly explored in clinical resources in what are sometimes called 'fluency' tasks (a use of the word 'fluency' that should not be confused with the term that relates to stuttering and other disorders); see, for example, the 'Word Associations' sub-test of CELF-4 (ages 9–16), 'Fluency Measures' in the MCLA or sub-test B of 'Naming and Word Finding' in the Western Aphasia Battery. In such tests, clients are given instructions like 'Name as many items of clothing as you can in one minute. For example, you might say *sock* and *shirt*'. In other words, the client is being asked to supply as many hyponyms as possible in response to the hypernym or superordinate term.

Exercise 3.3

In Chapter 2, we directed readers to the MacArthur Bates Communicative Development Inventories (http://www.sci.sdsu.edu/cdi/). List the superordinate categories into which their target words are grouped.

Synonymy. Synonyms are words with identical (or almost identical) meanings, for example, *friend* and *pal*, *seem* and *appear*, *little* and *small* or *quickly* and *fast*. Linguists and philosophers have spilt a great deal of ink over the question of whether there are any pairs of words that are completely synonymous. For example, though *friend* and *pal* can both be used to denote the same referent, they differ in terms of degree of formality, with *pal* being the more informal term, and they cannot be used completely interchangeably (**Boy pal*, **Pals of the Earth*). But SLTs are not usually concerned with detailed philosophical arguments of this kind. Examples of assessments that test the ability to identify synonyms are sub-test 3 (Spoken Analogies) in the TOAL-4, and 'Synonyms' in the TOWK.

Exercise 3.4

Produce five more pairs of synonyms. Are there subtle differences in the way that the two words can be used (as with the *friend* and *pal* example above)?

Opposition. There are many examples of words that have opposite meanings, such as *parent/child*, *buy/sell*, *married/single*, *under/over* and *quick/slow*. Assessments that contain items that target clients' understanding of this meaning relation include the 'Word Opposites' sub-tests of the TOWK and the TOAL-4, and sub-test 6 of the Bracken Basic Concept Scale (Expressive).

Linguists distinguish between different kinds of opposition. **Antonyms** are oppositions that indicate the two extremes at opposite ends of a scale of possibilities, such as *quick/slow*, *happy/sad*, *confirm/deny* and *wealth/poverty*. Because the two terms represent the extremes on the scale, with values in between, negating one of the terms does not automatically result in the opposite term. So saying that someone is *not happy* does not necessarily mean that they are *sad*; they may be neither *happy* nor *sad*; and it is not unusual to hear a newsreader say that someone 'would neither confirm nor deny reports' about something. Such opposites are said to be **gradable**; they can be modified with words such as *very* or *extremely* to indicate more extreme levels of the property that they express.

Directional opposites, as the name implies, involve terms that represent opposite directions relative to some reference point, such as *under/over*, *up/down* and *in front of/behind*. Some pairs of directional opposites describe movement in space, e.g. *come/go*, *ascend/descend*. Directional opposites may refer to time as well as space, as in *before/after* and *yesterday/tomorrow*. Extending this idea, we can classify the pair *buy/sell* as directional opposites; the meanings of the two words involve the transfer of an entity from one person to another, and they differ just in terms of direction relative to the reference point (or 'reference person'). Notice that when we employ the words in a sentence context we do in fact attach words that are more clearly directional: we *buy from* someone and *sell to* someone. Pairs of words that describe the bringing about of a state and return to the prior state are also considered to be directional opposites, e.g. *lock/unlock, open/close*. These are also called **reversives**.

Complementary opposites occur when there are just two alternatives in a set and referents can only be classified as one or the other. The terms for siblings are of this kind: a sibling is either a brother or a sister, a sibling who is not a sister is a brother and a sibling who is not a brother is a sister. The gender terms *male* and *female* are normally considered to be complementary opposites, as are *alive* and *dead*. Complementary opposites are said to be **non-gradable**; they are not usually preceded by words like *very* or *extremely* to indicate increased levels of a quality, and it does not make sense to refer to *more* or *less* of it. It is difficult to find examples that are truly non-gradable in linguistic terms, because usage depends so much on the individual speaker's world view or other considerations. For most people, in everyday language, *not male* would imply *female* and vice versa, but in a discussion of transgender issues this would not be the case. Consider also this example from the US TV show The Big Bang Theory: Stuart and Sheldon are having an argument, and Stuart challenges Sheldon's position, saying 'I'm afraid you couldn't be more wrong'. Sheldon, who is pedantic at the best of times, replies, 'More wrong? "Wrong" is an absolute state and not subject to gradation', but Stuart disagrees: 'Of course it is. It is a little wrong to say a tomato is a vegetable; it is very wrong to say it is a suspension bridge'.

Relational opposites are pairs like *parent/child* that describe converse or reciprocal relationships: if A is B's parent, then B is A's child. In fact, such pairs are sometimes called **converses**. Some of the pairs that we considered earlier also fall into this category: if X is *above* Y, Y is *below* X; if Ken *buys* something from Peggy, Peggy *sells* something to Ken.

Exercise 3.5

Consider the following pairs of words, and discuss each pair in terms of meaning relations. Be as explicit as possible.

above/below
odd/even
teach/learn
employer/employee
hero/villain
marry/wed
bus/vehicle
same/different

3.4.6 Lexical ambiguity

Many words in English are ambiguous in that they have more than one distinct meaning, such as *date* (whose many meanings include 'time period on a calendar', 'social interaction' and 'dried fruit'), *habit* ('customary behaviour', 'religious apparel' etc.), *trip* ('journey', 'drug-induced experience', 'stumble', etc.) or *light* ('weighing little', 'pale in colour', 'illumination', etc.). We refer to such cases as **lexical ambiguity**. In such cases, there are several superficially identical lexemes (to use a term introduced in Chapter 2) – we could refer to $DATE_1$, $DATE_2$ and so on.

This situation, where a lexically ambiguous word form has distinct alternative meanings, is called **homonymy**. **Homonyms** are words with distinct semantic representations, but identical pronunciations and spellings. This kind of multiple meaning is often exploited in children's jokes, such as, 'What's the difference between a well-dressed man and a dog?' 'One wears suits, the other just pants'. This joke depends in part on the homonymy of *pants*, though it also depends on aspects of sentence structure that will be considered in later chapters. The 'Only Connect' example in Section 3.4.4 relies on the fact that some of the words are homonyms, with the different senses belonging to different semantic fields.

Items where the ambiguity is confined to the spelling only but where the meanings are represented by distinct spoken forms (as in *bow* meaning 'bend the head and body forward', rhyming with *cow*, or 'decorative knot', rhyming with *low*) are called **homographs**. Conversely, forms with identical pronunciations but different spellings, such as *bare* and *bear*, are called **homophones**.

In other cases, the different meanings of the ambiguous word seem to be related, as in, for example, *mouth* ('facial opening bordered by the lips', or 'place where a river flows into the sea'). This is termed **polysemy**. The decision about whether a particular case of lexical ambiguity should be seen as homonymy or polysemy has traditionally depended on judgements about whether the present-day words are **cognate** (have the same historical origin). In practice, the two types of lexical ambiguity can be difficult to distinguish, and speakers may hold different opinions about the relatedness of the meanings of ambiguous words. In the context of speech and language therapy, the historical origin (**etymology**) of words is not usually relevant, although the Vocabulary Enrichment Intervention Programme does seek to develop clients' understanding in this area as a means of deepening their vocabulary knowledge.

It stands to reason that a homonym or a polyseme can have more than one opposite (see Section 3.4.5). The antonym of *light* would be *dark* on a scale representing level of illumination, but it would be *heavy* on a scale representing weight; the antonyms of *thin* could be *thick* or *fat*, depending on the relevant sense of *thin*. Similarly, the synonyms of such a word may relate only to one specific sense of the homonym/polyseme: *gaunt* could be a synonym of *thin* on the 'body-weight' scale, *narrow* on the 'width' scale, and *slender* could be a synonym relating to both senses.

Exercise 3.6

List three further examples of homonymy and three further examples of polysemy.

Healthy, mature speakers of a language usually find it easy to distinguish the alternative meanings of lexically ambiguous items. Some SLT clients, however, find it difficult to recognise these multiple meanings. Resources that investigate this ability include Understanding Ambiguity (Multiple Meanings in Context sub-test), the Vocabulary Enrichment Intervention Programme and the TOWK Multiple Contexts sub-test. For example, in the TOWK, a client could be asked, 'tell me two things that *light* means'.

Chapter summary

In this chapter, we have seen that

- Lexical semantics refers to the aspect of linguistics that is concerned with the meanings of individual words and other forms that are stored in the mental lexicon.
- There are at least two interpretations of the concept of 'meaning' in linguistics: reference, that is, the object, action, concept, etc. that a word refers to, and sense, the 'definition' of a word.
- There is a distinction between the lexeme, which is the 'dictionary entry' in the mental lexicon; category, the set of referents to which a lexeme refers; and concept, the 'sense' or 'dictionary definition' of a word. The relationship

between the lexeme and the category is abstract and indirect, being mediated by the concept. Except in rare cases of onomatopoeia, it is also arbitrary.

- A popular approach to the analysis of word meaning involves decomposition, the idea that word meanings are complex entities that can be analysed into more basic meaning components. Such basic components are called semantic primitives or semantic primes. A related approach in speech and language therapy involves the identification of so-called basic concepts, usually focusing on those that a child needs to acquire before they will be able to benefit from formal education.
- Semantic fields consist of semantic associates, words that are related in meaning.
- Linguists identify a number of key sense relations:
  - Hyponymy is a hierarchical relationship involving a superordinate term or hypernym and subordinate terms or hyponyms.
  - Synonymy involves items that have approximately the same meaning.
  - Opposition involves 'opposite meanings', and may take various forms, including antonyms, complementary opposites, heteronyms, directional opposites and relational opposites.
- Lexical ambiguity takes various forms:
  - In homonymy a single form (written and spoken) has multiple unrelated meanings.
  - Homographs are forms with a single spelling but different pronunciations associated with the different meanings.
  - Homophones have a single pronunciation but more than one spelling associated with the different meanings.
  - In polysemy, the multiple meanings are related.

Exercises using clinical resources

3.7. Examine the 'Word Classes' Expressive sub-test in the CELF-4 (ages 9–16). What concept(s) discussed in this chapter, does it assess?

3.8. In sub-test 49 of the PALPA (Auditory Synonym Judgements), clients have to indicate whether pairs of spoken words have similar meanings. There are two sets of items consisting of high and low imageability words (see Chapter 2). Think of two more word pairs for each set.

3.9. Sub-test 46 of the PALPA (Homophone Spelling) looks at the client's ability to spell homophones correctly to dictation, when given a disambiguating definition, such as *fare* – 'sum of money paid for travelling on a bus'. Think of five more homophones with disambiguating definitions that could be used in this task. At least one should be a spelling exception (see PALPA task).

3.10. Look at the sub-test 'Word Opposites' in the TOWK. Stimuli are grouped in age-appropriate bands, the lowest age band being 5–6 years and the highest, 13–17 years. Think of two more pairs of examples, one that would be appropriate to the lowest age band and the other that would be appropriate for the highest.

3.11. The Pyramids and Palm Trees resource is described in this chapter. Look at the assessments and come up with two more sets that could be used in the test, or as further items for intervention. Choose items that would be suitable for representing as pictures.

3.12. In the Semantic Links resource, the items consist of a central picture surrounded by at least two other pictures, and the client's task is to select the target (the picture that is most closely associated with the central picture) while ignoring the distractor(s) (the other picture(s)). The number and type of distractors vary. Think of an example of your own that could be used in these resources; your example should have a central picture, a target, a semantic distractor (less closely related to the central picture than the target), a phonological distractor (similar in sound but not meaning to the central picture) and an unrelated distractor.

Further reading

More comprehensive discussion of lexical semantics can be found in numerous linguistic texts on the subject, such as Löbner (2002) or Hudson (1995).

The historical background to the development of resources such as the Bracken Basic Concept Scale and the Bracken Concept Development Program is discussed by Bracken and Panter (2011).

4 Sentence Meaning

4.0 Introduction

In Chapter 3 we were concerned with the meanings of items that are stored in the mental lexicon, particularly words. But understanding the meaning of a sentence, even a sentence that is heard or seen out of context (as is often the case in clinical resources) involves more than understanding the meanings of the individual words. This is because of factors like word order and the presence of grammatical markers that do not have a readily identifiable meaning in themselves but perform an important function in terms of indicating the relationships between words in the sentence. For the majority of sentences, we do not store the meaning in the mental lexicon; instead, we compute their meaning as we encounter them. We will be having a detailed look at how we accomplish this in the next few chapters, but it will be worth looking in this chapter at the aspects of **sentence-level semantics** that are relevant in speech and language therapy resources.

4.1 Why do SLTs need this knowledge?

Clients with or without word-finding difficulties may find it hard to produce and understand sentences, or may have difficulties with mapping skills, that is, the ability

Introductory Linguistics for Speech and Language Therapy Practice, First Edition. Jan McAllister and Jim Miller.
© 2013 John Wiley & Sons, Ltd. Published 2013 by John Wiley & Sons, Ltd.

to integrate sentence structure with sentence meaning. For example, a person with receptive aphasia may understand the meaning of individual words in a particular sentence, but have problems understanding who carried out the action referred to in the sentence. Many clinical resources include items that target this ability.

4.2 Learning objectives

After reading this chapter and doing the exercises listed at the end, you should be able to:

- Analyse simple sentences in terms of semantic roles or semantic relations such as Agent, Patient, Source, Goal and Experiencer;
- Explain the point of using reversible materials in clinical assessments;
- Define, and give examples of, contradiction and syntactic ambiguity.

4.3 Sentence-level meaning

In the previous chapter we were concerned with lexical semantics, the meanings of individual words. For words that we already know, these meanings are stored in the mental lexicon. When we produce a multi-word sentence, the meanings of the individual words do of course contribute to the meaning of the sentence, but often additional layers of meaning emerge because of grammatical considerations that we will be exploring in later chapters. Consider (1).

1 a Eric is taller than Iain.
   b Iain is taller than Eric.

The meaning of (1a) is determined partly by the meanings of the five individual words in the sentence; but to understand what the <u>sentence</u> actually means – for example, to be able to draw a picture that represents the situation, or know that (1b) describes the opposite situation – we have to take into account more than word meanings. This idea, that in sentence meaning the whole is usually more than the sum of the parts, is called the **principle of compositionality**.

As another example, consider (2).

2 a The snake chases the tortoise.
   b The tortoise chases the snake.

Sentences (2a) and (2b) are similar to items that appear in many clinical assessments. One or the other of them might be presented in the context of a receptive (comprehension) task in which the client had to choose the picture, out of the four in Figure 4.1, that portrays the scenario that the sentence describes. The two sentences use identical words, and thus are identical in terms of lexical semantics. All four pictures include a tortoise and a snake, so the meanings of these words do not help at all. If we know the meaning of *chases*, we know that pictures (b) and (c) are candidates for the correct answer, but not (a) or (d).

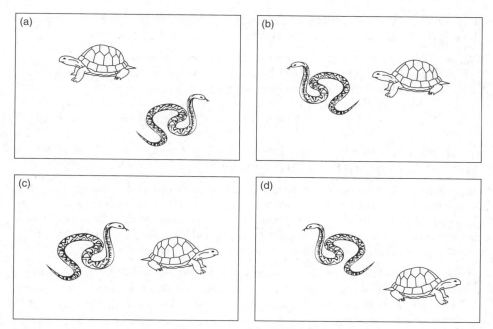

Figure 4.1 Picture selection. Adapted from Snodgrass and Vanderwart (1980). © American Psychological Association.

If we were presented with (2a) and the four pictures in Figure 4.1, we could only know that we should select picture (c) if we knew how to map the order in which the words occur on to the picture scenarios in terms of 'who did what to whom' or 'Doer, Action, Done-To'. The sentences in (2a) and (2b) have completely different meanings, for reasons that are nothing to do with the meanings of the individual words. The origin of the different meanings lies in syntax, the level of linguistic description that is concerned with the relationships between words in a sentence and the impact of syntax on sentence-level semantics. The meaning of sentences in terms of 'who did what to whom' or 'Doer, Action, Done-To' is called the **propositional meaning**. The propositional meaning is the factual situation that the sentence describes. Several different sentence forms can be used to convey the same propositional meaning; see (3).

3   a   The tortoise is chased by the snake.
     b   It is the tortoise that the snake chases.

The sentences in (3), as well as (2a), all convey the same propositional meaning. We will see in later chapters that these different sentence forms can be used to emphasise different aspects of the message, but for the moment we are only concerned with their propositional meanings.

Clients who are seen by speech and language therapists often have problems with sentence-level semantics, affecting their ability to interpret sentences even if they understand the meanings of the individual words involved. Consider the Semantic

Relationships sub-test in the CELF-4; here are examples similar to those used in the sub-test (with the two responses to be chosen from the list in brackets):

4   a   Days are shorter than (minutes; years; weeks; seconds).
    b   Sue hid the present on the top shelf of the cupboard under the window. The present was (above the window; under the cupboard; in the cupboard; under the window).
    c   Lucy helped John but not Barry or Rob. They helped her. Who was helped? (Lucy; John; Barry; Rob).
    d   In a year starting on 1st January, June comes between (April and May; March and September; May and November; July and December).

The client is given a sentence fragment and four options for completing it or answering a related question, and must choose the two options that are appropriate. To be able to carry out the task successfully, clients must identify the critical words and concepts in the sentence and synthesise or combine them into a mental image, draw on world knowledge and much more.

The kinds of relationships that are explored in the Semantic Relationships sub-test – comparison, spatial organisation, time, sequencing and passive (see Section 4.3.1) – may appear diverse at first sight, but they all require accurate processing of sentence-level meaning.

4.3.1   Semantic roles

One of the relationships that are explored in the Semantic Relationships sub-test, which was considered in the previous section, is 'passive'. The term passive refers to a particular syntactic structure that will be explained in detail in a later chapter. The reason that the passive sentence structure is included in the CELF-4 and in many other assessments is that people with language difficulties often have problems with determining its propositional meaning.

Consider the pairs of sentences in (5) to (8). In each pair, the first sentence has the **active** structure, while the second is **passive**.

5   a   Lucy punched Jane.
    b   Jane was punched by Lucy.

6   a   The pig pushes the donkey.
    b   The donkey is pushed by the pig.

7   a   Mary has iced the cake.
    b   The cake has been iced by Mary.

8   a   I will mark the essay.
    b   The essay will be marked by me.

For the moment, we will ignore the details of the syntactic relationship between active and passive sentences. Just think about the semantic dimension of these examples – what is their propositional meaning? What factual situation do they describe? As speakers of English, you can recognise that the two sentences within each pair have identical propositional meaning. They only differ in syntactic form. We can describe the relationship between each (a) sentence and its (b) counterpart in the following non-technical terms: In each of the sentences above we can identify an **action**, which is described by a different grammatical word form depending on whether it is in the (a) version (the active sentence) or the (b) version (the passive sentence) – *punches/was punched, pushes/is pushed, has iced/has been iced* and *will mark/will be marked*. In each active sentence, the doer of the action is presented before the action is mentioned. In each passive sentence, the doer of the action is mentioned after the action, following the word *by*.

Exercise 4.1

Below are four passive sentences. The structure of active and passive sentences will be explored in more detail in a later chapter, but speakers of English are usually intuitively aware of the relationships between the two types of sentence, and we have just described the relationship in non-technical terms. Based on the examples of active/passive pairs that are just discussed, as well as your intuitive knowledge of English, what are the equivalent active forms? *Hint* – start each sentence with the Doer of the action that is described in the sentence.

a. 'Death on the Nile' was written by Agatha Christie.
b. Lynette Ridgeway is shot by Simon Doyle.
c. Poirot had been drugged by the murderer.
d. The mystery will be solved by Poirot.

When linguists describe the semantic content of sentences like these, they relate each part of the sentence to a set of so-called **semantic roles** (or **participant roles**, or **thematic roles**) that allow the sentence to be described in terms of propositional meaning – Doer, Action, Done-To and so on.

The Doer of the action is usually referred to as the **Agent** (alternatively **Actor**). The Agent deliberately performs the action. In (5), the Agent is *Lucy* in both the active and the passive version; in (6), the Agent in both sentences is *the pig*; in (7), the Agent is *Mary*; and in (8), the Agent is expressed by *I* in the active sentence (8a) and *me* in the passive sentence (8b). Typically, agents are animate, that is, their referents are humans or other animals (see Chapter 3, Section 3.4.3).

A further role can be identified in (5) to (8), associated with *Jane* in the first pair of sentences, *the donkey* in the second, *the cake* in the third and *the essay* in the fourth. In traditional grammars this is the entity that 'receives or undergoes the action' and it is given various labels including **Patient**.

Exercise 4.2

In each of the passive sentences in Exercise 4.1 above, identify the Agent and Patient.

Linguists identify many different semantic roles. Consider (9):

9   a   The man opened the door.
     b   The key opened the door.
     c   The man opened the door with the key.
     d   The door opened.

Notice in particular the similarity between (9a) and (9b). These have identical syntactic structures, as we will see in later chapters. But it should be becoming obvious that they are not the same semantically. In (9a), we would assign the Agent role to *The man* and Patient to *the door*. Recall that we said that Agents are usually animate; so despite the syntactic similarity between (9a) and (9b), *the key* would not be assigned Agent in (9b). Its role is more obvious when we look at (9c) – it is the instrument that is used to achieve the action in the sentence, and **Instrument** is exactly the semantic role label that we give it. Having identified these three roles in the situation that is being described – Agent (*The man*), Patient (*the door*) and Instrument (*the key*), we can see that we do not have to express every role in every sentence – Agent and Patient in (9a), Instrument and Patient in (9b) and just Patient in (9c).

Beneficiary and Experiencer are two further roles. The **Beneficiary** is the entity for whose benefit the action occurs – *Chloe* in (10):

10   Martin wrote a poem for Chloe.

The **Experiencer** is the entity that receives emotional or sensory input – *his daughter* in (11a); *Chloe* in (11b).

11   a   Martin amused his daughter.
      b   Chloe watched.

The **Source** role indicates the starting point of an action, for example *the room* in (12):

12   She ran from the room.

The **Goal** of an action is its end point, such as *the library* in (13):

13   He returned a book to the library.

Some theories use the label **Theme** for the role played by an entity that moves or is moved from one location to another, such as *a book* in (13).

If you explore the Further Reading that is suggested at the end of this chapter, you will find many more semantic roles identified. However, in clinical resources the roles that are most often explored by far are Agent and Patient.

The semantic roles approach has also been used in the description of child language. This approach, which is sometimes called **semantic relations**, does not use exactly the same theoretical framework as the one just described, but there are some similarities. Examples of the labels that are used in this approach are Agent, Action, Object, Location, Entity, Possessor, Possession, Attributive and Demonstrative, and the use of the labels is demonstrated in (14) to (21), which could have been produced by a young, typically developing child. The text in brackets provides a context for each utterance, and the description of the utterance in terms of the standard roles is provided.

14   Mummy wash. (As her mother washes the child's hair) Agent + Action

15   Wash hair. (As her mother washes the child's hair) Action + Object

16   Mummy hair. (As her mother washes the child's hair) Agent + Object

17   Mummy hair. (As the child strokes her mother's hair) Possessor + Possession

18   Hair wet. (Pointing to the hair) Entity + Attributive

19   Put table. (Putting a cup on the table) Action +Location

20   Cup table. (Putting a cup on the table) Entity + Location

21   This cup. (Pointing to the cup) Demonstrative + Entity

The rudimentary 'sentences' that young children produce generally lack the grammatical markers that are present in the language of older children and adults, but it may be possible to infer the semantic role structure of what they say from context. If the child's cognitive and language processing capacities only allow her to produce two words at a time, she cannot represent the range of semantic roles that a mature speaker would. Notice how in (14) to (16), different roles are encoded to describe the same scenario, with no single utterance encoding the full set of roles that an older child would in a sentence like *Mummy is washing my hair*. Notice also that the same utterance is analysed differently in (16) and (17) because the different contexts suggest that the words are realising different semantic roles.

A similar framework is used in the Derbyshire Language Scheme to describe multi-word utterances.

4.3.2   Reversibility

Consider examples (5) to (8) again. Notice an interesting semantic distinction between the first and second pair of sentences on the one hand, and the third and fourth on the other. For example, in (6), the action is 'pushing' and the semantic roles are associated with *the pig* (Agent) and *the donkey* (Patient). Notice that although the Agent role is associated with *the pig* in the actual examples, the lexical semantics of both *pig* and *donkey* mean that either could be an appropriate Agent for the action 'pushing'; they are both entities that are capable of pushing because they are both animate. To put it another way, if I said that I wanted you to make a sentence out of the action 'pushing' and the entities *the pig* and *the donkey*, you could choose to make either *the pig* or *the donkey* the Agent. Using the active and passive structures that have been used so far, there are four possible sentences:

22   a   The pig pushed the donkey.
      b   The donkey was pushed by the pig.

23   a   The donkey pushed the pig.
     b   The pig was pushed by the donkey.

Sentences (22a) and (22b) have the same propositional meaning as each other. Sentences (23a) and (23b) have the same propositional meaning as each other. Sentences (22a) and (23a) are active sentences, and (22b) and (23b) are passive sentences.

We could make similar remarks about the sentences (5a) and (5b) – our knowledge of the lexical semantics of animate entities like *Jane* and *Lucy* indicates that either could be the Agent, since both are entities that are capable of 'punching'. So we could have

24   a   Lucy punched Jane.
     b   Jane was punched by Lucy.

25   a   Jane punched Lucy.
     b   Lucy was punched by Jane.

We refer to sentence structures like this, in which the lexical semantics of the entities are such that either entity could be associated with either semantic role, as **reversible**: for example, all the (b) sentences in (22) to (25) are all **reversible passives**. We could also say that all the (a) sentences in (22) to (25) are **reversible actives**; in the TROG-2, Block E (Reversible SVO) is of this type. For reasons that we will explain below, it is usually reversible passives that are of the most interest to clinicians, so these are more common in clinical resources than they are in everyday language.

Now consider (7) and (8) in the same way. Make a sentence involving the action 'icing' and the two entities *Mary* and *a cake*. This time only one pair of sentences is plausible – an active and a passive version which both have *Mary* as Agent and *a cake* as Patient, (i.e. sentences (7a) and (7b)). The alternative versions, with *a cake* as Agent and *Mary* as Patient, are syntactically possible but semantically implausible – **A cake has iced Mary* or **Mary has been iced by a cake*. Similarly, with regard to the (8a) and (8b), active and passive versions with *the essay* as the Agent are implausible: **The essay will mark me*; **I will be marked by the essay*. Structures like this, in which the assignment of the semantic roles is determined by the lexical semantics of the entities, so that only one of them can plausibly be Agent, are said to be **non-reversible**; so *A cake was iced by Mary* and *The essay will be marked by me* are both **non-reversible passives**.

Exercise 4.3

In Exercise 4.1, which sentences are reversible passives, and which are non-reversible passives?

We will discuss the active–passive distinction in more detail in a later chapter, but for the moment, notice that in the active examples given above, the Agent appears immediately before the action, while in the passive examples the Agent is introduced by the word *by*. There is much more to be said about the structure of passives, but this is a useful point to draw out in the present discussion.

The reason for devoting a relatively large amount of space to these examples is that some people with language difficulties (and all typically developing young children) make consistent mistakes with reversible passives like *The donkey is pushed by the pig*. They will, for example, interpret this sentence as though it said *The donkey pushed the pig*, with *the donkey* rather than *the pig* as agent, and in picture selection tasks they will accordingly make the wrong response. For this reason, many clinical assessments that target language abilities include reversible passive items. For example, the Sentence Processing Resource Pack has a whole booklet entitled 'Reversible Passives'.

Exercise 4.4

Identify Agent and Patient in the sentences below. Say whether each sentence is reversible active, reversible passive, non-reversible active or non-reversible passive.

a. A new law has been debated by MPs.
b. Chris shot Jamie.
c. The prime minister was attacked by the leader of the opposition.
d. The actress greeted the critic.
e. The composer has written a new piece.

The idea of semantic reversibility also crops up elsewhere. In the TROG-2, are items labelled 'Reversible in/on' which are similar to the following:

26   The circle is in the triangle.

27   The map is on the book.

In (26), the shapes have been chosen because either <u>could</u> be inside the other, and in (27) either object <u>could</u> be on the other. Other kinds of reversibility are possible – see the exercises at the end of this chapter.

Remember that concepts like reversible/non-reversible and the roles that we have discussed here are concerned with the <u>semantic</u> properties of sentences. Clients may encounter difficulties with deriving these semantic representations from particular syntactic structures. The syntactic structures themselves will be considered later in this book.

4.3.3   Contradiction

A further aspect of sentence-level semantics that we will consider here is **contradiction**. The Greek philosopher Aristotle formulated the Law of Contradiction which stated that 'The same attribute cannot at the same time both belong to and not belong to the same subject in the same respect'. For example, (28a) and (28b) cannot be true simultaneously:

28   a   *Mad Men* is my favourite TV show.
      b   *Mad Men* is not my favourite TV show.

Contradiction can also occur when the lexical semantics of two or more words in a sentence are in conflict. Consider (29).

29   The elderly man was very young.

This sentence is contradictory because the lexical semantics of *elderly* is such that it cannot apply to someone who is very young. One might argue that this is only the case for a literal interpretation of the sentence, where both *elderly* and *young* are being interpreted 'in the same respect', to use Aristotle's term. It is interesting that our drive to make sense of language is such that even when faced with such a contradiction, we instantly, and even unconsciously, identify plausible non-literal or indirect meanings (for example, perhaps *very young* refers to the man's mental attitude or similar). Indeed, psychologically registering such meaning conflicts is part of what we do when we realise that a sentence should be interpreted not literally, but figuratively or metaphorically, but that is a topic to be explored elsewhere. Here, we simply note that the literal interpretation of (29) is contradictory because of the semantic mismatch between *young* and *elderly* when it is supposedly describing one and the same referent.

The ability to recognise that such a sentence is contradictory requires sophisticated processing on the part of the listener, in terms of retaining semantic descriptions of several words in memory simultaneously, and comparing them to identify discrepancies. Contradiction is therefore sometimes used in clinical resources. In the 'Verbal Message Evaluation' sub-test of the LIST, clients are asked to identify 'bad' items, some of which contain contradictions along the lines of *The tall boy is very short* or *Every girl got a prize but one girl got no prize*.

4.3.4   Syntactic ambiguity

When we considered lexical semantics, we recognised that lexical ambiguity can occur when a particular lexeme is associated with more than one meaning. For completeness, a similar observation can be made about other linguistic structures such as phrases and sentences when the ambiguity resides not in the meanings of the individual lexemes, but in the grammatical relationships between them. This kind of ambiguity is called **syntactic ambiguity**, because, as we saw in Chapter 1, syntax is the aspect of linguistics that is concerned with grammatical relationships between words. Syntax will be explored later in this book, but syntactic ambiguity should be mentioned here because its key characteristic is the existence of multiple meanings associated with a single syntactic structure. Here are some examples:

30   Highly qualified men and women will be successful.

31   Vomiting bug closes three wards.

In each of the examples, the ambiguity arises from the existence of more than one possible syntactic interpretation, not from multiple meanings of individual lexemes. In (30), it is not clear whether both the men and women, or just the men, are highly qualified; the fact that syntax is the cause of the ambiguity is apparent if we compare (30) with the similar, but unambiguous, sentence (32):

32   Women and highly qualified men will be successful.

Sentence (31), a real headline from the BBC news website, is syntactically ambiguous because one interpretation involves a bug that causes vomiting while the other involves a bug that is vomiting.

Syntactic ambiguity is difficult to study in the kinds of resources that are typically used in the clinic, but it has often been the subject of experimental studies in people with aphasia.

Chapter summary

- Linguists describe the propositional meaning of sentences in terms of semantic roles such as Agent, Patient, Source, Goal and Experiencer.
- A similar approach has been used to describe children's early attempts at producing multi-word utterances, using the labels Agent, Action, Object, Location, Entity, Possessor, Possession, Attributive and Demonstrative.
- To explore sentence processing, clinical resources often use reversible materials, such as those in which either participant could in theory be the Agent. This means that clients are not able to exploit semantic cues in comprehension, so they would have to rely on syntax.
- A sentence is contradictory when there are discrepancies between the meanings of individual words.
- Even if no individual word in a sentence is lexically ambiguous, a sentence may still be syntactically ambiguous.

Exercises using clinical resources

4.5. Look at the Grammaticality Judgement sub-test of the Verbs and Sentences Test (VAST) and pick out the sentences that are labelled P (passive). Use the concepts covered in this chapter and previous chapters to explain the difference between the 'good' and 'bad' sentences as defined in the instructions to the test.

4.6. Identify reversible passives in the following clinical resources:
    a. TROG-2
    b. PALPA
    c. TAPS-R

4.7. Look at sub-test 58 of the PALPA, Auditory Comprehension of Locative Relations. This concerns reversible relations similar to 'reversible in/on' from the TROG-2 that was discussed above. Make up four more items that could be used in this sub-test, choosing four different locative prepositions (but you can use ones that are already used in the PALPA).

4.8. Look at the Boston Diagnostic Aphasia Examination, section D, Syntactic processing (p17 of the response booklet). The items in Section 2 are labelled 'reversible possessives'. Explain why.

Further reading

More comprehensive discussion of semantics can be found in numerous linguistic texts on the subject, such as Lyons (1995) or Löbner (2002).

For a more detailed discussion of semantic roles that are particularly relevant to the work of SLTs, see the manual of the *Sentence Processing Resource Pack* (Marshall, Byng and Black, 1999). A more extensive set of roles is discussed in more traditional linguistic texts such as Brown and Miller (1991).

The historical background to the development of resources such as the Bracken Basic Concept Scale and the Bracken Concept Development Program is discussed by Bracken and Panter (2011).

5 Parts of Speech

Clinical resources that will be referenced in this chapter:

A-STOP-R – Advanced Syntactic Test of Pronominal Reference
CAT – Comprehensive Aphasia Test
CELF-4, CELF-Preschool – Clinical Evaluation of Language Fundamentals
DASS – Dorset Assessment of Syntactic Structures
ERB – Early Repetition Battery
LARSP – Language Assessment, Remediation and Screening Programme
RDLS – Reynell Developmental Language Scales
STASS – South Tyneside Assessment of Syntactic Structures
TOAL-4 – Test of Adolescent and Adult Language
TROG-2 – Test for the Reception of Grammar
VAN – Verbs and Nouns Test

5.0 Introduction

In this chapter we consider a fundamental concept in linguistic description, the system of labels for different types of words. We recognise different classes of words partly because of the way they behave in the grammar of English and partly because of the differences in their meanings. The different classes are traditionally known as **parts of speech**. The label **word classes** is in general use in linguistics but we avoid that term as it has another meaning in one of the commonly used SLT assessments. The parts-of-speech framework involves labels like noun, verb, adjective, etc. You will find the framework given other names as well, including **lexical and grammatical categories** and **syntactic categories**.

Some students join speech and language therapy courses with no knowledge of these labels. Others arrive believing that they already know how to identify the

---

Introductory Linguistics for Speech and Language Therapy Practice, First Edition. Jan McAllister and Jim Miller.
© 2013 John Wiley & Sons, Ltd. Published 2013 by John Wiley & Sons, Ltd.

different parts of speech. Unfortunately, it is often the case that the traditional criteria that they have been taught are potentially misleading. So even if you think that you already know your parts of speech, please read on!

In English, identifying the part of speech of a word in a particular sentence context often involves a process of elimination and the use of multiple clues in a search for patterns. This can initially be confusing and laborious for students. A full account of distributional criteria needs the concepts of 'phrase' and 'clause', which will be explored in detail in Chapter 7 and subsequent chapters. In this chapter, we try to stick to simple examples to make the learning process easier; if you work your way through each exercise in turn, you should learn the rudiments of the parts-of-speech system, and be able to build on this knowledge in future chapters. There is a great deal more that could be said about parts of speech than we have space for here, but the level of detail that we provide is sufficient for introductory purposes; for a more comprehensive picture, consult the references given in Further Reading.

5.1   Why do SLTs need this knowledge?

As usual, we need to consider the clinical resources that SLTs use when they are assessing and treating people with language problems. Many assessments make explicit reference to part-of-speech labels. For example, the South Tyneside Assessment of Syntactic Structures (STASS) and the Dorset Assessment of Syntactic Structures (DASS) are used in many paediatric clinics. Take a look at the Rapid Assessment Score Sheet of these assessments; in particular, examine the boxes labelled PHRASE. Notice that these contain symbols such as AUX or PRON, or sequences of labels such as PREP D N or ADJ ADJ N. These symbols refer to parts of speech such as auxiliary verb, pronoun, preposition, determiner, adjective and noun. The clinician has to listen to what the client says and write down which of these parts of speech (or sequences of parts of speech) occur. For a clinician who had not already mastered the parts of speech, filling in this Rapid Assessment Score Sheet would be anything but rapid!

Or take an assessment that is used with clients with aphasia, the Verbs and Nouns Test (VAN). As the name of this test indicates, it is concerned with the processing of two distinct parts of speech – verbs and nouns. Suppose that you use the VAN and discover that your client can cope with nouns, but has problems with processing verbs. How will you be able to design therapy materials that focus on verbs if you do not know what a verb is?

5.2   Learning objectives

After reading this chapter and doing the exercises, you should be able to identify the following in some simple sentences: nouns, pronouns, verbs (full and auxiliary) adjectives, adverbs, determiners, prepositions and conjunctions.

5.3   Identifying parts of speech

5.3.1   Content words and function words

The part-of-speech labels that we will explore in this chapter are as follows: determiner, preposition, auxiliary verb, pronoun, conjunction, noun, full (or lexical) verb, adjective and adverb. The first five of these – determiner, preposition, auxiliary verb, pronoun and conjunction – belong to a larger group that goes by various names. We will refer to them as **function words**, but they are sometimes called **grammatical words** (because they have a grammatical role in the sentence, rather than contributing to 'dictionary' meaning), **closed class words** (because they are a relatively fixed set of items that is 'closed to new members' – it is unlikely that a new word that enters the language will belong to one of these parts of speech), or **minor** or **form words**. The last four parts of speech in the list – noun, full verb, adjective, adverb – belong to a larger group that we will call **content words**. They are also called **open class words** (because membership is 'open' to the extent that new words entering the language will almost always be nouns, full verbs, adjective or adverbs), **lexical words** (because their definition in the dictionary, or lexicon, contains an interpretable meaning rather than just referring to a grammatical role), or **major** or **full words**.

The distinction between content words and function words is of interest to SLTs because clients may experience problems with one broad class more than the other. For example, different forms of aphasia may affect one or other class more seriously, and when asked to repeat sentences, children with language problems may make more errors on function words than content words.

5.3.2   Why is it sometimes difficult to identify parts of speech in English?

If it is so important to know the part-of-speech label for words, you might wonder why you cannot simply learn the label for each word. There are a few reasons why this approach will not work. First, there are so many words. A typical adult knows tens of thousands of words, so learning the part-of-speech label for each one would be a challenging task, even if it were possible in English – but, as we will show in this section, it is not. Still, if you are prepared to learn the parts of speech of individual words, that is good news, because, as we will see later on, one of the most useful things you can do to master parts of speech is to sit down and learn the labels of around 200 words that provide relatively reliable information about parts of speech (see the end of this section).

Another reason that you cannot acquire part-of-speech knowledge just by learning to associate every word with a single part-of-speech label is that new words constantly enter any language, and English is no exception. The technical term for these new words is **neologisms**. Hundreds, or more likely thousands, of neologisms enter the language each year – think of words like *chav* or *retweet*, which have entered the language relatively recently. Oddly enough, though, speakers of the language know how to use the word correctly after hearing it only once or twice, even if they are not absolutely certain about the meaning. Consider (1) and (2).

1 a   He's a chav.
   b   Look at that chav.
   c   *He's chavving it.
   d   *He looks quite unchav.

2 a   Can you ask him to retweet that?
   b   He's retweeting it.

If a native speaker of English encounters the word *chav* for the first time in the context of (1a), they would immediately know that it would be (grammatically, if not socially!) acceptable to say (1b) but probably not (1c) or (1d). On the other hand, a speaker who heard *retweet* for the first time in the context of (2a) would know that it would probably be grammatically acceptable to say (2b), which appears to be similar to the unacceptable sentence in (1c). This is because native speakers have an implicit knowledge of the grammatical rules of their language, even though they may not have explicit, conscious knowledge of labels like *noun* or *preposition*; so when a new word is encountered in a particular sentence context, speakers can use that context to work out what part of speech the new word belongs to, and this enables them to infer other ways in which the word could be used.

A further difficulty that we face with English is that even the existing words of the language can often belong to more than one part of speech, and we can only tell which one we are dealing with in a particular sentence by taking into account multiple piece of information. Take the word *fast*. It can belong to four parts of speech (admittedly involving two different meanings, one relating to abstaining from food and the other to speed – but that is beside the point):

- Verb: *Some Jewish people fast for six days of the year.*
- Noun: *If a fast is not broken, starvation can occur.*
- Adjective: *I like driving fast cars.*
- Adverb: *I like driving fast.*

Linguists would treat these four versions of FAST as different lexemes.

The fact that many (probably most) words of English can belong to more than one part of speech is another reason that it is completely infeasible to try to learn 'the' label for every word. Instead, you need to master some criteria that will enable you to identify the part of speech of a particular word in a particular sentence context. This can be a complicated process which depends on factors that will not be explored until later in this book. But if we confine ourselves to fairly simple, straightforward examples (and many clinical resources do just that) we can make a start in this chapter, and will then be in a position to use this information to help us to explore other concepts in the next. When we try to assign part-of-speech labels we often have to form a hypothesis (in other words, an educated guess) about the most likely solution, and then use some tests to see whether the hypothesis is confirmed.

One last point – though it is true that many or most words of English can belong to more than one part of speech, there are some that are less ambiguous, and because they can be used as relative 'islands of reliability' in the swirling sea of the English language, it pays students to learn them. We will point out such islands of reliability as we go along. For the most part they are drawn from the function word/closed class categories, but there are some common unambiguous content words that it will be useful to remember, either because they occur very frequently or because they are used so often in assessments. We have listed about 200 such words in total in Appendix A. Learn it!

5.3.3   Traditional, meaning-based criteria

At school, many students learn traditional, meaning-based criteria for assigning words to parts of speech; for example, they have been told that 'a noun is the name of a person, place or thing', while a verb is 'a doing word'. Unfortunately, these traditional, meaning-based rules are insufficient. They apply only to a small number of central nouns and verbs: it is true that the noun *girl* denotes a type of person and the verb *decorate* denotes an action or 'doing', but for many nouns and verbs, these are not helpful criteria. For example, though *tolerance* and *absurdity* are both nouns, it is difficult to think of either of them as the name of a person, place or thing. Consider (3).

3   The assassination of a president is a punishable offence.

When students who are beginning to learn about parts of speech in an SLT course are asked to underline any verbs in (3), many will underline *assassination* and *punishable*, which are both 'doing words' in some sense, though neither is a verb; they typically miss the only verb in the sentence, *is*.

Traditional, meaning-based criteria like these do not allow us to identify parts of speech accurately, at least when they are the only information being used. The most we can say is that <u>some</u> nouns are the names of people, places or things, that <u>some</u> verbs are 'doing words' and so on. Linguists use more reliable evidence to identify parts of speech; they use form-based criteria.

5.3.4   Form-based criteria

As we know from Chapter 1, the form of a piece of language refers to the way it looks or sounds. In the present context, we want to consider, for example, what letters or sounds occur at the end of a word, or what words precede it. There are two kinds of form-based evidence that are useful for identifying parts of speech in English: suffixation and distribution.

Suffixation refers to endings on a word. For example, the **suffixes** *-ity* (e.g. *severity*), *-ance* (*abundance*) and *-ation* (*alienation*) usually indicate that a word is a noun, while *-able (laughable)*, *-ic (strategic)* and *-ous (numerous)* usually indicate adjectives and *-ise (theorise)* usually indicates a verb. Suffixation will be considered in more detail in the next chapter, but since suffixes can provide valuable information for part of speech identification, a list of suffixes that are useful in this respect is given in Table 5.1. These are not without exceptions: some examples will be given under 'Tests for Parts of Speech' (Section 5.3.5). Some of the suffixes that we include here are fairly unlikely to turn up in clinical resources, but we are including them here because noticing when they turn up, and using them to help you to recognise parts of speech, will consolidate your understanding of these categories.

Many of the suffixes in Table 5.1 provide fairly reliable signals of part of speech, but some are of limited usefulness if we only focus on individual words. Unfortunately, some of the most common suffixes only give a partial answer to the part-of-speech puzzle. For example, the apostrophe in the relatively common suffix -'s/-s' is of course only present in the written form, so this suffix is of less help when we are trying to identify parts of speech in spoken language. Consider also the suffix *-s* (without an apostrophe). This is one of the most common word endings in English, but sometimes it signals nouns and sometimes it signals verbs. We have suggested in Table 5.1 that it is worth considering whether it has the meaning 'more than one'. Consider (4).

4 a   He overpowered the guards.
   b   He overpowered the guard.
   c   He guards the Prime Minister.

In (4a), *guards* is a noun; we can tell this partly from distributional evidence (see Section 5.3.5.4), but we can also consider the meaning. A native speaker of English would know that in (4a) more than one guard was overpowered. What happens when we remove the *-s*? In (4b), only one guard was overpowered. This suggests that the suffix *-s* in (4a) contributes the meaning 'more than one', and this fact is a clue that *guards* could be a noun in (4a). In (4c), we cannot make this case about the *-s* on *guards* meaning 'more than one', so here *-s* does not point us towards a noun label. This reasoning does not work well in every case, but until students are in a position to use syntactic analysis to identify parts of speech (and many are not in this position at the start of a course in speech and language therapy), it is often not possible to find a single piece of evidence that points unambiguously to one label. Instead, it is a question of assembling several pieces of evidence that, when taken together, strongly suggest a particular label. Each individual piece of evidence therefore has the status of a **heuristic** (a 'rule of thumb') that frequently gives the right answer but may be wrong, hence the need to take into account other pieces of information. However, some students have found this kind of heuristic useful when they are learning to identify parts of speech.

Distribution refers to the other words that occur in the context of the word whose part of speech we are trying to determine. This information is useful because we can identify common patterns or sequences of parts of speech that occur in English. For example, a word that occurs right at the end of a sentence and is immediately

Table 5.1   Some suffixes that may be useful for identifying parts of speech

Suffix	Examples	Cautionary notes
(a) *May indicate nouns*		
-age	Luggage	
-ance	Performance	
-ancy	Tenancy	
-(at)ion	Location, version	
-dom	Kingdom	
-ence	Licence	
-ency	Complacency	
-ee	Employee	
-ery	Delivery	
-ess	Duchess	
-ette	Suffragette	
-er, -eer, -or -ar	Worker, engineer, doctor, registrar	Only when it means something like 'doer of' something; otherwise it can signal an adjective or adverb
-ics	Linguistics	
-ism	Racism	
-ist	Violinist	
-ity, -ty	Quantity, safety	
-let	Piglet	
-ment	Enjoyment	
-ness	Happiness	
-'s, -s'	Worker's, workers'	-'s for a single entity, -s' for more than one; must mean something like 'belonging to'. Check first that -'s is not an contracted form such as *is* or *has* (e.g. *Where's he gone; He's a chav*) because this is not the suffix, and the word that it is attached to may not be a noun.
-s, es	Workers, classes	Only if it means 'more than one' – otherwise it can signal a verb, e.g. *likes*
-ship	Friendship	
-tude	Gratitude	
(b) *May indicate verbs*		
-ate	Locate	May also indicate a noun, e.g. *delegate* or adjective, e.g. *delicate* – use other tests to check
-ed	Wanted	May also indicate an adjective – use other tests to check
-en	Moisten	
-ify	Testify	
-ise, -ize	Advertise	
-s	Seems	Only if it does NOT indicate 'more than one' – if it does have this meaning, it signals a noun

(*continued*)

Table 5.1   (*Continued*)

Suffix	Examples	Cautionary notes
(c) *May indicate adjectives*		
-able, -ible	Laughable, audible	
-al, -ial	Local, special	May also indicate a noun, e.g. *recital* – use other tests to check
-an	Texan	
-ant, -ent	Militant, penitent	May also indicate a noun, e.g. *assistant* – use other tests to check
-er	Louder	Only when it means 'more' and appears on a word that describes a verb
-est	Loudest	Only when it means 'most' and appears on a word that describes a verb
-ful	Wonderful	May also indicate a noun when a quantity is indicated, e.g. *spoonful*, *cupful*
-ic	Athletic	
-ish	Selfish	
-ive	Restrictive	
-less	Mindless	
-like	Childlike	
-ory	Sensory	
-ous	Ridiculous	
-some	Irksome	
-th	Tenth	Only when added to numbers; otherwise may indicate a noun, e.g. width, length
-y	Rubbery	
(d) *May indicate adverbs*		
-er	Louder	Only when it means 'more' and appears on a word that describes a noun
-est	Loudest	Only when it means 'most' and appears on a word that describes a noun
-ly	Extremely	Usually indicates an adverb, but may indicate an adjective, e.g. *cowardly*. Use other tests to check.

preceded by the word *the* or *a* will be a noun. This is another piece of evidence that confirms our hypothesis about *guards* in (4a) and *guard* in (4b). Consider also (5).

5   a   I am going for a swim.
    b   I swim every day.

In (5a), because the context is consistent with the heuristic that we just presented, *swim* is a noun. It is a verb in (5b); we will explain why later when we consider the tests for verbs.

We can think of the distributional evidence as a sort of pattern identification. A common pattern that we find in English at the end of a sentence is *the* or *a* followed by a noun. Indeed, this pattern is found elsewhere in sentences; it just happens to be very clear at the end of sentences. The existence of these patterns is explicitly recognised in the STASS and DASS, two assessments that were mentioned earlier in this chapter (as well as the LARSP, on which they are based). The STASS and DASS list common sequences such as D N, PREP D N and PREP D ADJ N, where PREP stands for preposition, D stands for determiner, ADJ stands for adjective and N stands for noun. We will say more about these patterns later.

In the following sections we list some useful heuristics that will help you to label words with their parts of speech. These tests will consist mainly of information about suffixation and distribution.

5.3.5   Tests for parts of speech

5.3.5.1   *Determiners*

Determiners are a small set of function words that will be useful to learn because they can often act as islands of reliability that are extremely useful for categorising more ambiguous words:

– *the, a, an* (also called 'articles')
– *this, these, that, those* (also called 'demonstratives')
– *my, your, his, her, its, our, their* (also called 'possessives')

The determiner *the* is also referred to as the definite article, while *a* and *an* are indefinite articles.

The words *the, a, an, your, its, our* and *their* are <u>always</u> determiners, and *my* is also nearly always a determiner (in fact it always is, apart from when it occurs in the exclamation *My oh my!*). The others can belong to other classes: *his* and *her* can also be pronouns, as can all of the demonstratives *this, these, that* and *those*; and *my* is sometimes used as an exclamation or interjection (as in *My oh my!*), though it is usually a determiner.

When you encounter words that have more than one part-of-speech label, use other tests to work out which one you are dealing with. A useful test in these cases is **substitution**. Consider (6) and (7):

6   a   I like this book.
    b   I like the book.
    c   I like their book.

Table 5.2   Some common English prepositions

About	Behind	In	Since*
Above	Below	Inside	Through
Across	Beneath	Into	Throughout
After*	Beside	Near	To*
Against	Between	Of	Towards
Along	Beyond	Off	Under
Amidst	By	On	Up
Around	Despite	Onto	Upon
At	During	Of	Via
Because of	For	Over	With
Before	From	Past	Without

Note: Those words marked with an asterisk also function as other categories.

7   a   I like this.
    b   *I like the.
    c   *I like their.

You might want to know the part of speech of the word *this* in (6a). As we just noted, *this* can be a determiner, but it can also be a pronoun (see Section 5.3.5.4). If it is a determiner, it should be possible to substitute another, unambiguous determiner such as *the* or *their* without the sentence becoming ungrammatical, and as (6b) and (6c) show, we can do so. We thus have evidence consistent with the hypothesis that *this* is a determiner in (6a). The fact that the same substitution test fails in (7b) and (7c) suggests that *this* is not a determiner in (7a). When you reach Section 5.3.5.4, you will see some examples of words that are unambiguous pronouns and you can try substituting those to see whether the word *this* really is a pronoun in (7a).

In some texts, and indeed in some clinical resources, you will find the words *my*, *your*, *her*, *its*, *our* and *their* listed as 'possessive pronouns'. We will return to this point when we cover pronouns later.

5.3.5.2   Prepositions

Prepositions also consist of a larger closed class set that can provide useful islands of reliability. Table 5.2 shows some common prepositions. Learn them! The forms that are marked with an asterisk may also turn up as other categories; for example, *after* can be a subordinating conjunction as well as a preposition (see Section 5.3.5.9). But the majority are reliably prepositions.

Sometimes prepositions occur as part of multiword verbs (see Section 5.3.5.6) such as *shut up* or *sit down*. Under these circumstances the preposition is often labelled a particle. We will return to this point in Section 5.3.5.6.

Exercise 5.1

Check that you have learned the determiners and prepositions mentioned so far in this chapter. Underline all the determiners and highlight all the prepositions in the following passage:

This paragraph concerns the novel 'David Copperfield', which was written by Charles Dickens. It was published in the form of a novel in 1850, a year after its serialisation in a magazine. It is about the life of David Copperfield. He was orphaned at a young age and for a time worked in a factory under cruel conditions. During this time he lodged with a family called Micawber who were sent to prison because of their debts. Facing a life without financial or emotional support, our hero eventually escaped from those miserable conditions and was raised by his aunt, Betsey Trotwood. Through her kindness he completed his education and later began a legal career. Mr Micawber came into the story again when he provided evidence against an evil character, Uriah Heep. Over the years, David developed a talent for storytelling and observation, and later became an acclaimed writer.

Now that you have mastered some determiners and prepositions to use as islands of reliability, we can exploit this information when we consider categories that are sometimes more difficult to classify.

5.3.5.3   Nouns

Many words that can be **nouns** can also turn up as other parts of speech. The following tests can be useful for determining whether a word is a noun in a particular context. Remember that they are only heuristics or rules of thumb, and that a definitive answer will depend on syntactic analysis that we will cover in later chapters.

Suffixation can provide useful evidence for nouns. Check whether the word ends in one of the noun suffixes listed in Table 5.1. As we noted earlier, some of the evidence provided by suffixes is pretty reliable even when we are considering a word in isolation. For example, the presence of the suffix *-ist* should make us pretty certain that *archaeologist* is a noun, even out of context. We also pointed out earlier that some suffixes are a bit more ambiguous. For example, although the suffix *-s* can signal other parts of speech, if it contributes the meaning 'more than one', it is likely to be a noun. In *The archaeologists found several wells*, the presence of *-s* with the meaning 'more than one' indicates that here, *well* is a noun (and so is *archaeologists*, as we noted earlier).

The suffix that is written *-'s* (apostrophe -s), with a meaning something like 'belonging to', also signals a noun, so if we had *The well was the engineer's greatest achievement*, we could also hypothesise that *engineer* was a noun in this sentence. Note that the form *-'s* does not always have signal 'belonging to' or anything similar. For example, it can be an abbreviation for *is* (e.g. *That's fine*), *has* (He's gone) or *us* (e.g. *Let's do it!*). In such cases, the word that it is attached to is not necessarily a noun, though it can be, as in *Britain's Got Talent*.

Notice that both of these endings can be added to words that already have endings that indicate nouns; for example, in the phrase *their Royal Highnesses*, the last word has the ending *-ness* that indicates a noun, followed by the ending *-s* meaning 'more than one', and this word is indeed a noun.

We have just stated that we can add the suffix *-s* meaning 'more than one' (or **plural**, to use the term that linguists use) to most nouns, but there are exceptions to this general observation. Some nouns, such as *child* and *mouse*, form their plural in a more idiosyncratic way (*children, mice*), and we will return to such forms in Chapter 6. Other nouns do not usually have plural forms at all. These **mass nouns** refer to entities in which we cannot identify individual sub-units (e.g. substances, such as *porridge*) or do not choose to do so (e.g. *footwear*). Nouns that do have a plural form, such as *chair, child* or *mouse*, are called **count nouns**. Some forms that are typically used as mass nouns can be used as count nouns in a specialised sense; for example, *wine* is normally used as a mass noun, but a wine merchant might refer to *the wines of Australia*, referring to different varieties.

Distributional evidence is often useful for nouns. Categories that frequently precede nouns are determiners, (see Section 5.3.5.1), prepositions (Section 5.3.5.2) and adjectives (Section 5.3.5.5), or sequences of these. For example, *look* can be a noun or a verb, but it is a noun in *Take a look* (Determiner + Noun), *He silenced her with a look* (Preposition + Determiner + Noun), *He gave her an angry look* (Determiner + Adjective + Noun) and *He silenced her with an angry look* (Preposition + Determiner + Adjective + Noun). Note that in the STASS and DASS, you are asked to record the occurrence of sequences like this in the client's speech, using the labels DN, PrDN, DAdjN and PrDAdjN, respectively.

If the target word is the very last one in a sentence, and is immediately preceded by a determiner (especially those unambiguous ones *the, a, an, my, your, its, our* and *their*), it is probably a noun; to continue the example above, in *The archaeologists found a well*, the last word is probably a noun because the word *a* preceding it is unambiguously a determiner. Also, the presence of the first word *The* alerts us to the fact that the next word, *archaeologists*, could be a noun. When we take into account the fact that *archaeologists* also ends in *-s* and that the *-s* means 'more than one', we can feel pretty confident that *archaeologists* is a noun here. Nouns are also often directly preceded by a preposition (see Table 5.2) as in *The well was found by archaeologists*, or a sequence of preposition followed by determiner as in *The well was found by the archaeologists*. If the target word is the very last one in a sentence and is preceded by a preposition, it is a noun.

A noun can be an appropriate one-word answer to a *What . . . ?* or *Who . . . ?* question, e.g. *Who found the wells? Archaeologists*, or *What did the archaeologists find? Wells*. In these two examples, we can see that the one-word answers both refer to 'more than one' (see the discussion of the plural suffix earlier in this section); for cases where the target word refers to a single entity, we could precede it in the answer with a determiner: *Who found the wells? An archaeologist*, or *What did the archaeologists find? The wells*.

The names of people and places are nouns, such as *Martin* and *London* in *Martin lives in London*. These sorts of nouns are also called **proper nouns**.

Though we said above that the traditional criterion that defines a noun as 'the name of a person, place or thing' was not very helpful as the only test of a word's part of speech, it is worth bearing in mind as an additional piece of confirmatory evidence if the other clues point towards this category.

Exercise 5.2

Underline any nouns in the following sentences. Remember to look out for (i) words that end in the suffixes that signal nouns (see Table 5.1), and/or (ii) words that are preceded by determiners or by a sequence of preposition + determiner. Therefore, *begin by identifying determiners and prepositions and noun-signalling endings*, and use these as islands of reliability.

a. Procrastination is the thief of time.
b. The Queen is a believer in the sanctity of marriage.
c. This wine tastes of blackcurrants.
d. Your attitude causes problems.
e. The magician astonished us with his performance.
f. The activist's heroism led to a change in the law.
g. A horse, a horse, my kingdom for a horse!
h. The company's employees voted for a strike.
i. Levels of employment must rise.

5.3.5.4 Pronouns

A **pronoun** is an example of a **pro-form** – it is a word that can be substituted for another word, or for a group of words. Consider (8).

8   a   Ted liked Sue, but she didn't like him.
     b   Ted liked Sue, but Sue didn't like Ted.
     c   That man liked the girl, but she didn't like him.

In the second part of (8a), *she* has been substituted for *Sue* and *him* has been substituted for *Ted*. A sentence like (8b) that does not involve this substitution would be acceptable, but perhaps sounds a little stilted. The words *she* and *him* are both **pronouns**, and though they replaced individual words in (8a), they could replace certain groups of words instead. For example, we could have (8c), in which the pronouns replace both the sequence Determiner + Noun (*That man*; *the girl*). Later, there will be further discussion on the groups of words that pronouns can replace.

As we just noted, pronouns typically refer back to something that has been mentioned earlier in the sentence. The terms **anaphora** or **anaphoric reference** are used to refer to this situation. The technical term for the more specific word (or group of words) that was mentioned earlier is **antecedent**. So in (8a) the antecedent

Table 5.3 Personal pronouns

	Number	
Person	**Singular**	**Plural**
First person	I	We
	Me	Us
Second person	You	You
Third person	He, she, it	They
	Him, her, it	Them

of *she* is *Sue* and the antecedent of *him* is *Ted*. In (8c) the antecedent of *she* is *the girl* and the antecedent of *him* is *that man*. Occasionally, the pronoun may precede rather than follow the more specific word or groups in the sentence, as in (9).

9   As soon as I saw <u>him</u>, I knew that <u>John Smith</u> was guilty.

This is an example of the **cataphoric** use of pronouns, which is more common in written than spoken language.

There are several different types of pronouns. Some can offer islands of reliability, so they should be learned. The various types of pronoun frequently turn up in clinical resources. For example, look at the items in CELF-4's Word Structure section, in particular those labelled 'subjective pronouns' and 'objective pronouns', 'reflexive pronouns' and 'possessive pronouns'.

We will start by considering **personal pronouns**, which are shown in Table 5.3, along with their labelling system. This requires a little explanation. Consider first the three cells in the column labelled 'Singular'. Each pronoun listed here refers to a single individual, which is why the number label 'Singular' is applied. The three 'Person' labels, first person, second person, and third person, can best be thought of as a way of referring to the participants in a conversation involving a rather egotistical speaker. When the speaker wants to refer to himself or herself, the forms 'I' or 'you' will be used; this egotistical speaker considers themselves to be the 'first person', so 'I' and 'me' are first person forms. From the speaker's point of view, the second most important person in the conversation, the 'second person', is the person they are talking to; the speaker will refer to this person with 'you', the second person form. Anyone or anything else that these two talk about will be referred to using the third person forms *he, she, it, him* and *her*.

Where two lines are shown in a cell, the upper line gives the **subjective form** and the lower gives the **objective form**. Consider (10), in which the examples contain two pronouns and the verb *like*.

10   a   I like her.
     b   *Me like she.

The subjective form goes before the verb in (10a), and the objective form follows the verb; switching them around, as in (10b), results in an ungrammatical sentence. The 'second person' row only contains the word *you*, which does not vary in the way that the first person pronouns do. The 'third person' row again has some distinctions between subjective and objective forms, though the form *it* does not vary. For the moment, just learn to label each form as subjective or objective, as appropriate. Knowing these labels will help you later when we come to consider sentence structure in Chapter 7.

Inspection of the pronouns labelled 'Plural' reveals that all of these items refer to more than one individual, but otherwise the remarks that were made previously about Person and subjective and objective forms also apply here. For example, the speaker, when referring to a group of people of which he or she is a member, will use first person forms *we* (subjective) or *us* (objective), and so on.

Each of the two rows in the 'Third person singular' cell contains three items, corresponding to the 'gender' dimension. In each row, the first form is used to refer to male individuals, the second to female individuals, and the third to genderless entities. Look at the 'Pronoun gender/number' items in the Test for the Reception of Grammar (TROG-2), which assess clients' ability to understand these aspects of personal pronouns in a picture selection task.

Exercise 5.3

Consult the personal pronoun table in this chapter and produce the appropriate label for the following personal pronouns. For example, 'me' would be labelled 'first person singular, objective form'.

Pronoun	Person	Number	Form
Me	First person	Singular	Objective form
They			
He, she, it			
We			
Them			
Him, her, it			
I			
Us			

Let us now consider **reflexive pronouns**, which are shown in Table 5.4. Consider (11).

11 a Eric sent a photo of himself.
   b *Eric sent a photo of Eric.
   c Eric sent a photo of him.

Table 5.4   Reflexive pronouns

Person	Number	
	Singular	Plural
First person	Myself	Ourselves
Second person	Yourself	Yourselves
Third person	Himself, herself, itself	Themselves

In (11a), *himself* is a reflexive pronoun. As this example illustrates, reflexive pronouns refer to the same entity as a noun that has been mentioned earlier in the sentence. Notice that (11b), with the noun repeated, could have the same meaning as (11a), but it is not the way a native speaker would express this concept. In fact (11b) is ambiguous because the two tokens of the word *Eric* might denote two different individuals (though under such circumstances, it is likely that the speaker would differentiate them, by adding their surnames for example). Alternatively, in (11c), where a personal pronoun is used instead of a reflexive pronoun, the pronoun has to be referring to someone other than *Eric*.

We turn now to **possessive pronouns**. Remember that we said earlier that pronouns substitute for a noun or a sequence of words containing a noun, such as (Determiner + Noun). Consider (12).

12   a   That Ferrari is John's.
     b   That Ferrari is his.
     c   I like John's Ferrari.
     d   I like his Ferrari.

Notice that in (12a), *John's* carries the suffix -'s that contributes the meaning 'belonging to' (see Table 5.1). Since forms that end in -'s are often called **possessive** forms, we could refer to *John's* as a **possessive noun**, a term that is used in the CELF-4 Word Structure section. The sort of word that substitutes for a noun is a pronoun, so *his* in (12b) would be a possessive pronoun. Further possessive pronouns are shown in Table 5.5.

Table 5.5   Possessive pronouns (pronoun use – see text)

Person	Number	
	Singular	Plural
First person	Mine	Ours
Second person	Yours	Yours
Third person	His, hers	Theirs

To continue our analysis of (12), if *John's* in (12a) is a possessive noun, and by virtue of this we call the substituted form *his* in (12b) a possessive pronoun, what about *his* in (12d)? This form also substitutes for *John's* in (12c), a possessive noun, so presumably we should call this token of *his* a possessive pronoun as well, and indeed, this is the traditional label that would be applied to *his* in both (12b) and (12d). Now consider (13).

13 a   That Ferrari is mine.
    b   *That Ferrari is my.
    c   My red Ferrari is fantastic.
    d   *Mine red Ferrari is fantastic.

In traditional grammars, and indeed in some clinical resources such as the STASS and DASS, in (13) both *mine* and *my* would be labelled possessive pronouns, just like *his* in (12). How do we explain the ungrammaticality of (13b) and (13d)? Look back at examples (6) and (7), which illustrated the way that substitution could be used to identify the part of speech of *this* in (6a) *I like this book*. The fact that we could substitute unambiguous determiners *the* and *their* in (6b) *I like the book* and (6c) *I like their book* led us to conclude that *this* was a determiner in (6a). So by the same criterion, in both (14a) and (14b), *his* should be a determiner.

14 a   I like his book.
    b   I like his Ferrari.

So one approach seems to call *my, your, his*, etc. determiners, and the other calls them pronouns. How do we resolve these conflicting labels? The compromise that is sometimes adopted (see Further Reading) is to call all the forms in Table 5.5, plus *my, your, his, her, its, our* and *their* 'possessives' and to identify two sub-groups based on function (according to the criterion of substitutability): the forms in Table 5.5 are possessives with the '**pronoun function**' or '**independent function**' and the rest are possessives with the '**determiner function**'. Be conscious of this distinction when you encounter the term 'possessive pronoun' in textbooks and assessments.

Interrogative pronouns occur in question forms and comprise the words *who, whom, whose, which* and *what*, as in the following sentences:

15   Who was that masked man?
16   To whom should this letter be addressed?
17   What is your name?
18   Which is your office?
19   Whose office is this?

Because they all begin with the letters wh- they are often called **wh-forms**. We have been using the notion of substitution to explain what pronouns are. Interrogative pronouns are substituted in cases where the full form is not known, and that is why the speaker is asking a question in the first place. For example, it is obvious that the person who asks *Who was the 35th US president?* or *What is Joanna Lumley's middle name?* does not have the information that would be required to provide the specific form of reference (e.g. *John F. Kennedy was the 35th US president* or *Lamond is Joanna Lumley's middle name*). For example (19), we could have a discussion similar to the one around 'possessive pronouns'.

The form *whom* is nowadays associated with quite formal language; in less formal interactions we might restructure the sentence and use *who* instead, for example, *Who should this letter be addressed to?*

The **relative pronouns** *who, whom, whose, which* and *that* sometimes have the same form as interrogative pronouns, but they are not necessarily used in question forms. Here are some examples of relative pronouns:

20   Tim Berners-Lee is the person <u>who</u> invented the World Wide Web.

21   He is Tim Berners-Lee, <u>whose</u> name is associated with the invention of the World Wide Web.

22   The manager is the person to <u>whom</u> letters should be addressed.

23   There are various ways in <u>which</u> we can identify parts of speech.

24   This is the house <u>that</u> Jack built.

In (20), the speaker presumably is not asking to be told the identity of the person who invented the World Wide Web when they use the word *who*. Instead, *who* is being used here to introduce a particular syntactic structure called the relative clause, which will be considered in Chapter 8.

The use of the **demonstrative pronouns** is illustrated in the following sentences:

25   I like <u>this</u>.

26   I like <u>that</u>.

27   I like <u>these</u>.

28   I like <u>those</u>.

The forms *this* and *that* are used to refer to singular entities, while *these* and *those* are plural forms. *This* and *these* are used when the entity that is being referred to is relatively close to the speaker in space or time, while *that* and *those* refer to more distant entities. For example, (29) and (30) refer to the place where the speaker is currently, or the current time, respectively:

29   I love places like <u>this</u>.

30   I love moments like <u>these</u>.

But in (31) and (32), the speaker must be referring to places or times other than those that they are currently experiencing:

31   I love places like <u>that</u>.

32   I love moments like <u>those</u>.

A final group of forms that we will identify are called **indefinite pronouns.** These include *no one, someone, anyone, everyone, nobody, somebody, anybody, everybody, nothing, something, anything, everything,* etc.

Exercise 5.4

Underline any pronouns in this passage. For each pronoun that you identify, indicate its type (personal, reflexive, possessive, interrogative, relative), and if relevant, its label in terms of Person, Number and subjective/objective.

Snow White's stepmother, the Evil Queen, had a Magic Mirror which could speak. Every day she looked at herself in it and asked, 'Who is the fairest in the land?'. The Mirror usually replied, 'You are, my Queen'. But one day the Mirror replied, 'Snow White is the fairest'. The Queen was furious. She would do anything to be rid of Snow White. She called for the woodcutter and ordered him to take Snow White into the forest and kill her. The woodcutter was deeply shocked by this. He did take Snow White into the forest, but he let her escape.

Snow White met seven dwarves, who allowed her to live with them. 'Will you look after this house for us while we are at work?' they asked. They went off every day to work in a gold mine. One day while they were out the Queen came along in disguise. She tricked Snow White into eating a poisoned apple. At first Snow White was reluctant, saying, 'The dwarves told me not to take anything from strangers. I am not sure whether I should eat that'. But the Queen said, 'See, I have cut the apple in half and we will each take half. You eat yours, and I will eat mine'. But the half that she gave Snow White contained poison. As soon as Snow White bit the apple she fell into a deep sleep.

When they saw her, the dwarves persuaded themselves that she was dead, and placed her in a glass coffin. But a year later a Handsome Prince saw the sleeping Snow White and fell in love with her. He awakened her with a kiss, and said at once, 'Will you marry me?' Snow White agreed, and they were married, and lived happily ever after.

5.3.5.5 Adjectives

The traditional definition of an **adjective** is 'a describing word'. As we noted earlier, these traditional definitions are sometimes misleading, and even when they are not, they often only tell part of the story. Although it is true that many adjectives do describe something, other parts of speech could also be said to have a describing role. It may, however, help us to identify the part of speech 'adjective' if we bear in mind that what adjectives 'describe' are nouns. For example, consider (33) and (34).

33   The runner is fast.

34   The fast runner won the race.

In (33) and (34), *fast* is an adjective, and it describes (or as linguists would say, **modifies**) *runner*. *Runner* has characteristics that should make us suspect that it is a noun: It ends with the suffix *-er* which here has the 'doer of' meaning mentioned in Table 5.1, and it is preceded by the determiner *the* in (33). If we have the sequence (Determiner + Noun) in *The runner* in (33), that is reassuring, because that is one of the sequences that the STASS and DASS tell us to record (DN); and if *fast* is indeed an adjective, in *The fast runner* in (34) we would have D ADJ N, another sequence specified by the assessments. So in both (33) and (34) the evidence points to *fast* being an adjective. Notice that in both of these examples, *fast* refers to a characteristic of the runner, not of the manner in which they ran on this occasion – for example, they may have run at a moderate speed on the occasion when they ran the race, if the other runners ran even more slowly.

Here are some further comments about tests for identifying adjectives.

- Suffixation: Some suffixes that may signal adjectives are shown in Table 5.1. This should be self-explanatory, but notice in particular the suffix *-er*. A suffix that signals nouns and that has exactly the same form appears elsewhere in the table; for example, when *-er* is added to *work*, it indicates a noun, because *worker* means 'someone who works' so the *-er* suffix here has the meaning 'doer of'. The suffix *-er* only signals an adjective if it has the meaning 'more' (and if the word that ends in -er modifies a noun); for example, in *That noise is louder* or *That is a louder noise*, *louder* modifies the noun *noise* and it means 'more loud' not 'someone who louds'.
- Distribution: As noted earlier, adjectives can turn up in two contexts, illustrated by the examples just used. *That noise is loud* is an example of the so-called **predicative** use of the adjective *loud*, while *That is a loud noise* or *A loud noise startled me* are examples of the **attributive** use. Similarly, *fast* is used predicatively in (33) but attributively in (34). Notice that the adjective occurs between a determiner and a noun in the attributive examples just given. In fact, it is possible for the determiner to be omitted in certain structures that include attributive adjectives. For example, we may have *The fast runners won the race* or *Fast runners won the race*. The latter would conform to the ADJ N pattern that the STASS and DASS identify.
- An adjective can modify a pronoun if the adjective is used predicatively, as in *She is famous*. There are some cases where attributive adjectives modify pronouns, such as *silly me* or *poor you*, but they are in the minority.
- An adjective can be modified by adverbs (see Section 5.3.5.8).
- A noun can be modified by a sequence of adjectives, as in *He was carrying a large, heavy suitcase*, in which the noun *suitcase* is modified by the two adjectives *large* and *heavy*. Sequences of adjectives can occur attributively, as in the previous example, or predicatively, as in *The suitcase was large and heavy*. Notice that in the predicative usage, the word *and* occurs between the adjectives (see Conjunctions, Section 5.3.5.9). The word *and* can occur between the adjectives in the attributive usage (e.g. *He was carrying a large and heavy suitcase*), but it is perhaps less common.

Exercise 5.5

Underline any adjectives in the passage below. Remember to look out for words that modify nouns. They may end in one of the adjective suffixes listed in Table 5.1; they may occur in a sequence containing other adjectives; they may appear between a determiner and a noun if used attributively, though the determiner may be omitted. It therefore makes sense to start by identifying any islands of reliability in the form of determiners and prepositions, as well as nouns.

La Pedrera is the name of a building designed in the twentieth century by the Catalan architect Antoni Gaudi. Its basic design was controversial because of the curvaceous forms of the façade. Architecturally it is considered innovative because of original methods used in its construction. Other innovations were the construction of separate lifts and stairs for the owners and their servants. It was built for a wealthy couple, Roser Segimon and Pere Milà, whose lifestyle was extremely lavish and flamboyant. Gaudi held strong religious beliefs and tried to incorporate Christian symbols in the design of the building, but the local government objected to this. Today La Pedrera is a venue for various activities and exhibitions.

5.3.5.6 Full verbs

In standard English, all grammatical sentences contain a **verb**. We can respond to a question, for example, with a single word that is not a verb (e.g. *What is your favourite ice-cream? Strawberry*) but the response is not technically a sentence. Verbs have traditionally been defined as 'action' words or 'doing' words. The verb in (35) is *walk*:

35   The children *walk* in the park.

In this sentence, it is true that the verb *walk* does denote an action which the children perform – the action of walking in the park. However, in (36), *walk* is not a verb, but a noun – it is preceded by the determiner *a* (see Section 5.3.5.3):

36   The children took a *walk* in the park.

There are many verbs that do not denote an action at all. For example, in (37), we cannot say that the verb *seems* denotes an action.

37   The evidence seems undeniable.

It would hardly be accurate to say that the evidence is performing any action when it 'seems' undeniable. So the notion of verbs as 'action' words is somewhat limited.

We can go some way towards identifying verbs by looking at the suffixes that commonly appear on this part of speech (see Table 5.1). Some of the items listed there, such as *-ify*, *-ise* and *-ize*, are fairly strong indicators of a word's status as a verb. One suffix to note, because it is not a straightforward indicator, is *-s*, which we have discussed earlier. A suffix with this form was mentioned previously as signalling nouns, with the important proviso that when it signalled this part of speech it should have the meaning 'more than one'. As we will see when we discuss suffixes in more detail, the -s that signals a verb <u>never</u> has the meaning 'more than one', so this is a useful way of distinguishing between the two forms. For example, consider (38) and (39).

38   He fears spiders.

39   He has many fears.

The word *fear* can be a noun or a verb. In (38), the -s on *fears* does not mean 'more than one', so *fears* is not a noun here – in fact it is a verb. The -s on *spiders*, however, does mean 'more than one', and *spiders* is a noun. By contrast, in (39), the -s on *fears* does indicate 'more than one', so here, *fears* is a noun. As we noted earlier, these are only simple heuristics to help you to hypothesise what part of speech you might be dealing with until you have a proper understanding of syntax, but they can be useful while you are learning.

Distributional evidence can also help us to identify verbs. Verbs are often preceded by pronouns, or by groups of words that can be replaced by pronouns; for example, *start* is a verb in *They start on Monday* or *The new students start on Monday*. We can also use distributional evidence as a signal that a word is <u>not</u> a verb; for example, verbs are not directly preceded by determiners, so *start* is <u>not</u> a verb in *The start of term is Monday* (here it is a noun).

We can identify two kinds of verb: **full** (or **main**, or **lexical**) and **auxiliary** verbs. An example of a full verb is *decorate* and an example of an auxiliary verb is *should*. The majority of verbs that are listed in a dictionary are full verbs – that is, drawing on terminology that we encountered in Chapter 2, among verbs, the majority of lexemes or word <u>types</u> are full verbs. On the other hand, the <u>frequency</u> of full verbs tends to be much lower than that of auxiliary verbs.

The dictionary entry for a full verb will consist of meaningful, interpretable definitions and synonyms. For example, the dictionary entry for the full verb *appear* might include 'to seem; to be obvious or easily perceived; to perform publicly, as in a play, film, etc'. This is why full verbs are sometimes called lexical verbs – because they have an interpretable meaning in the dictionary (or lexicon). Contrast this with the dictionary entry for an auxiliary verb such as *is*, which will consist instead of a definition couched in grammatical terms such as 'used with the present participle of another (full) verb to form the progressive tense'. It will by now come as no surprise that many forms can function as either full or auxiliary verbs, depending on context. The verb *has* is one such form: it is a full verb in (40), with the lexical meaning 'owns', but an auxiliary in (41).

40   She has a red Ferrari.

41   She has appeared in 'Chicago'.

To give you a feel for what lexical verbs are like, complete the following exercise, in which the only verbs that are used are lexical verbs. Before you try it, go to Appendix A and make sure that you have learned the verbs that are shown there as islands of reliability.

Exercise 5.6

In the following sentences, the only verbs that we have used are full verbs. Underline them. Remember that (i) you should consult Table 5.1 for a list of suffixes that signal verbs; (ii) you should have learned a list of common verbs from Appendix A as 'Islands of Reliability'; if any of these appear in the examples below, they are being used as full verbs; and (iii) when completing this task you should be taking into account the part of speech of other words in the sentence as well, to help you in the process of elimination, so look out for (and label) determiners, prepositions, nouns and adjectives as well as verbs.

a. This exercise seems easy.
b. Towards the finish, the runners quicken their pace.
c. We celebrate Christmas in December.
d. The party was a great success.
e. Henry has measles.
f. Voters often criticise the government.
g. Those flowers are gorgeous.
h. *The Iron Lady* concerns the life and career of Margaret Thatcher.
i. He explained his concerns about the plan.
j. She became an MP in 1966.
k. Leaves change their colour in autumn.

As we noted earlier, several verb forms can either be full verbs or auxiliary verbs, depending on the context in which they appear. Auxiliary verbs will be described in the next section. One form that can be a full or auxiliary verb is 'to be', which includes the forms *am, is, are, was* and *were*. When one of these forms is being used as a full verb it is sometimes referred to as a **copula** or **copular verb**. There are other copular verbs, including *appear, seem* and *become*. However, in some assessments (such as the STASS) you will see references to 'the copula' or 'Cop', and unless you are told otherwise you can assume that the verb 'to be' is intended. The reason for using this specific name for the lexical verb function of 'to be' is that it is such a common verb and that it often turns up in its alternative function, as an auxiliary verb, so it is useful to have a special label for it when it is being a full verb.

The forms *am, is* and *are* are sometimes used in a contracted form, written with an apostrophe, as in (42) to (44):

42 I'm sorry.

43 He's an idiot.

44 They're here.

You will see such forms referred to in language development textbooks and clinical resources as the **contractible copula**. Such forms are indicated in the STASS and DASS using the symbol 'cop. Similarly, when the verb appears in its full form, e.g.

45 I am sorry.

46 He is an idiot.

47 They are here.

it is referred to as the **uncontractible copula**. These labels seem to imply that the forms 'can' or 'cannot' be contracted, which may be a little misleading; better labels might be 'contracted copula' and 'uncontracted copula', but the other labels are conventionally used. The uncontractible copula is labelled Cop in the STASS and DASS.

In Section 5.3.5.2 we mentioned that prepositions sometimes occur alongside full verbs to form multiword verbs such as *cross out* or *turn on*, and that in these circumstances the preposition is often called a **particle**. Assessments such as the STASS, DASS or LARSP note these forms and label them 'V Part'. Notice that with such forms, the particle can occur immediately after the verb, as in (48a) and (49a), or other words can intervene, as in (48b) and (49b).

48   a   She crossed out her name.
     b   She crossed her name out.

49   a   He turned on the radio.
     b   He turned the radio on.

5.3.5.7   *Auxiliary verbs*

In the previous exercise, we confined ourselves to examples that contained only full verbs. Often, however, a full verb will be accompanied by an auxiliary verb. For example, consider (50).

50 They have arrived.

In (50), *have* is an auxiliary verb, and the full verb is *arrived*, which includes the suffix *-ed*. Auxiliary literally means 'helping', and the role of an auxiliary verb (or just 'auxiliary') is to help the full verb by providing grammatical support.

As we noted earlier, many of these auxiliary verbs can be full verbs as well. See (51) to (53).

51 They have money.

52 She is crying.

53 She is sad.

In (51), *have* is an auxiliary verb; contrast this with (50). In (52), *is* is an auxiliary verb, but in (53) it is a full verb.

In the sorts of examples that turn up in clinical resources, auxiliaries almost always turn up with their full verb. This does not have to be so; for example, an auxiliary may turn up without its lexical verb in a reply to a question such as *Who is crying? She is*. But such examples are not typical of SLT resources, so if you suspect that a particular form is an auxiliary rather than a lexical verb, you should check whether another word in the item could be the full verb; if so, this strengthens the hypothesis that the ambiguous word (the one whose label you want to know) is an auxiliary. If there is no other word that is a candidate for the full verb in an item in a clinical resource, then most likely the ambiguous item is a full verb. Since *crying* fulfils criteria for being a full verb, we can feel confident that *is* is an auxiliary in (52). If the word in question is followed by an adjective, determiner or noun, it will be a full verb.

We can identify three kinds of auxiliary verb.

Primary auxiliaries are forms of the verb BE (*am, is, are, was, were, been, being*) and HAVE (*have, has, had, having*). They are the most common auxiliaries. Primary auxiliaries have a purely grammatical role.

The auxiliary verb DO (*do, does, did, doing*) is also sometimes called the **dummy auxiliary** because it is used when an auxiliary is needed and there is no other one available. Consider, for example, what happens when a question is formed from a statement in modern English, as in (54).

54   a   You are reading a book.
    b   What book are you reading?

The question may need to contain an auxiliary, and if the statement version contains an auxiliary already, this is used. So here, since *are* is a primary auxiliary, it is used in the question. But what happens if there is no auxiliary in the statement, as in (55)?

55   a   You prefer vanilla.
    b   What flavour do you prefer?

In (55b) the dummy auxiliary *do* is used. We will consider question formation in more detail in Chapter 8.

By contrast with primary auxiliaries, **modal auxiliaries** have a meaning dimension in addition to a grammatical role. The modal auxiliaries are *can, could, may, might, shall, should, will, would* and *must*. Semantically they express permission, ability, obligation or prediction. For example, the verbs in (56) express no lexical meaning beyond that in the full verb *writing*, but (57) expresses the additional meaning of obligation, which the word *must* conveys alongside its grammatical role.

56   I am writing.
57   I must write.

As we noted earlier, a sentence may contain only a full verb, or it may contain a full verb accompanied by one or more auxiliaries. For example, consider (58).

58   a   He goes.
      b   He went.
      c   He has gone.
      d   He was going.
      e   He may go.
      f   He has been going.
      g   He may have been going.

(58a) and (58b) contain only full verbs; (58c) and (58d) contain one primary auxiliary in addition to the full verb; (58e) contains one modal auxiliary in addition to the full verb; (58f) has two primary auxiliaries followed by the full verb; and (58g) has a modal auxiliary followed by two primary auxiliaries followed by the full verb. Though sequences of verbs like those in (58) may contain more than one primary auxiliary, it can only contain one modal auxiliary.

Exercise 5.7

Underline any auxiliary verbs in these sentences. Note that some of the sentences contain no auxiliaries. Remember that in the examples we use here, in common with most clinical assessments, if an auxiliary is used, the full verb will also be present. So if you think you see an auxiliary, check that you can find its full verb.

For each auxiliary that you identify, say whether it is modal, dummy or primary.

a. I am a fan of *The Big Bang Theory*.
b. *The Big Bang Theory* is about Leonard, Sheldon, Howard, Raj and Penny.
c. Leonard has glasses.
d. Penny is working as a waitress.
e. Penny and Leonard have been dating.
f. Sheldon and Leonard share an apartment.
g. Why do Sheldon and Leonard share an apartment?
h. Howard is an engineer.
i. Sheldon should have been awarded the Nobel prize by now.
j. Raj is usually shy with women.

5.3.5.8   Adverbs

We noted earlier that although adjectives are traditionally defined as 'describing words', this is true of other categories as well, and that it is more accurate to say that adjectives describe or 'modify' nouns. Another category that could be thought of as 'describing' is **adverbs,** which describe, or modify, verbs, adjectives and other adverbs. Consider (59) and (60).

59   a   Louise sings.
      b   Louise sings loudly.

60   a   Tom ran.
      b   Tom ran fast.

(59a) consists of a noun followed by a verb; in (59b), *loudly* is an adverb because it describes the manner in which the singing happens, not *Louise*. The same is true of *fast* in (60b); *fast* is describing the action of the verb *ran*, not *Tom*, who might habitually be slow. When adverbs modify verbs they can add a wide variety of meanings, relating to time, place, manner and so on, as illustrated in (61) to (63):

61   She left early.

62   She lives here.

63   She sings beautifully.

Adverbs can also modify adjectives, as in (64a) and other adverbs, as in (64b).

64   a   Her departure was unnecessarily abrupt.
      b   She left unnecessarily early.

More, most, less and *least* can also be used as adverbs modifying adjectives or other adverbs, as in (65) and (66).

65   He chose the less complex solution.

66   This is the most eagerly awaited episode.

Some resources refer to **intensifiers** (also known as **adverbs of degree**) such as *very* and *extremely*. See (67) to (69). The use of intensifiers is recorded by the label 'Int X' in the STASS, DASS and LARSP.

67   She is a very fast runner.

68   She runs very fast.

69   *She runs very.

Other adverbs of degree are called **qualifiers,** such as *rather* and *quite*.

Consider the following when you think a word might be an adverb:

- Common adverbs: see the list of adverbs that can be islands of reliability in Appendix A.
- Suffixation: Although *-ly* usually indicates an adverb (e.g. *slowly, beautifully*), this is only the case when it is added to an adjective (*slow, beautiful*). But there are a few exceptions (words that end in *-ly* but are not adverbs) such as the adjectives *friendly* and *cowardly*. That can be accounted for by a rule: if *-ly* is added to a noun, the resulting word is an adjective. Like adjectives, adverbs can have the suffix *-er* meaning 'more than' and *-est* meaning 'most' (e.g. *She ran faster; She ran fastest*).
- Many words that are commonly used as adverbs do not end in -ly, e.g. *more, most, less, least, not, never, very, quite, now, then, often, sometimes, always, here, there, fast, slow, loud.*

Exercise 5.8

Identify the adverbs in the following:

Boiling an egg

Never boil an egg that you have taken straight from the fridge because it will immediately crack in the boiling water. Always use a small saucepan. Fill the pan with water, and when it is just simmering, quickly but gently place the egg in the water using a spoon. After one minute remove the pan from the heat. Use a timer to measure the next stage exactly. After 6 minutes the yoke should be fairly liquid and the white will be quite wobbly; after 7 minutes the white will be completely set and the yolk should be lightly cooked but still soft.

5.3.5.9   Conjunctions

Conjunctions are used to join linguistic elements together. There are two kinds of conjunction: **coordinating** and **subordinating**. We will consider coordinating conjunctions first.

The most commonly used coordinating conjunctions are *and, but* and *or*. These can be used to join two linguistic units of the same kind, as in (70) to (74).

70   My favourite fruits are oranges and bananas. (two nouns)

71   I cried and cried and cried. (three verbs)

72   She spoke slowly and clearly. (two adverbs)

73   He was poor but honest. (two adjectives)

74   He was poor but he was honest. (two sentences)

Some conjunctions are used in pairs; examples of these **correlative conjunctions** are *either/or, neither/nor, not only/but (also), not just/but (also)* and *both/and*, as illustrated in (75).

75   a   He was either poor or honest.
      b   He was neither poor nor honest.
      c   He was not only poor but also honest.
      d   He was both poor and honest.

While coordinating conjunctions are used to link linguistic units that have the same grammatical status as each other, when a **subordinating conjunction** is used, it is signalling that one of the units is grammatically 'subordinate to' the other. For example, *because* is a subordinating conjunction in (76).

76   Rosa Parks was arrested because she would not give up her seat on the bus.

To anticipate a more detailed discussion that will occur in later chapters, notice that in the previous sentence we can identify two strings of words that could stand alone as sentences: *Rosa Parks was arrested*, and *she would not give up her seat*

Table 5.6   Some common subordinating conjunctions

After	Since
Although	So that
Because	Though
Before	Till
Even if	Unless
Even though	Until
If	While

on the bus, which is introduced by the subordinating conjunction. The presence of the subordinating conjunction indicates that the sentence *she would not give up her seat on the bus* has a lesser (grammatical) status than the 'main' part of the sentence, *Rosa Parks was arrested.* The part of the sentence that is introduced by the subordinating conjunction may occur after the 'main' part of the sentence, as in the previous example, or before it, as in (77).

77   a   Because she would not give up her seat on the bus, Rosa Parks was arrested.
     b   Because Rosa Parks would not give up her seat on the bus, she was arrested.

The issue of subordination is a complex one that will be considered in more detail in later chapters. For the moment, look at Table 5.6, which lists some forms that are commonly used as subordinating conjunctions in English.

Notice that some of the forms can also be prepositions (see Table 5.2). For example,

78   a   I go for a run before breakfast.
     b   I go for a run before I have breakfast.

In (78a), *before* is a preposition which is followed by the noun *breakfast*; but in (78b), *before* is a subordinating conjunction because it is followed by a set of words that could be used as a stand-alone sentence. Use distributional information to determine whether you are dealing with a preposition in a particular example.

Exercise 5.9

Identify the conjunctions in the following, and say whether they or coordinating, correlative or subordinating:

John Fitzgerald Kennedy ('JFK') was the 35th President of the United States. He served from 1961 until he was assassinated in 1963. After he completed military service, he represented Massachusetts in the US House of Representatives. In the presidential elections he defeated Richard Nixon even though he had far less experience than his opponent. His success was partly due to his skilful use of television. While JFK looked young and handsome in televised debates, Nixon looked tense and uncomfortable and perspired freely. Radio listeners to the same debates thought that Nixon had either won or performed equally well.

JFK was assassinated on 22nd November, 1963, in Dallas, Texas. Lee Harvey Oswald was charged with the crime, but he was shot and killed two days later by Jack Ruby before he could be tried. JFK's assassination has been the subject of many conspiracy theories, not just in the United States but elsewhere in the world.

5.3.5.10   *Putting it all together*

Now that you have learned to recognise various parts of speech – nouns, pronouns, full verbs, auxiliary verbs, adjectives, adverbs, determiners, prepositions and conjunctions – you should be able to have a go at assigning labels to all of the words in simple sentences.

We noted early on in this chapter that one source of information about parts of speech concerned the distribution of the category, that is, the parts of speech that often occur in its immediate context. Where relevant we have included information about distribution among the tests for particular parts of speech. Another way of thinking about these distributional characteristics is that there are certain patterns or sequences of part-of-speech labels that you can look out for in sentences that you are trying to analyse. For example, common patterns involving nouns are

- Determiner + Noun
- Preposition + Noun
- Preposition + Determiner + Noun
- Adjective + Noun
- Determiner + Adjective +Noun
- Preposition + Determiner + Adjective + Noun
- Adjective + Adjective + Noun

Full verbs are often preceded by one or more auxiliaries. The STASS, the DASS and the LARSP explicitly identify such sequences as part of the language profile of clients. Review the distributional information in the sections of this chapter and think about this when you are trying to identify parts of speech. We will have more to say about these common patterns in later chapters.

Exercise 5.10

Use the information that you have learned in this chapter to assign a part-of-speech label to each word in the sentences below. Choose the most explicit label that you can; for example, 'modal auxiliary' rather than just 'auxiliary', or 'reflexive pronoun' rather than just 'pronoun'.

a. The children crossed the very busy road.
b. She was becoming rather cross.
c. The teacher put a cross beside the answer.
d. Raise your hand if you can answer.

e. The cook added the juice of an orange to the mixture.
f. He was wearing an orange suit, which he bought at Primark.
g. Long hair suits you.
h. What were they doing?
i. You should cook the eggs until they are very firm.
j. The firm's accountant demanded immediate payment from us.
k. I received a final demand in the post.
l. I must post this letter.
m. Would you prefer fish or meat?
n. We could fish in the sea.
o. The road that leads to my home is completely straight.
p. These are mine and those are yours.
q. That might have been the best solution for this problem.
r. Who's there?
s. It's me.

Chapter summary

In this chapter, we have seen that if we wish to identify parts of speech such as determiner, preposition, auxiliary verb, pronoun, conjunction, noun, lexical verb, adjective and adverb:

• apart from a smallish number of exceptions, it is infeasible to learn the part-of-speech label of the many thousands of words that we know;
• we need to use information about endings on the word (suffixation) and the context in which the word occurs (distribution).

We can use a variety of tests to check our hypotheses about a word's part of speech. These include:

• Suffixation – the presence of particular word endings;
• Distribution – the presence of other nearby words.

Exercises using clinical resources

5.11. Look at the CAT, Section 9 'Comprehension of Spoken Sentences'. Give a part-of-speech label to each word of the 16 target items there (i.e. the sentences in bold).

5.12. In the TOAL-4, subtest 4 (Word Similarities), which of the 40 target items could be
   a. Nouns
   b. Verbs
   c. Adjectives
   d. Adverbs

Just base your answer on the written form of the target as shown on the response booklet – ignore other materials.

5.13. Identify the types of pronouns that are examined in the following resources:
a. CELF-4
b. CELF-Preschool
c. TROG-2
d. ERB
e. New RDLS

5.14. In the CELF-4 sub-test Formulated Sentences, identify lexical items that can be used as the following (i.e. ignoring any picture stimulus):
a. Verb (which kind?)
b. Adjective
c. Adverb

5.15. What kinds of pronouns are tested in the A-STOP-R? Be as specific as possible.

5.16. Which modal auxiliaries are listed under AUX on the STASS/DASS Rapid Assessment Score Sheet?

Further reading

A more comprehensive coverage of parts of speech is provided by Greenbaum and Quirk (1990). See Table 6.2 and Section 6.6 for the treatment of possessive forms.

The clinical differences between content words and function words are explored in the manual of the Early Repetition Battery (ERB).

6 Word Structure

Clinical resources that will be referenced in this chapter:

ACE – Assessment of Comprehension and Expression 6-11
CAT – Comprehensive Aphasia Test
CELF-4, CELF-Preschool – Clinical Evaluation of Language Fundamentals
DASS – Dorset Assessment of Syntactic Structures
ERB – Early Repetition Battery
LARSP – Language Assessment, Remediation and Screening Programme
Living Language
PALPA – Psycholinguistic Assessment of Language Processing in Aphasia
PPT-2 – Past Tense Test
STASS – South Tyneside Assessment of Syntactic Structures
TALC – Test of Abstract Language Comprehension
TOAL-4 – Test of Adolescent and Adult Language
TROG-2 – Test for the Reception of Grammar
VATT – Verb Agreement and Tense Test
Vocabulary Enrichment Intervention Programme

6.0 Introduction

An item on a teen magazine website invites readers to *Blair-ify your headbands!*, apparently referring to a style of hair ornament worn by a character called Blair Waldorf in the TV series Gossip Girl. Even without ever encountering the novel form *Blair-ify* before, and even if we are unfamiliar with the TV series, we can still interpret it because we know that *Blair* probably refers to a person and *-ify* turns up in words whose meaning includes 'to make', as in *purify* 'to make pure' or *clarify* 'to make clear'. So we interpret the novel word as meaning something like 'to make (into something having qualities associated with) Blair'. The fact that we can do this must mean that we have stored the sub-word unit *-ify* and linked this kind of meaning to it. This example highlights the fact that a common mechanism

---

Introductory Linguistics for Speech and Language Therapy Practice, First Edition. Jan McAllister and Jim Miller.
© 2013 John Wiley & Sons, Ltd. Published 2013 by John Wiley & Sons, Ltd.

for creating new words in English is the novel recombination of existing elements. It follows that words in English have an internal structure and that the rules that govern this structure are part of native speaker competence.

This chapter introduces the frameworks that linguists and SLTs use when discussing the internal structure of words. We first look at some general concepts to do with word structure, and then examine in more detail the main mechanisms for forming new words in English.

6.1   Why do SLTs need this knowledge?

Typically developing children, children experiencing language difficulties and people with agrammatic aphasia often produce utterances that violate the rules of word structure, or apply the rules in cases where they are inappropriate. You have probably heard a typically developing child producing forms like *goed* instead of *went* or *childs* instead of *children*. Although such errors are characteristic of typical development, persistent difficulty with these sorts of grammatical markers is a key feature of specific language impairment.

Many clinical resources are designed to target clients' knowledge of word structure. Some assessments, such as the TROG-2, CELF-4, DASS or STASS, cover a range of structures. Other resources, such as the VATT and PPT-2 focus on very specific areas that are often problematic, and as a clinician you need to understand the structures concerned in order to read the literature and to be able to identify further examples. When you have completed the assessments with a client and are interpreting the results, you need to be familiar with the terminology that is used for grouping related items, and once you have identified areas that you need to work on, you need to have a mastery of these concepts so that you can select appropriate materials for use in intervention. The manual of the Vocabulary Enrichment Intervention Programme points out that improving children's ability to analyse word structure is also beneficial for their vocabulary development.

6.2   Learning objectives

After reading this chapter and trying the exercises, you should be able to:

- Explain the terms morpheme and morphology;
- Carry out morphological analysis (morphological segmentation) to identify roots and affixes;
- Discuss allomorphy, including listing some allomorphs;
- Identify some allomorphs for which there are morphophonological rules;
- Identify the components of compound words and discuss their structural and semantic characteristics;
- Distinguish between prefixes and suffixes;
- Distinguish between inflectional and derivational suffixes.

6.3 Words and morphemes

Consider the word *unbuttoned* as in *He unbuttoned his jacket*. We can identify another word, *button*, inside it; while this element carries the main semantic content of the larger word, the elements that precede and follow *button* also contribute to the meaning of the word as a whole. The element *-ed* that follows *button* indicates that the action took place sometime in the past, and the element *un-* that precedes *button* indicates a negation or reversal of an action of buttoning. The three elements that have been identified in this analysis are called **morphemes**[1]. A morpheme is the smallest unit of meaning. The aspect of linguistics that is concerned with morphemes is called **morphology**, and we would say that when we identified the morphemes in *unbuttoned* we were carrying out a **morphological analysis** or **morphological segmentation** of the word. The word *morphology*, which turns up in other academic disciplines besides linguistics, is itself amenable to morphological segmentation: the morpheme *-ology* is found in many words with the meaning 'study of' (e.g. *biology, psychology*), while the *morph-* part is seen in several related words including *morpheme* with the meaning 'structure' or 'form'. Morphology is thus the study of the structure or form of words, although as we will see, when we carry out morphological analysis, meaning and grammatical function are taken into account as well as form.

As speakers of English, our knowledge of morphology tells us not just what the constituent morphemes of a word are but also how they can be combined. So even though we can attribute the meanings to *un-* and *button* and *-ed* that we have just suggested, we cannot put the morphemes together in any old way and expect people to know what we are talking about: **edunbutton, *buttonedun*, etc., are not acceptable. Similarly, although *button* can occur in isolation (e.g. *They button their jackets*) or with either of the other two elements (*unbutton, buttoned*), neither of the other morphemes can occur on their own or in a combination that does not include *button* or a similar morpheme: **un, *ed* and **uned* are all unacceptable. This alerts us to an interesting point about the differing status of these morphemes. *Button* is in some sense more central to the word *unbuttoned* than the other two elements, and linguists would classify it as its **root**. All words contain at least one root. The other two morphemes can only occur in combination with a root. They are both termed **affixes**; an affix like *un-* that occurs before the root is called a **prefix,** and one like *-ed* that occurs after the root is called a **suffix.** We encountered the term suffix in Chapter 5, where we saw that suffixes can provide useful information about a word's part of speech. It is handy to have a term that can be used when talking about the morphological element to which a suffix is being added. Sometimes, this is just a simple root; for example, in *selfish*, the suffix *-ish* has been added to

---

[1]Linguistics texts use a variety of notational conventions to indicate morphemes. Sometimes capitalisation is used to represent morphemes at an abstract level of representation with italics to represent the variant that actually appears (compare with the lexeme/word form distinction introduced in Chapter 2). Sometimes curly brackets are used for the abstract representation. We will adopt the first of these conventions, but only if it is necessary to make a distinction between the abstract representation and the form that is realised in a particular word.

the simple root *self*. Sometimes, however, the suffix is being added to a form that already contains a suffix; for example, in *selfishly* the suffix *-ly* is being added to the root + suffix form *selfish*. Here we would say that *selfish* is the **base** to which *-ly* is added.

From the fact that we identified the two-syllable word *button* as a morpheme, it should be clear that morphemes are not the same things as syllables. We can have morphemes that consist of one syllable (*take, sky, hot*), two syllables (*grovel, dragon, little*), and three or more syllables (*abolish, caterpillar, magenta*). Equally, we can think of one-syllable words that consist of more than one morpheme, such as *picks*.

Some words do not have internal structure – they are **monomorphemic**. Apart from *picks*, all of the italicised words in the previous paragraph are monomorphemic. A word that consists of two or more morphemes is termed **polymorphemic**. Some words look as though they may be polymorphemic, but on closer inspection they turn out to be monomorphemic. The monomorphemic word *wicked* meaning 'evil' is very similar in its written form to the polymorphemic word *picked*, which consists of two morphemes (*pick* + *ed*). Why do we not divide *wicked* into *wick* + *-ed*? The reason has to do with consistency of meaning and/or function. The meaning of *wick* (e.g. 'fibres in the centre of a candle') is completely unrelated to the meaning of *wicked*. Similarly, the *-ed* at the end of *picked* can indicate past time, as in *Yesterday the farmer picked the strawberries*, or have the grammatical function of marking past tense or past/passive participle (see Section '*Inflectional suffixes*'), but the letter sequence *ed* does neither of these things in *wicked*.

As we saw in Chapter 5, assigning part-of-speech labels to words in a sentence often involves checking whether several criteria have been met. The same is true when doing morphological analysis, where the criteria are as follows:

- All parts of the word should be accounted for, with no 'leftovers';
- For polymorphemic words, it should ideally be possible to give examples of other words that contain the hypothesised morphemes;
- Morphemes should have the same or vaguely similar meanings or grammatical functions wherever they occur. This third criterion may need to be rather loosely applied; sometimes the meaning of a morpheme is very obvious, but sometimes it is more abstract.

So, applying these criteria, *pencil* is monomorphemic because although we can identify the letter sequence *pen*, which might lead us to think that this is a morpheme meaning 'writing implement', the sequence *cil* would be a 'leftover' because it could not be found with a consistent meaning in any other word. The word *button* cannot be analysed as *but* + *ton*, because neither the meaning nor the function of these two hypothesised morphemes are consistent with that of *button*; for the same reason it cannot be *butt* + *on*; it is monomorphemic. *Misreading* is polymorphemic, consisting of *mis* + *read* + *ing*; *mis-* occurs in many other words, including *misdirect* and *misquote*, with the meaning 'false(ly)' or 'inappropriate(ly)'; *read* is able to occur as a word in its own right as well as in other combinations such as *reads, reader* etc; and *-ing* occurs in many words as a marker of grammatical function, e.g. *going, singing*.

Exercise 6.1

Identify the morphemes in the following examples by putting a + between each morpheme. For example, *unbuttoned = un + button + ed*:

Dirty; firstborn; ketchup; oddity; offering; offloading; paperback; repayment; singer; stubborn; unit; uncle; unclean; uncommonly; upmarket; waiter; water.

6.4   Free and bound forms

When considering the word *unbuttoned* earlier, we noted that the root, *button*, was able to occur in isolation, as a word in its own right, but that neither the prefix *un-* nor the suffix *-ed* could do so. Forms that can occur in isolation are called **free morphemes** or **free forms**; *button* is a free root. Forms that cannot occur in isolation but have to occur in combination with other morphemes are called **bound morphemes** or **bound forms**; all affixes, including *un-* and *-ed*, are bound.

If all roots were free and all affixes were bound, the free/bound distinction would be redundant (that is, it would not provide any information over and above the root/affix distinction itself). Since we have already mentioned that all affixes are bound, you should be suspecting that there must be bound roots, and if so, your suspicion is correct!

Consider the words *disrupt* and *rupture*. In both words the letter sequence *rupt* appears, and both words are loosely to do with 'breaking'. Remember that all words must contain at least one root. If the root in these two words is RUPT, it must be a bound root, because **rupt* is not a valid free form. We know that *dis-* can be a prefix (e.g. *disagree, disallow, disappear*) and *-ure* can be a suffix (e.g. *departure, portraiture*), so this analysis does seem to work. Similarly, *construct* and *structure* have the bound root STRUCT, which has a meaning relating to 'building'. There are many such roots in English, inherited from Latin. The meaning relationships between words that share the same bound root may sometimes be a little tenuous but where there is distributional evidence to support it, it may be appropriate to postulate a bound root.

Exercise 6.2

Consider the words *consume*, *pervert*, *receive* and *detract*. What evidence is there that they contain bound roots?

Notice that some bound forms are identical to free forms that have a different meaning and that are in fact quite different morphemes. The bound root DENT that appears in *dentist* and *dental* has nothing to do with the free root DENT that means 'a hollow or depression in a surface'; we might refer to them as $DENT_1$ and $DENT_2$, respectively. The free root ABLE (e.g. *I am able to do that*) is quite distinct from the suffix with the same spelling (e.g. *comfortable*). Even though their meaning and spelling overlap, their pronunciations are different – the free form ABLE rhymes with *table* and *label*, whereas the suffix does not. The suffix *-able* has more in common with *-ible* in words like *flexible* and *accessible* and the less common *-uble* (e.g. *voluble*). A similar example concerns the free form LESS and the suffix LESS (e.g. *useless*) – despite the similarity of spelling, they are pronounced differently and their meanings are not quite the same, with the free form meaning something like 'not quite as much' but the bound form meaning 'completely lacking in'. Finally, compare the free form FULL and the bound form FUL (e.g. *thankful, beautiful*); here, we can again perceive a meaning similarity, but the slightly different spellings and pronunciations alert us to the fact that these are different morphemes.

6.5   Allomorphs

A complicating factor in the morphology of English (and most other languages) is the existence of alternative forms, or **allomorphs**, for many morphemes. The *allo-* morpheme in *allomorph* means 'other', 'alternative' or 'different', and as we noted above, *morph* itself means 'form' or 'shape', so **allomorphy** is concerned with the alternative forms that a morpheme can take. If you are studying phonetics and phonology you may have encountered the comparable term *allophone*. In the previous section, we noted that the suffix *-able* had much in common with the suffixes *-ible* and *-uble*; in fact, all three are identical in meaning, and *-ible* and *-able* have the same pronunciation, and it makes sense to think of them as three alternative manifestations of the same morpheme. The exact form that appears in any given word is determined by the etymology (source language) of the root; *-ible* and *-uble* are only added to roots derived from Latin (e.g. *possible, soluble*) whereas *-able* can be added to roots from any language (e.g. *suitable, capable*).

Exercise 6.3

Think of words ending in *-able* and *-ible*. Is there another tendency that you can identify about the roots?

We will start with an example that only affects the written form of a set of words. Consider what happens when the suffix *-ing* is added to the base form *make*, resulting in the form *making*. If you were asked to say what the constituent morphemes were, you could identify the suffix *-ing* straightforwardly, but you would have to say that either the lexical base was *mak-*, or that the 'word-final e' of *make* was deleted when the *-ing* was added. Whichever way you look at it, the form to the lexeme MAKE to which *-ing* is added is not absolutely identical to *make*, otherwise we would get **makeing*. Rather, *mak-* is an alternative form that is used when certain suffixes are added – that is, it is a bound form of MAKE.

As we noted above, the previous example affects only the spelling of the morphemes, but not their pronunciations. A similar phenomenon occurs in *dissect/dissection*, but here pronunciation rather than spelling is affected.

Exercise 6.4

Identify the morphemes in the words *electric, electrify, electricity, electrician*.

In still other cases both spelling and pronunciation can be affected. The morphologically related words *romance* and *romantic* illustrate such a case. If we hypothesise that *romantic* contains a bound counterpart of *romance*, namely *romant-*, we need to be able to identify other words that contain *-ic* in which it has a similar meaning or performs a similar function, and there are plenty of these: as we noted in Chapter 5, *-ic* turns up in many words (*athletic, scenic, acidic, classic,* etc) marking them as adjectives, and that is its function here. We can therefore conclude that the free form *romance* and the bound form *romant-* are allomorphs of the same morpheme. Another way of saying this is that *romance* and *romant-* **alternate** with each other, or we could say that they are morphological **alternants**. Allomorphy is a very common feature of English.

Exercise 6.5

What happens when suffixes such as *-ive, -ion* or *-ual* are added to words containing CEIVE (see Exercise 2)?

Some morphological alternations in English follow distinct patterns involving pronunciation change. Think about pairs like *brief/brevity, obscene/obscenity, metre/metrical, nation/national, explain/explanatory, vain/vanity, ferocious/ferocity, verbose/verbosity, precocious/precocity* and many more. In these pairs, there is a systematic shortening of the vowel that is stressed in the form with the additional suffix. This kind of process, where there is a systematic relationship between the levels of morphology and phonology, is called **morphophonology**.

Exercise 6.6

Each item in this exercise consists of a word followed by a sentence in which you must supply the appropriate form to fill in the gap. For each item, say whether the word you supply contains a distinct allomorph of the related word. If so, do they differ in terms of spelling, pronunciation or both?

a. (confess) The criminal made a _____ to the police.
b. (secret) The minister was sworn to _____ about the plan.

c. (deep) The engineers measured the _____ of the pit.
d. (decide) Think carefully before you make your _____.
e. (sign) In linguistics, an asterisk _____ an unacceptable form.
f. (define) What is the _____ of the word 'allomorph'?
g. (swim) My favourite sport is _____.
h. (able) This test will assess your spelling _____.
i. (qualify) She is a newly _____ therapist.
j. (compose) A new piano _____ by Mozart has been discovered.

6.6   Common mechanisms of word formation in English

In the introduction to this section we gave an example of the way that speakers of English recombine the existing stock of meaning elements in the language to form new words. This process of new word formation is possible because knowledge of the word structure of English is part of the competence of every mature healthy speaker of the language. So word formation and word structure are opposite sides of the same coin.

Many clinical resources include a section about word structure. For example, look at the Record Form 1 and Examiner's Manual of the CELF-4, and turn to the section 'Word Structure'. You will see that we have already dealt with some of the structures that are covered here. We introduced pronouns (items H, J, O and P) and discussed the different forms that pronouns can take in Chapter 5, where we also explained the contractible and uncontractible copula (items F and M). All the other forms from the Word Structure section of the CELF-4 are discussed in the remainder of this chapter. Most other clinical resources that deal with this area cover these same concepts, so these are the ones that we will concentrate on here. There is a great deal more that can be said about word formation in English; for a more comprehensive account, see the references at the end of the chapter.

6.6.1   Compounding

Compounds (or compound words) are created by combining free forms, for example *fire-engine, food poisoning, catfish*. As these three examples show, the elements in a compound may have a hyphen, space or nothing at all between them, and one or more of the elements may be morphologically complex, as in the second example where the second element consists of a root plus a suffix. The compound may function as various parts of speech, including noun (e.g. *There was a traffic jam*), verb (e.g. *The workers who went on strike were blacklisted*) and adjective (e.g. *He read it in a singsong voice*). Given the ambiguity inherent in parts of speech in English, it is difficult to be certain what categories the component parts of speech are, but many combinations seem possible, including noun–noun (e.g. *suicide pill*), preposition–verb (*overact*), adjective–noun (*bluebell*) and verb–noun (*tell-tale*).

The elements of compounds may display a variety of meaning relationships, which can be summarised by descriptions in which the first element is labelled A and the second B. These include:

A causes B: *bullet-wound, brushstroke*
B causes A: *love potion, smallpox virus*
B prevents A: *flood barrier, draught excluder*
B resembles A: *mushroom cloud, wingnut*
B is appropriate at time A: *birthday cake, evening meal*
B is made of A: *haystack, carrot cake*
B is part of A: *shoe buckle, car engine*

Notice that different meanings are possible despite superficial similarities between compounds. We have suggested above that *smallpox virus* should be interpreted as 'a virus that causes smallpox', but we could not say that a *computer virus* causes computers, or that the *Yosemite virus* causes the Yosemite National Park in the USA.

In compounds, one element is generally more dominant semantically, and this element is labelled the **head** of the compound, and the other element is a **dependant**. A *mushroom cloud* is a kind of cloud, not a kind of mushroom, so *cloud* is the head of this compound, and a *bullet-wound* is a kind of wound, not a kind of bullet, so *wound* is the head here. The dependant usually precedes the head in compounds.

Exercise 6.7

For each of the meaning relations in compounds listed above, list one more example.

So far we have only given examples of compounds consisting of two elements, but they can be more complex than this. Consider *diamond earring* or *talent show host*. Each seems to consist of three morphemes. In *diamond earring*, the position of the space reflects the fact that there is a closer relationship between *ear* and *ring* than between *diamond* and *ear*. In the parallel example *diamond nose ring*, where spaces are inserted differently, we could indicate the close relationship between the second two elements by using brackets: (*diamond (nose ring)*). In these two examples, this seems to be the appropriate grouping, as the alternative would seem to suggest an ear or a nose made of diamonds, which is not the usual interpretation of these forms. The bracketing would be different in *talent show host*, where the closer relationship is between the first and second elements ((*talent show) host*), not (*talent (show host)*. We could use a similar approach for four-element compounds such as *bank holiday week end* – ((*bank holiday)(week end)*).

Exercise 6.8

How would you analyse the compound *wrist watch strap shop* (that is, a shop that sells wrist watch straps)? Indicate the structure with brackets.

Compounds are not often examined in clinical resources, but in the LARSP noun–noun compounds are recorded with the symbol NN.

6.6.2   Affixation

Affixation, the addition of prefixes and suffixes to a form, is the most common word formation mechanism in English, and certainly the mechanism that is most often included in clinical resources. As we noted earlier, prefixes precede the root and suffixes follow it. A word that contains affixes is called a **complex** form.

6.6.2.1   More on prefixes

Table 6.1 shows some common prefixes of English. We have come across various examples of prefixes so far. They can attach to free roots (e.g. *unbutton, misread*), or bound roots (*consume, pervert, detract*). A word may contain several prefixes, e.g. *unreconstructed*.

Some prefixes, typically those that can be attached to free roots, are relatively **productive** – that is, they can be added to existing forms of the appropriate part

Table 6.1   Some common prefixes of English

Prefix	Examples	Meaning
Anti-	Anti-semitic, antichrist	Against
De-	Dematerialise, de-ice	Reverse, undo
Dis	Discontinue, discount	Reverse, undo
Ex-	Ex-husband, ex-army	Former
Il-, im-, in-, ir-	Illegal, immaterial, inappropriate, irrational	Negative
Inter-	International, inter-racial	Between
Intra-	Intramural, intranet	Within
Mis-	Mis-inform, misapprehension	False(ly)
Pre-	Pre-ordained, prepaid	Before
Pro-	Pro-conservative, pro-life	In favour of
Re-	Redo, retread	Again
Trans-	Transatlantic, transfer	Across
Un-	Unlikely, unfasten	Negative, reverse

of speech to create new words. For example, *un-* can be attached to verbs, such as *unpack* or *undress*, to indicate a reversal of the action expressed in the verb, or to an adjective with meaning X to create a form that means 'not X' (*just/unjust, kind/unkind*). If we invent a new verb or adjective such as *fost*, we would generally expect to be able to add *un-* to it and expect it to contribute the same sort of negative meaning to the new word. We would not be able to add *un-* to a noun, however: *unladylike* but **unlady*.

Exercise 6.9

Notice that one prefix listed in Table 6.1 has multiple allophones. What determines which allophone will be selected? What happens if the prefix is added to the word *constant* or *capable*?

In English, prefixes do not usually change the part of speech of a word to which they are attached. An exception is the prefix *be-* (e.g. *befriend, bedew*) which, when added to a noun, creates a verb.

Clinical resources focus much more on suffixes than prefixes. The TOAL-4 (subtest 2, Word Derivations) is one resource that does look at prefixes, focusing on the more productive examples.

6.6.2.2 More on suffixes

In English, we can identify two kinds of suffix – inflectional and derivational. Clinical resources mainly concentrate on the inflectional suffixes, a small set that can easily be learned. All other suffixes are derivational. As with many aspects of English, there are ambiguous cases where we need to take other information into account in order to be sure which kind of suffix we are dealing with, but we will draw attention to these when we come to them.

In some texts you will see the term **stem** used to refer to the base to which an inflectional suffix is added, so in *singers* the inflectional suffix *-s* is being added to the stem *singer*.

Inflectional suffixes

In the 'Word Structure' section of the CELF-4, the items that are listed include 'Regular Plural', 'Irregular Plural', 'Third Person Singular', 'Possessive nouns', 'Regular Past Tense', 'Irregular Past Tense' and 'Comparative and Superlative'. These items are members of a set called the **inflectional suffixes.** Because the inflectional suffixes are theoretically and clinically important, the word structure aspects of clinical resources such as the CELF-4, DASS, STASS and TROG-2 devote more space to them than to other suffixes, and we will do the same. Each major part-of-speech category (noun, verb, adjective, adverb) has specific inflectional suffixes associated

Table 6.2   Common irregular forms in English

Plural Nouns	Past Tense		Past/Passive Participle	
	Verbs			
Children	Ate	Got	Been	Gone
Feet	Blew	Had	Blown	Got
Geese	Bought	Hit	Bought	Had
Men	Broke	Made	Broken	Hit
Mice	Brought	Put	Brought	Made
People	Built	Ran	Built	Put
Sheep	Came	Read	Chosen	Read
Teeth	Chose	Rode	Come	Ridden
	Cut	Sat	Cut	Run
	Drank	Slept	Drawn	Sat
	Drew	Smelt	Driven	Seen
	Drove	Spent	Drunk	Slept
	Dug	Stood	Eaten	Smelt
	Fell	Swung	Fallen	Spent
	Flew	Was, were	Found	Stood
	Found	Went	Flown	Swung
	Gave		Given	Taken
				Thrown

with it. There are only eight in total, and they are so important to the work of a speech and language therapist that you should learn what they are and their properties. They are detailed below, grouped according to the type of content word that they are associated with.

Every suffix has a typical or **regular** form, that is, the form that it takes in the majority of words. For example, the plural morpheme that indicates 'more than one' is most often represented in written language by the addition of -s (e.g. *two days, two dogs, two ducks*), so this is the regular form of the plural. Some other words do not form the plural in this way, so their plural form is **irregular**. In such cases, the suffix may take an unusual form, e.g. *two children*, or it may consist of an alteration to a vowel in the word, e.g. *two mice*, or it may not differ from the **citation form** of the word (the form that would be listed as the heading of a dictionary entry), e.g. *two sheep*. A list of common irregular forms is shown in Table 6.2.

Although the main function of the inflectional suffixes is grammatical, for some we can give an approximate meaning, which should help you to identify which suffix you are dealing with (because, unfortunately, several of the suffixes have exactly the same form).

Noun inflectional suffixes

Plural

- Regular form: -s
- Example: *There are many students in the class.*
- Meaning: 'more than one'.
- Examples of irregular forms: *people, men, women, children, mice, oxen, sheep* and many more.
- Further points:
  - A form that refers to only one entity is called a Singular form, but in English this is not marked with a specific suffix (it is '**uninflected**'): Singular *student*, Plural *students*.
  - There are many irregular forms, and these often involve high-frequency words. See also note about Third Person Singular Present Tense.

Possessive

- Regular form: singular -'s (apostrophe s), or, if the noun is plural and usually takes the regular form, -s' (s apostrophe).
- Examples: Singular: *The cat's fur is black.* Plural: *Many students' marks were high.*
- Meaning: 'belonging to'.
- Examples of irregular forms: none.
- Further points:
  - Notice that in spoken English, in which the apostrophe is not represented, this suffix is identical to Plural and Third Person Singular Present Tense, but if the suffix contributes a meaning something like 'belonging to', it is the Possessive.
  - In written English, when the Possessive suffix attaches to an Irregular Plural such as *people*, it takes the form -'s, not -s': *The People's Princess.*
  - The written singular Possessive suffix -'s should not be confused with contracted forms (see Chapter 5), such as *that's nice, he's gone* or *let's go*. In these forms, -'s is not a suffix but a contraction of *is, has* and us, respectively.

Verb inflectional suffixes

Third Person Singular Present Tense

- Regular form: -s.
- Example: *He likes chocolate.*
- Meaning: This suffix has a grammatical function rather than a meaning.
- Examples of irregular forms: none, but note that in some dialects, such as that spoken in Norfolk, this suffix is omitted and utterances like *He work here* are heard.
- Further points:
  - Notice that Regular Plural has exactly the same form as Third Person Singular Present Tense, and in spoken English, so does Possessive. But these have quite distinctive meanings, as discussed above. If the word that the suffix is attached to is a noun, then the suffix is Plural or Possessive rather than Third Person

Singular Present Tense. If the word that the suffix is attached to is a verb, it is Third Person Singular Present Tense.

o We encountered the label 'Third Person Singular' when considering the various personal pronouns in Chapter 5. This suffix and the Third Person Singular subjective pronouns share a label because they occur together. Notice how the suffix Third Person Singular Present Tense is attached when there is a Third Person Singular subjective pronoun (*He laughs*), but not when there is a Third Person Plural subjective pronoun (*They laugh*). (See also Chapter 7 on 'number agreement'.)

Past Tense/Simple Past

- Regular form: *-ed*.
- Examples: *After trying to find a new job for ages, yesterday I succeeded.*
- Meaning: Refers to the past.
- Examples of irregular forms: *made, wrote, thought, took, knew, built, sang, flew* and many more.
- Further points:
  - o Compare with the Past Participle. The form that occurs in the context "*Yesterday, I ____ ...*" is the Past Tense: *Yesterday I learned a new song*; *Yesterday I flew to Paris*.
  - o Difficulty with past tense is considered to be a key behavioural marker of specific language impairment.

Past Participle/Passive Participle

- Regular forms: *-ed, -en*.
- Example: *After trying to find a new job for ages, at last I have succeeded. This photo was taken last year.*
- Meaning: refers to the past.
- Examples of irregular forms: *made, thought, known, built, sung, flown* and many more.
- Further points:
  - o Compare with the Past Tense. The form that occurs in the context "*In the past, I have ____ ...*" is the Past Participle: *In the past, I have flown to Paris.*
  - o The same form also occurs in a structure called the passive, which has been mentioned already and will be explored further in later chapters. The passive is included in many clinical assessments as it can be very difficult for a person with language problems to understand. Examples: *This photo was taken last year*; *Benedictine liqueur is made by monks*; *The contestants will be introduced by Terry Wogan.*
  - o In the LARSP, the past participle is indicated with '-en'.

Exercise 6.10

List five verbs that have not been mentioned so far that have an irregular past tense and a past/passive participle is a different form in standard English (e.g. *took/taken*).

Progressive

- Regular form: *-ing.*
- Example: *I am cooking dinner; He was eating rice.*
- Meaning: Ongoing action.
- Examples of irregular forms: none. Its regularity makes it among the first suffixes to be acquired by typically developing English-speaking children.
- Further points:
  - *-ing* is only the progressive suffix when used with an auxiliary verb. Sometimes a suffix with the same spelling is used to form a noun from a verb (e.g. *I swim → I like swimming*). The latter suffix is derivational (see Section below on derivational suffixes).
  - This form has alternative names. It is sometimes called the present participle, but this is inaccurate as it can be used to indicate non-present time, e.g. *I was cooking* (past progressive); *I will be cooking* (future progressive). See the discussion of tense and aspect in the next paragraph. The *-ing* form is also referred to as continuous (present continuous *I am going*, past continuous *I was going*, future continuous *I will be going*).

To complete our discussion of verb inflections, we need to introduce a distinction between **tense** and **aspect**. The central tense system in English rests on the contrast between, e.g. *works* and *worked*. The inflections *-s* and *-ed* signal information about the location of an event or action in time. We locate objects in space with reference to some landmark, as in *Our house is opposite the Post Office*, where *the Post Office* refers to the landmark. When locating events, actions or states in time, the landmark, or **reference point**, is the **moment of speech**. *Wynne works at the mill* locates the event in present time, that is, in a stretch of time that includes the moment of speech. The past tense inflection, as in *Wynne worked at the mill,* locates the event in past time, that is, at a time before the moment of speech.

To locate an event in future time, speakers of English use *will* or *be going to*: *Wynne will work in the mill, Wynne is going to work in the mill*. The concept of future tense is controversial. The difficulty is that *will* is a modal auxiliary whose original meaning had to do with intention or volition: *I'll come round at 5pm* is to be interpreted as 'I intend to come round at 5pm'. In many examples, it is impossible to distinguish between intention and reference to future time. The alternative form *be going to* is in origin a verb of movement: doing something in the future can be conceived of as moving towards an event. In spite of the controversy, the label 'future tense' remains in general use and we continue to use it here. It is also a standard term in SLT clinical resources. We continue to classify *will* as a modal auxiliary. The form BE + *going to* is sometimes referred to as a **semi-auxiliary**.

Aspect refers to a different dimension: the distribution of an event or action over time. The fundamental contrast that is conveyed by aspect is whether the event or action is ongoing and spread over time (**progressive aspect**) or has been completed. The distinction is signalled in English by the contrast between, e.g., *wrote* and *was writing* and between *writes* and *is writing*.

To construct the progressive aspect, we use the auxiliary BE and the progressive form of the lexical verb. Consider the following:

1 a They were writing a book. (Present Progressive)
   b They wrote a book. (Simple Past)

The use of the past tense of the auxiliary *were* in (1a) locates the action of writing in past time. The progressive suffix *-ing* on the lexical verb *writing* focuses on the ongoing nature of the writing.

(1b) presents the event as completed. (1a) presents the event as ongoing. Consider (2):

2 They were writing the book when I left. (I'm surprised they haven't finished it.)

The event of book-writing is spread over time. The time occupied by the book-writing contains within it the time of leaving.

(1b) refers to a single event of book-writing and this is its default interpretation. In (3), a different interpretation is required:

3 They often wrote books about Welsh geology.

In (3), *often* indicates that *wrote books* is to be interpreted as referring to repeated events, possibly to events that were habitual.

The Simple Present differs from the Simple Past; its default meaning is 'habitual event' or 'repeated event', as in (4):

4 They write letters home every week.

The Simple Present refers to a single completed event only in special contexts such as sports commentaries or stage directions, as in (5) and (6):

5 Nogood <u>places</u> the ball, <u>walks</u> back, <u>pauses</u>, <u>runs up</u>, <u>shoots</u> – and the ball <u>goes</u> high over the bar.
6 The detective <u>exits</u> stage left. The butler <u>enters</u> centre stage.

The **Perfect Tense** construction is based on the primary auxiliary HAVE and the past participle, as in the following:

7 a They have written a book. (Present Perfect)
   b They had written a book. (Past Perfect)

Location in time is signalled by the primary auxiliary: *have* is present tense and *had* is past tense. What is called the past participle, here *written*, was originally a **resultative participle** denoting the result of some action. Putting it rather crudely, the Perfect came historically from a resultative construction: *They have written the book* came from a structure that can be glossed as 'They possess a result: The book is written'. That is, the Perfect does not refer to a completed action directly but we infer that in order to have a result, some action must have been completed.

The Present Perfect is said to have four major interpretations: the **Result Perfect,** as in (8); the **Experiential Perfect,** as in (9); the **Hot-News Perfect,** as in (10); the **Extended-Now Perfect,** as in (11).

8   Lucie has cooked the meal.

9   We have visited Troy. (Note the interrogative Have you ever visited Troy?)

10   The Queen has just arrived.

11   We've been working on the book for ten years.

The last type of Perfect is a combination of the Perfect and the Progressive: the Perfect is *have been* and the Progressive is *been working.*

Note that the Simple Past as in (1b) denotes an event that took place in past time and was completed. The Present Perfect focuses on present time and presents the result of an action in the past. You can say *I built a snowman* even if the snowman thawed and vanished some days ago. You can't say *I've built a snowman* unless the snowman is still in existence (or unless you are merely claiming to have had the experience of building snowman: *Who here has (ever) built a snowman? – I have built a snowman. It was some years ago but I still know how to do it.*)

The forms discussed above represent only a sample of the possible ways in which auxiliaries and verb inflections can combine. In addition to the aforementioned simple forms they convey a range of subtle meaning differences. The choice of these different forms is governed by complex rules that are relevant to the expression and reception of narrative, which we will consider in Chapters 14–16.

Adjective and adverb inflectional suffixes

Adjectives and adverbs have the same inflectional suffixes.

Comparative

- Regular form: *-er.*
- Example: *He is tall<u>er</u> than me. She ran fast<u>er</u> than the rest.*
- Meaning: can be paraphrased as 'more X', e.g. *taller = more tall.*
- Examples of irregular forms: *better, worse, more, less.*
- Further points:
   - Words of more than one syllable tend to have *more* added rather than the suffix -er, e.g. *more rapid,* not **rapider.* There are quite a few exceptions, e.g. *cleverer* (at least for some speakers), *easier, deadlier, mightier, holier.*
   - Notice that the suffix with the form *-er* is not always the comparative. In *painter,* the -er suffix is derivational, with a meaning along the lines of 'doer of action'.

Superlative

- Regular form: *-est.*
- Example: *The fastest runner won. She ran fastest.*
- Meaning: can be paraphrased as 'most X', e.g. *tallest = most tall*
- Examples of irregular forms: *best, worst, most, least.*

- Further points:
  - ○ In standard English, the same words that would form the comparative by adding *more* rather than *-er* also form the superlative by adding *most* rather than *-est*: **beautifullest, *quickliest*.

Exercise 6.11

In Chapter 2 we introduced the notion of lexemes and grammatical word forms, and have made this distinction a few times since then. Review the concept of grammatical word forms. Alternative grammatical word forms are produced when inflectional suffixes are added to a stem or when the root is altered in some other way (for example, when the plural of *mouse*, *mice*, is formed by altering the vowel). List the distinct grammatical word forms that are associated with the following lexemes and give them their labels (e.g. plural, superlative). Note that there may be several lexemes with the same form but different meanings and/or different parts of speech. Which lexemes have the largest number of distinct grammatical word forms?

BLACK
DECORATE
HARD (adverb)
FROG
MAN
SEE

Derivational suffixes

If a suffix is not inflectional, it is derivational. So the easiest way to distinguish between the two is to learn the eight suffixes listed above, including the distributional information that allows you to identify them, because then you will know that any other suffix that you encounter is derivational. Note, however, that some derivational suffixes have the same form as inflectional suffixes. An important example (because it turns up in various resources) is *-er*, which is inflectional in *He is fatter* but derivational in *He is a farmer*; the derivational suffix, which means 'doer of' something, has a special name, the **agentive** suffix. Similarly, *-ing* is inflectional in *He is drinking* but derivational in *I am concerned about his excessive drinking*). Differences between inflectional and derivational suffixes are summarised below.

A few assessments explicitly examine clients' ability to produce derivational suffixes. The CELF-4 includes a couple of derivational suffixes in the 'Word Structure' section. Sub-test 2 'Word Derivations' in the TOAL-4 examines a wider range of derivational affixes, which has a structure similar to that used in Exercise 6 of this chapter. The PALPA includes derivational suffixes in several sub-tests.

A list of some common derivational suffixes in English, with comments, is given in Table 6.3.

Table 6.3 Some common derivational suffixes in English (further examples are given in Table 5.1)

Suffix	Examples	Notes
-er also –or	Dancer, sender, sprinkler, printer, listener, vendor, author	This is called the agentive suffix. When added to a verb, it adds the meaning 'doer of action' and changes the verb to a noun. Do not confuse with the Comparative suffix, which is inflectional.
-ly	Quickly, suddenly	When added to an adjective, it creates an adverb. Note that when -ly is added to a noun, e.g. coward + ly, it creates an adjective. But there are only a few such words, that are lowish in frequency, and when assessments use -ly it is usually the 'adjective to adverb' sort.
-ic	Scenic, basic, gastric	Added to nouns and bound roots to create adjectives.
-ise, -ize	Familiarise, recognize	Added to adjectives and bound roots to create verbs. Some common verbs that end in -ise, e.g. surprise, are monomorphemic.
-ish	Reddish, boyish	Added to adjectives or nouns; the resulting word is an adjective.
-ity	Familiarity, chastity	Added to adjectives and bound roots to create nouns.
-ness	Kindness, darkness	Added to adjectives to create nouns.
-y	Lucky, watery, flowery	Added to nouns to create adjectives.

Differences between inflectional and derivational suffixes

Derivational suffixes differ from inflectional suffixes in several ways.

- Category change: It is clear from Table 6.3 that the addition of a derivational suffix often changes the part of speech of a word, though this is not always the case. Notice that inflectional suffixes never do this – the plural form of a noun is still a noun, and the superlative form of an adjective is still an adjective.
- Set size: There are far more derivational suffixes than inflectional suffixes.
- Productivity: Each inflectional suffix can be used with practically every member of the grammatical category that it is associated with – for example, there is a Possessive form of every noun, and a Progressive form of every verb. Derivational suffixes vary in terms of their degree of productivity.
- Selectivity: This is related to the previous point. While inflectional suffixes attach to pretty much every member of the content word class that they belong to, derivational suffixes tend to be more fussy. For example, -ness and -ity are both derivational suffixes that form nouns from adjectives, and their meanings are pretty similar too: for a given adjective X they produce a word with the meaning 'the quality associated with being X' (e.g. harsh + ness → harshness; severe + ity → severity). But -ity will generally only attach to Latinate roots and -ness to Germanic roots (*harshity; *severeness).

- Sequences of suffixes: a word can contain more than one derivational suffix (e.g. *structurally – struct + ure + al + ly*) but generally only one inflectional suffix (*likesed). The only exception to this is the addition of the possessive inflectional suffix to irregular plural forms, e.g. *children's*.
- Order: When a word contains several suffixes, derivational appear before inflectional, e.g. *allow + ance + s*, not **allow + s + ance*.
- Effect on stress: some derivational suffixes cause stress to move about in a word (compare *algebra*, stressed on the first syllable, and *algebraic*, stressed on the third), or attract stress to themselves (compare *Japan*, stressed on the second syllable, and *Japanese*, stressed on the suffix). Inflectional suffixes have no effect on stress.

Exercise 6.12

Identify the suffixes in the following sentences and indicate whether they are inflectional or derivational. Where appropriate provide a more specific label for the suffix, e.g. irregular plural, superlative, agentive.

A number of things surprise me about the way that we categorise words.
The children's shouts were becoming louder.
I hope you will be healthy, wealthy and happy.
The builder misled me about the cost of the improvements.

6.7   Mean length of utterance in morphemes

A practical application of morphological analysis is the calculation of a measure called **Mean Length of Utterance (MLU)**. Sometimes this is calculated in words (MLU_w); we count the number of words in the set of utterances, and then divide by the number of utterances. The problems with calculating MLU using words is that, especially in the early stages of language development, this method fails to reflect subtle and important differences. For example, we might observe two children who have started to produce two-word utterances. One child says things like *Mummy go* and *See car*, while the other says things like *Mummy going* and *See cars*. The MLU_w measure does not reflect the fact that the second child is more linguistically advanced than the first. If we calculate **Mean Length of Utterance in morphemes** (MLU_m) instead, we can reflect this difference: we count the number of morphemes in the set of utterances, and then divide by the number of utterances. To do this, we need to gather a large number of utterances and follow a set of rules about what to count as one and two morphemes in child language, which are given in most introductory language development texts.

Chapter summary

- Morphemes are the smallest unit of meaning.
- Morphology is the study of the system underlying word structure.

- Morphological analysis (morphological segmentation) must
  - Account for all parts of the word
  - Hypothesise morphemes that are observed in other words
  - Ideally find meaning relationships between morphemes in related words.
- Monomorphemic words consist of a single morpheme, and polymorphemic words consist of several morphemes. Polymorphemic words contain at least one root and possibly affixes as well (prefixes before the root, suffixes after it).
- Allomorphy occurs when a single morpheme has several variants (allomorphs or alternants); the different allomorphs may be subject to morphophonological rules that determine the pattern of sounds that occur.
- Compound words consist of at least two roots that may be characterised by a wide range of semantic relationships and parts of speech.
- Affixation is a more common word formation process.
- In English we can distinguish prefixes, which occur before the root, from suffixes, which occur after it.
- Inflectional suffixes have a main grammatical role. Each major part of speech has a set of inflectional suffixes that apply to its members.
- Other suffixes are derivational.

Exercises using clinical resources

6.13. In the ACE, which of the structures that we have discussed in this chapter are tested in the Syntactic Formulation (SF) subtest?

6.14. In the CAT, which sections contain only morphologically complex items? Do a morphological analysis of the target words that are used.

6.15. In the ERB, look at the Sentence Scoresheet and identify items that contain the following suffixes:
  a. plural
  b. progressive
  c. past
  d. third person singular, present tense

6.16. What suffixes are examined in the CELF-Preschool?

6.17. Examine the Syntax Summary of the Living Language programme. At what level are irregular plurals listed? Third person singular present tense forms of verbs? Progressive forms of verbs? Irregular past tenses? Irregular past participles?

6.18. Which of the verbs that are listed in Table 6.2 relate to test items in the PTT-2 and the VATT?

6.19. In the STASS, which of the items on the response sheet (i.e. the one showing 'TARGET RESPONSE' and 'ACTUAL RESPONSE') contain the following in the target response?
  a. Plural
  b. Possessive

c. Third person singular present tense
d. Progressive
e. Past tense
f. Past participle
g. Comparative
h. Superlative
i. A derivational suffix

6.20. Look at the manual of the TALC. At what level is the child expected to be able to explain the logic of compound words?

Further reading

Bauer (1983) gives a comprehensive account of this area.

Coates (1999) is more succinct than some other introductions to this area of this resource, but it nonetheless covers a broader range of concepts than this chapter. (The additional material that this source provides is not usually used by SLTs but could provide a more in-depth understanding of the topic.)

Fudge (1984) is mainly concerned with how word stress is allocated in English words, but this text contains useful lists of compounds and affixes as well.

7 Sentence Structure 1: Phrases and Clauses

7.0 Introduction

The previous chapter has looked at the way in which many words of English are constructed out of smaller bits – bases, prefixes and suffixes. We also saw that some words, such as *brick* and *dog*, consist of a single bit. In this chapter, we will be looking at how words are combined to produce phrases and how phrases combine to build clauses. We realise that many readers will come to this book with only a vague understanding of what a 'phrase' or a 'clause' is, but we will explain what we mean by these terms shortly.

Before you embark on this chapter, it would be advisable to check that you have understood the material in Chapter 5, Parts of Speech, and Chapter 6, Word Structure. In Chapter 5, we were able to give only a preliminary account of parts of speech, because a full account depends on an understanding of sentence structure, which we will begin to address here. But you will need to have a basic grasp of

Introductory Linguistics for Speech and Language Therapy Practice, First Edition. Jan McAllister and Jim Miller.
© 2013 John Wiley & Sons, Ltd. Published 2013 by John Wiley & Sons, Ltd.

parts of speech if you are to be able to understand what we say here. In Chapter 6, you should review the material about inflectional suffixes, because there is a close relationship between sentence structure and inflectional morphology.

As we noted in Chapter 1, the level of linguistic description that is concerned with sentence structure is called syntax. Syntax (from Classical Greek *sun* 'with, together' and *taksis* 'placing') is the study of phrases and clauses, and the key concept, a very traditional one, is that of construction – something that is 'built together' out of different pieces. When we examine constructions, we pay attention to the kinds of bits that combine to build them, the order in which the bits are arranged and the links between the bits – between words in phrases, between phrases in clauses and between clauses in sentences. These basic structural relationships will be our focus in this chapter. In later chapters, we will extend these fundamental concepts to explain how more complex syntactic structures are formed and how these are used communicatively.

7.1   Why do SLTs need this knowledge?

A client who could not use syntax would only be able to produce absurdly limited messages. Contrast the child who can produce the isolated words *pictures* and *book* with the child who can say *the pictures in the green book* or *Show me the pictures in the green book* or even *not the green book, the blue book – with the Gruffalo*. Or think how an adult's communicative ability would be restricted if, as a result of an acquired language disorder, they could produce content words but could not link these together in properly structured sentences.

Syntax is a central (many would say *the* central) component of the ability to produce and understand language. SLTs need an understanding of syntax in order to analyse the language produced and understood (or not produced and not understood) by clients, whether children or adults. People with agrammatic aphasia may produce short phrases with fewer words than one might expect and have trouble with grammatical words such as determiners and auxiliaries (see Chapter 5), word order and production of subordinate clauses (see Chapter 8). Typically developing children acquiring their first language also have problems with grammatical words at first, but acquire them in the course of normal development. (One of the second author's granddaughters, newly three at the time, announced *I cutting* as she expertly reduced sheets of coloured paper to tiny pieces.) Children with specific language impairment may struggle with production and/or comprehension of particular sentence structures.

As a result, many of the clinical resources that SLTs use target syntax. The Psycholinguistic Assessment of Language Processing in Aphasia (PALPA) has several sections that focus on Sentence Processing and that examine the use of quite sophisticated sentence structures. SLTs who work with children will routinely use assessments such as the South Tyneside Assessment of Syntactic Structures (STASS) and the Dorset Assessment of Syntactic Structures (DASS), which are concerned with syntax and morphology, or the Clinical Evaluation of Language Fundamentals

(CELF), which has Sentence Structure sub-tests in the versions for preschoolers and for older children. The STASS, the DASS and the LARSP (the Language Assessment, Remediation and Screening Program, on which the STASS and DASS are based) make explicit reference to the Phrase and Clause levels of description that will be the focus of this chapter.

7.2   Learning objectives

After reading this chapter and doing the exercises, you should be able to:

- List some tests for determining whether a group of words is a phrase;
- Explain what is meant by the head of a phrase;
- Recognise and give examples of the following kinds of phrases:
  - Noun Phrase
  - Prepositional Phrase
  - Adjective Phrase
  - Adverb Phrase
  - Verb Phrase;
- Define the concept of the clause as it is used in this chapter;
- Identify the following elements of the clause in some simple examples:
  - Subject
  - Verb
  - Direct object
  - Indirect object
  - Complement
  - Adverbial.

7.3   Syntax, morphology and the lexicon

In Chapter 2, we drew a distinction between lexemes, which we could think of as the heading on an entry in the mental lexicon (e.g. SAY) and the grammatical word forms that are associated with it (e.g. *say, says, saying, said*). When we produce sentences, we must ensure that the grammatical word form that is inserted is appropriate given the particular syntactic context in which the lexeme occurs. For example, a combination such as (1) comes out as either (2) or (3).

1   The chunky CHINCHILLA CHEW some chicory.

2   The chunky <u>chinchilla is</u> chewing some chicory.

3   The chunky <u>chinchillas are</u> chewing some chicory.

The singular noun *chinchilla* combines with the singular verb *is (chewing)* and the plural noun *chinchillas* combines with the plural verb *are (chewing)*. Any other combination is incorrect, at least in standard English.[1] This example demonstrates

---

[1] There are varieties of English where *The chinchillas is chewing* is the accepted pattern and SLTs will undoubtedly have dealings with speakers of such varieties.

the close link between syntax and morphology. Because of this close link, the term **morpho-syntax** is often used to cover the aspects of language description that straddle the two areas.

Another example of the syntax–morphology link is provided by verbs such as CONSIDER. Suppose our sentence begins *We considered . . .* and we wish to follow this with the appropriate form of the lexeme DEMOLISH. CONSIDER demands a word with the suffix *-ing*, as shown in (4) but excludes other forms such as *to demolish* or *demolish* by itself. In contrast, INTEND and PLAN allow *to demolish* but do not allow *demolish* on its own, and PLAN excludes the *-ing* form, as shown in (5) and (6).

4　a　The officials considered <u>demolishing</u> the building.
　　b　*The officials considered <u>to demolish</u> the building.
　　c　*The officials considered <u>demolish</u> the building.

5　a　The officials intended <u>to demolish</u> the building.
　　b　*The officials intended <u>demolish</u> the building.

6　a　The officials plan <u>to demolish</u> the building.
　　b　*The officials plan <u>demolish</u> the building.
　　c　*The officials plan <u>demolishing</u> the building.

Examples (4)–(6) point to the connection between syntax, morphology and the lexicon. Particular lexemes require particular constructions. Like *consider*, *regret* requires verbs with the suffix *-ing*, as in (7), whereas *refuse* requires *to*, as in (8). The adjective *enthusiastic* requires the preposition *about* and an *-ing* form, as in (9).

7　They regretted <u>demolishing</u> the building.

8　They refused <u>to demolish</u> the building.

9　They are enthusiastic <u>about demolishing</u> the house.

There are many interconnections between individual lexical items and particular syntactic constructions.

We turn now to a consideration of two fundamental levels of syntactic structure: phrases and clauses.

7.4　Phrases

Words are combined into phrases. Consider the sentence in (10).

10　Surprisingly large mice very rapidly built an exceedingly comfortable nest behind the cupboards during the winter.

The biggest and most obvious phrases in (10) are

surprisingly large mice
very rapidly
an exceedingly comfortable nest

behind the cupboards
during the winter
built an exceedingly comfortable nest behind the cupboards during the winter.

Smaller and not so obvious phrases are

the winter
behind the cupboards
the cupboards
exceedingly comfortable.

The two lists illustrate an important point: words do combine into phrases, as stated above, but phrases, or a word and a phrase, may combine to produce larger phrases, such as the word *during* combining with the phrase *the winter* to produce the larger phrase *during the winter* or the phrase *surprisingly large* combining with the word *mice* to produce the larger phrase *surprisingly large mice*.

The phrases that we have identified here are of many different kinds. Let us first explain how we know that they are phrases, and then we will explain how we know what kind of phrase each one is.

7.4.1   Criteria for phrases

How can we tell when two or more words hang together to make a phrase? There are two major criteria, **transposition** and **substitution**.

7.4.1.1   *Transposition*

The term 'transposition' refers to the idea of groups of words being moved around when a given example is rearranged. For instance, we can think of (11) as being rearranged to give (12).

11   That large black dog never catches our nimble cat.

12   Our nimble cat is never caught by that large black dog.

You will remember from Chapter 3 that sentence 11 is an active sentence and sentence 12 is a passive sentence; 11 and 12 convey the same propositional meaning but do so using different constructions. It so happens that we can think of active sentences as being dismantled and put together as passive sentences; in this context, transposition essentially has to do with the same words turning up in the same order in different constructions. To form the passive sentence from the active one, the words *that + large + black + dog* are moved to the end of the sentence all together. You can't leave any of them behind and you can't change the order of these words. And the words *our + nimble + cat* are moved to the front of the sentence all together. Similarly, the examples in (13) all show transposition at work.

13   a   I gave the bone to that large black dog.
     b   I frightened that large black dog.

    c   It is <u>that large black dog</u> that chases our nimble cat.
    d   There is <u>that large black dog</u> in our garden again.
    e   They have a Rottweiler, never mind <u>that large black dog</u>.

In all of these examples, the group of words *that large black dog* functions as a coherent unit – a phrase.

7.4.1.2   Substitution

The second criterion is simply whether one word can be substituted for a group of words.

14   a   <u>That large black dog</u> chased <u>our nimble cat</u>.
     b   <u>It</u> chased <u>her</u>.

It is substituted for *that large black dog* and *her* for *our nimble cat*. This is evidence that each of these groups of words forms a phrase in (14a).

Exercise 7.1

In the following examples, do the underlined words form a phrase? You need to consider the criteria that we just discussed. For example, if the sentence is turned from active into passive, or passive into active, do the words all move together as a unit (transposition); is it possible to substitute a single word for the group and still end up with a grammatical sentence (substitution)?

1. <u>Neil Armstrong</u> led the Apollo 11 mission.
2. Neil <u>Armstrong led the</u> Apollo 11 mission.
3. Neil Armstrong <u>led the Apollo 11</u> mission.
4. Neil Armstrong led <u>the Apollo 11 mission</u>.
5. <u>The mission</u> was funded by NASA.
6. <u>The mission was</u> funded by NASA.
7. The mission was <u>funded by NASA</u>.
8. The mission <u>was funded by NASA</u>.
9. The mission was funded by <u>NASA</u>.

7.4.2   Types of phrases

When discussing (10), we noted that we could identify a large number of phrases. In (15), we give the conventional label for the phrases that we have underlined (sometimes there are several examples within the sentence).

15   a   <u>Surprisingly large mice</u> very rapidly built <u>an exceedingly comfortable nest</u> behind <u>the cupboards</u> during <u>the winter</u>. (Noun phrases)
     b   Surprisingly large mice very rapidly built an exceedingly comfortable nest <u>behind the cupboards</u> <u>during the winter</u>. (Prepositional phrases)

c   Surprisingly large mice very rapidly built an exceedingly comfortable nest
    behind the cupboards during the winter. (Adjective phrases)
d   Surprisingly large mice very rapidly built an exceedingly comfortable nest
    behind the cupboards during the winter. (Adverb phrase)
e   Surprisingly large mice very rapidly built an exceedingly comfortable nest
    behind the cupboards during the winter. (Verb phrase)

We will consider each of these phrase types in turn in Sections 7.4.3–7.4.8, including
the extent to which the criteria of transposition and substitution work for each
phrase type. But first, we will explain how we know which label to apply to a
particular phrase.

7.4.3   Heads, modifiers and phrase types

A key property of any complete phrase is that it contains a central and obligatory
word known as the **head**. In fact, we encountered the concept of the head of a
structure in Chapter 6 when we were looking at the word formation process called
compounding. We noted that in compounds we could identify a dominant element
which was the head of the compound. For example, in the compound *mushroom
cloud* the head is *cloud*, because the compound refers to a kind of cloud, not a
kind of mushroom. In our discussion of compounds we focused on the semantic
properties of heads, but this is not a useful way to think about the heads of phrases;
we need to pay attention instead to parts of speech. The part of speech of the head
appears in the phrase's label.

Exercise 7.2

Look back at (10) above, and list the part of speech of each word. Now look
at the parts of speech that make up each underlined phrase in (15).

Consider the phrases that we identified in (15) and notice that each noun phrase that
we underlined contains a noun, each prepositional phrase contains a preposition,
each adjective phrase contains an adjective and so on. We have selected the examples
so that there is only one word in each underlined phrase that has the appropriate
part-of-speech label, and that word is the head. So in the noun phrases, the words in
bold are the heads: *the **winter**, surprisingly large **mice**, an exceedingly comfortable
nest, the **cupboards***. The heads are also in bold in the prepositional phrases ***during**
the winter* and ***behind** the cupboards*, the adjective phrases *surprisingly **large*** and
*extremely **comfortable***, the adverb phrase *very **rapidly*** and the verb phrase *very
rapidly **built** an exceedingly comfortable nest behind the cupboards during the
winter*.

Heads control not only what type a given phrase is but also the presence of
modifiers – words that add to its meaning. Some words require modifiers, other
words exclude modifiers and yet others allow modifiers but do not require them.

For example, the prepositions *during* and *with* require at least a following noun. (16a,b) are acceptable, whereas (17a,b) are not.

16   a   We went skiing during the Christmas break.
    b   The doctor is with a patient.
17   a   *We went skiing during.
    b   *The doctor is with.

Modifiers can occur before or after the head. In the noun phrase *three big bears*, the modifiers *three* and *big* precede the head noun *bears*; here, the head noun is said to be **premodified** and the modifiers are known as **premodifiers**. In the phrases *bears with brown fur* or *bears eating marmalade* or *bears that come from darkest Peru*, the head of each phrase is still *bears*, but now the head is **postmodified**, and the modifiers are known as **postmodifiers**. The term 'postmodified' is used in some SLT resources, including the TROG-2 and the LARSP.

We will now consider each type of phrase in turn.

7.4.4   Phrases: noun phrases

As its name suggests, the head of a **noun phrase** (**NP**) is a noun. The head noun can be modified by many different types of words and phrases: adjectives, as in (18); prepositional phrases, as in (19); phrases with participles, as in (20); and relative clauses, as in (21).[2]

18   a   muddy **fields**
    b   bright **lights**
    c   unbelievable **stupidity**
19   a   the **lid** of the box
    b   **fields** under water
    c   a **book** about reptiles
20   a   some **walls** destroyed by the storm
    b   **shoes** bought for the children
    c   **programmes** watched by teenagers
21   a   the **roads** that were blocked by snow
    b   the **people** who stole the car
    c   the **paintings** which she admired

As some of the above examples show, the head noun in a noun phrase can be preceded (or premodified) by items such as *the*, *a* and *some*. As we established in Chapter 5, these are called determiners. Other examples are *this*, *that*, *all*, *few*, *no* as in (22).

---

[2]For a description of relative clauses, see Chapter 9 (Section 9.4.1) and for phrases with participles see Chapter 10.

22 a <u>This</u> **film** [is rubbish].
    b <u>All</u> **bets** [are off].
    c <u>Few</u> **people** [understand his theory].

Adjectives can also premodify nouns. In *long black curly hair*, the noun *hair* is premodified by three adjectives.

Under the substitution criterion for phrases, noun phrases can be replaced by pronouns, as we have already seen. In terms of transposition, we can see examples of noun phrases behaving as coherent units whenever we change an active construction into its passive counterpart and vice versa. Thus, applying the transposition criterion to (23) confirms that *My brother* and *this email* are both noun phrases.

23 a My brother sent this email.
    b This email was sent by my brother.

In the first sentence of this section we noted that the term 'noun phrase' is often abbreviated to NP. You will find this abbreviation turning up in **expansion statements** in the STASS, DASS and LARSP, as a shorthand way of indicating that the client is realising a particular syntactic function using more than one word. This notation draws attention to the fact that, for example, a child who says *the car*, *red car* or *the red car* is more linguistically advanced than a child who can only say *car*. This is not to say that in linguistic analyses a noun phrase has to consist of more than one word. For example, in (24), all of the underlined portions are noun phrases, but the one in (24a) consists of only one word.

24 a I like <u>bread</u>.
    b I like <u>brown bread</u>.
    c I like <u>fresh brown bread</u>.

For linguists it is useful to have a level of representation where *bread, brown bread* and *fresh brown bread* in (24) are all given exactly the same label (i.e. noun phrase) because in many respects they behave in the same way. For example, they can all be replaced by the same pronoun *it*. Giving all three the same label captures the fact that at the phrase level they are the same thing. In clinical resources, however, you will most often see the terms noun phrase or NP used to refer to multi-word sequences.

7.4.5 Phrases: prepositional phrases

The underlined groups of words in (25) are **prepositional phrases (PPs)**.

25 a They are going <u>to France</u>.
    b They are leaving <u>on Saturday</u>.
    c They are travelling <u>by train</u>.
    d They are staying <u>for a week</u>.
    e They are staying <u>with relatives</u>.

The head of a prepositional phrase is a preposition: *to* in (25a), *on* in (25b), *by* in (25c), *for* in (25d) and *with* in (25e).

Often the substitution criterion for identifying phrases does not work well for PPs. Although we can sometimes find a single word to substitute for a PP, such as *there* in (25a) and *then* in (25b), and we might be able to substitute *thus* at a stretch in (25c), it does not seem possible to use this criterion in (25d) and (25e). The transposition criterion is more effective; consider (26) to (28).

26   a   They are travelling to France by train.
    b   They are travelling by train to France.
    c   They are staying in France for a week.
    d   They are staying for a week in France.

27   a   The clock is on my mantelpiece.
    b   On my mantelpiece is the clock.
    c   The clock on my mantelpiece is five minutes fast.
    d   It's on the mantelpiece that you'll find the clock.

28   a   The children ran into the gloomy wood.
    b   Into the gloomy wood ran the children.

Notice that in each of these examples of prepositional phrases, the head is followed (modified) by a noun phrase. Sometimes the NP consists of a single word, e.g. *France*, and sometimes it consists of more than one word, e.g. *the gloomy wood*. In the STASS, DASS and LARSP the phrase level does not explicitly capture this regularity (i.e. the fact that these are all noun phrases); instead, the possible phrase structures are listed as sequences of part-of-speech labels such as PREP N, PREP D N and PREP D ADJ N.

7.4.6   Phrases: adjective phrases

The underlined words in (29) are **adjective phrases**, consisting of an adjective *dry* premodified by an adverb *exceedingly*.

29   a   Australia's climate is exceedingly dry.
    b   Australia's exceedingly dry climate causes droughts.

Using terminology introduced in Chapter 5, we can identify the predicative use of the adjective phrase in (29a) and the attributive use in (29b).

Examples (29a) and (29b) fulfil the transposition criterion for these adjective phrases. The substitution criterion is illustrated in (30):

30   My cousin is very brusque and so is her daughter.

So substitutes for *very brusque*.

7.4.7   Phrases: adverb phrases

The examples in (31) illustrate the transposition of *very carefully*, which is an **adverb phrase** consisting of an adverb *carefully* premodified by another adverb, *very*.

31 a She put the brooch in the box <u>very carefully</u>.
   b She <u>very carefully</u> put the brooch in the box.
   c <u>Very carefully</u> she put the brooch in the box.

As with adjective phrases, *so* substitutes for adverb phrases in certain constructions:

32 My cousin speaks very loudly and <u>so</u> does her daughter.

In (32), *does* replaces *speaks* and *so* substitutes for *very loudly*.

7.4.8 Phrases: verb phrases

The final type of phrase that we need to look at is the **verb phrase (VP)**. There are two different interpretations of this label. In some clinical resources, the label refers to sequences of auxiliary and main verbs. Thus, *will lend, might lend, has been lending, has been lent* all count as verb phrases. This concept of verb phrase turns up the Comprehensive Aphasia Test (CAT) Sections 9 and 10, as well as the STASS, DASS and LARSP. This interpretation equates verb phrases with the 'verbal element' in 'elements of the clause' (see Section 7.5.2).

An interpretation that is common in linguistic descriptions, but which is less widely used in clinical resources, is illustrated in (33), in which the verb phrases (according to this interpretation) are underlined.

33 a Charles Dickens <u>wrote many novels</u>.
   b Susan <u>seemed fairly cheerful</u>.
   c Wimbledon <u>started today</u>.
   d Her face <u>suddenly turned white</u>.

The head of this type of phrase is a verb. The head can be modified by a wide variety of structures including noun phrases (33a), adjective phrases (33b,d) and adverbs (33c,d). As (33d) shows, premodification (*suddenly*) and postmodification (*white*) are both possible.

Continuing with this second interpretation, we can say that verb phrases are the weakest kind of phrase. Substitution only applies to the entire verb phrase in cases of ellipsis (the omission of elements in the clause that is made possible because they have been mentioned previously). Consider (34).

34 a Kirsty writes poems and <u>so</u> does James.
   b Kirsty lends money to Amelia and James <u>does</u> too.
   c Who lends money to Amelia? James <u>does</u>.

In (34a) *does* substitutes for *writes* and *so* for poems. In (34b), *does* can be taken as substituting for *lends money to Amelia*. In (34c) *does* certainly seems to substitute for *lends money to Amelia*. Transposition likewise can only be applied with difficulty. Consider (35).

35 <u>Came right in</u> she did, without bothering to knock.

Sentence (35) seems to be related to *She came right in, without bothering to knock*. The problem is whether *without bothering to knock* is part of the verb phrase. If it is, the criterion does not apply, since only a bit of the verb phrase is moved to the front. Even if it does apply, this construction is a minor one and rather uncommon. Evidence from central, regularly occurring constructions carries more weight than evidence from infrequent and peripheral constructions. Other attempts to justify this interpretation of the verb phrase also run into problems.

In spite of these difficulties, verb phrases remain popular with many linguists.

Exercise 7.3

What type(s) of phrases are underlined in the following examples? For instance, in (1), *the new house* is a noun phrase and *very impressive* is an adjective phrase.

1. The new house is very impressive.
2. Into the secret drawer, he put a bundle of notes.
3. The dog chewed the edge of the carpet.
4. The documents were all destroyed by the shredder.
5. These exceedingly expensive houses have no insulation worthy of the name.
6. New components can be delivered tomorrow.
7. The storm blew a number of slates right across the street.
8. Not surprisingly, the silk-wool carpets cost a bomb.
9. I found the coffee very strong.
10. Which committee members do you think he bribed?

7.5 Clauses

In Section 7.4 we looked at the phrase level of description, identifying noun phrases, prepositional phrases and so on. We now move to a different level of description, where we will be concerned with the functions that particular phrases take on. To this extent there is a mapping between the phrase and the clause level, but it is quite a complicated mapping, as we will see. Before we get to that, however, we need to clarify what we mean by a clause.

The Test of Adolescent and Adult Language (TOAL) and the syntax workbook of the Clinical Language Intervention Program (CLIP) each have a subsection called 'Sentence Combining', in which the client is given two or more sentences and is asked to make them into a single sentence. To take a very simple example, we could combine (36a) and (36b) to produce (36c):

36 a   The road was icy.
    b   I slipped.
    c   Because the road was icy, I slipped.

Linguists would say that while (36a) and (36b) each consist of a single **clause**, (36c) consists of two clauses, which have been combined in such a way as to indicate the causal relationship between them. We will have a great deal more to say about clauses in the next two chapters, but for the purposes of the present chapter, we can define a clause as a sequence of words like (36a) or (36b), which contains a verb (*was* or *slipped* in our examples) and can stand alone as simple sentence. The main verb may be modified by one or more auxiliaries, and the clause may also contain a variety of phrases.[3]

Exercise 7.4

How many clauses do the following sentences contain?

1. Linguistics is important although it is sometimes complicated.
2. What is your name and age?
3. What is your name and when were you born?
4. Measure two ounces of butter, melt it in a pan and add the onions.

7.5.1   Elements of the clause

Descriptions of typical and atypical language development and of language impairment in acquired disorders often include analysis at the level of the clause, because a person who is struggling linguistically may find it difficult to process (produce or understand) all of the constituent parts of the clause accurately. Consequently, many language assessments that SLTs use investigate the clause level; so SLTs need to be able to recognise the **elements of the clause**.

In Section 7.4.8 we noted that on one interpretation the 'verb phrase' consists of a main verb plus any associated auxiliary verbs and that this corresponded to the verbal element at the clause level. In the context of a discussion of elements of the clause, we often refer to the verbal element simply as the 'verb', but be aware that this may be more than a single word. When analysing a clause, we have to specify what this verbal element is, and also identify any other phrases in the clause, the order in which they occur and the relationship between each phrase and the verbal element. Verbal elements combine with the sorts of phrases described in Section 7.4: noun phrases, adjective phrases, prepositional phrases and adverb phrases. At this clausal level of analysis, the phrases are said to have various functions: subject, object, complement and adverbial. The complete set of clausal elements that we are interested in is therefore Subject, Verb, Object, Complement and Adverbial, often abbreviated to SVOCA (see Section 7.5.8 for the notation conventions).

---

[3]The term 'simplex sentence' has also come into use; it appears to have been coined by analogy with 'complex sentence', a term that will be explored in later chapters.

We will see in the next two chapters that clauses can have complicated structures, but for the moment we will make two simplifying assumptions (which in fact allow us to analyse a substantial number of the items that are used in clinical resources that target language). First, we will limit the structures to be covered by setting aside many of the clause constructions that are to be found in real speech and writing. In particular, we will not attempt to deal with fragments of clauses but will focus on complete clauses. So, although someone might respond to an accusation that they have not cleaned their room by protesting *I have!*, this is only a fragment of the complete clause *I have cleaned my room!*, and as such we will not be attempting to analyse it here. Second, we will confine ourselves to the basic type of clause illustrated in the following examples:

37   a   The wall collapsed.
     b   The car hit the wall.
     c   Catriona gave her brother the keys.
     d   Soon we will go home.

Examples (37a–d) are all active, as opposed to passive, and they are positive, as opposed to negative. Furthermore, they are all **main clauses**. A main clause can stand on its own as a sentence; in (36c) above, *I slipped* is the main clause, but *Because the road was icy* is not, since it cannot stand alone as a sentence. Taking this type of positive, active, main clause as basic we can handle the syntax of any other type of clause by describing how its structure relates to our basic clause structure, and we can deal with the meaning of any other type of clause. We will not try to deal with more complicated kinds of clauses like the following in this chapter, though we will address them in subsequent chapters:

38   a   The wall did not collapse.
     b   The wall was hit by the car.
     c   Did Catriona give her brother the keys?
     d   When will we go home?
     e   Go home!

To summarise so far: in clauses, verbs are central. They are related to and control the other elements, which are represented by various types of phrases – noun phrase, prepositional phrase, adjective phrase and adverb phrase. Following the standard descriptions of English grammar in SLT, we recognise four functions: subject, object, complement and adverbial. A particular type of phrase is not limited to one function. Noun phrases, for instance, can function as subject, object or complement. In a given clause, exactly which functions the noun phrases have depends on the individual verb and on which construction the clause has.

We have already discussed the different types of phrase. Here we move on to the various types of relationship between the verbs and the phrases that modify them in a clause. The STASS, the DASS and the LARSP explore the full range of functions that are outlined here, but many resources that are concerned with sentence structure, including the TROG-2, CELF, Reynell and PALPA, include items that relate to Subject and Object.

7.5.2 Elements of the clause: verb

As we noted earlier, the verbal element of the clause may consist of a single word (a main or lexical verb) or the main verb may be supported by one or more auxiliary verbs. The verbal element is underlined in the four examples in 39:

39 a My dog <u>chases</u> cats.
    b My dog <u>is chasing</u> cats.
    c My dog <u>has been chasing</u> cats.
    d My dog <u>may have been chasing</u> cats.

The verbal element may consist of more than one word in another sense – it may consist of a verb plus a particle, as, for example, in *ran away* in 40.

40 My dog ran away.

The sequence *ran away* would be labelled VPart (Verb + Particle) in the LARSP.

We are introducing the verbal element early in our discussion because it is so fundamental to the clause. We will now move on to considering the other elements, but will need to refer back to the verbal element many times because of the close relationships that it has with the other elements. In keeping with the approach that is generally adopted, we will often refer to this element simply as the 'verb', but bear in mind that it may consist of more than one word.

7.5.3 Elements of the clause: subject

A popular misconception is that the subject of a clause is 'the doer of the action'. As we know from Chapter 3, the correct term for this semantic role is the agent. Subject is not a semantic role, but a grammatical function. Subjects have several important grammatical properties.

Subject nouns are closely linked to the verb, for instance by being involved in **number agreement**. A singular subject noun combines with a singular verb and a plural subject noun combines with a plural verb. In (41), we see forms that are acceptable and unacceptable in standard English.[4]

41 a My dog chases cats.
    b My dogs chase cats.
    c *My dog chase cats.
    d *My dogs chases cats.

---

[4]SLTs are used to encountering non-standard varieties of English in which forms that are 'starred' here are acceptable. But what we are trying to do here is to explain the thinking behind items that readers will commonly encounter in clinical resources that focus on clients' abilities with regard to clause structure. In such items, the target is the standard-English form, unless the client's usual variety of English makes this inappropriate.

In the unacceptable forms (41c) and (41d), the subject and verb fail to agree in number.

A second property of subject noun phrases in standard English is that they are replaced by subjective forms of pronouns such as *he*, *she* and *they* (see Chapter 5), whereas noun phrases functioning as objects (see Section 7.5.4) are replaced by objective forms such as *him*, *her* and *them*. In (42a) the subject noun phrase is *Catriona* and is replaced by *she* in (42b). In (43a) the subject noun phrase is *many people*. It is replaced by *they* in (43b).

42   a   Catriona enjoyed the film.
      b   She enjoyed the film.
43   a   Many people enjoyed the film.
      b   They enjoyed the film.

At the start of Section 7.5 we mentioned the 'Combining Sentences' subtask of the TOAL and the CLIP, in which the client's task is to turn two or more sentences into a single sentence. This can be accomplished in various ways, but for some of the items the appropriate mechanism is to link the original sentences using a coordinating conjunction such as *and* or *but* (see Chapter 5). We call this mechanism **conjoining**. The subject noun phrase plays an important part when clauses are conjoined. Sentences (44) and (45) can be conjoined to give (46).

44   The flood wrecked the houses +

45   The flood carried off many cars.

46   The flood wrecked the houses and [ ] carried off many cars.

During the conjoining, *the flood* in the second clause is deleted. Only the subject noun can be deleted, precisely because it is central in both clauses. The brackets in bold in (46) show where the subject noun phrase has been removed. In the TROG-2, the items in block L illustrate this construction.

The first two grammatical properties that we outlined are obligatory rules in formal, standard English. In such forms of English, number agreement has to be implemented in the way illustrated in (41) and subjective forms of pronouns must be substituted for grammatical subjects as in (42). We will just mention a couple of less hard-and-fast tendencies that we can observe in everyday language – but there is a payoff here; so keep reading to the end of the section and make sure that you take away the full message!

We will see in the chapters on narrative that grammatical subjects often come first in clauses and perform an important function in narrative, that of theme. In narrative text, grammatical subjects typically refer to animate creatures, mostly humans, performing actions in the role of agent. In other words, for much of the everyday language that clients encounter, grammatical subject and agent refer to one and the same entity. Does this mean that SLTs can ignore the distinction between subject and agent? Certainly not! Clinical resources that target sentence processing do not necessarily try to reflect the patterns that occur in everyday language, because this is not their purpose. Their task is to pinpoint areas of difficulty in a client's language processing, and when we are trying to find out about a specific ability such as syntactic processing, it is often necessary to present clients with test items that appear less frequently in everyday language.

Recall our discussion of reversible active and passive sentences in Chapter 3. A reversible passive sentence is shown in (47a), and the result of substituting pronouns for the two noun phrases in (47b) (appropriate substitution) and (47c) (inappropriate substitution). Sentence (47a) is the sort of sentence that could appear as part of a picture selection task that included one picture in which a woman chases mice and another picture in which mice chase a woman.

47   a   The farmer's wife was chased by the mice.
     b   She was chased by them.
     c   *Her was chased by they.

The number agreement and pronoun substitution criteria that we outlined earlier indicate that *The farmer's wife* is the subject, but it is not the agent, and if a client thought that it was, they would select the wrong picture in the task. Passive sentences go against the trend of everyday language by representing the semantic role of agent and the grammatical role of subject in different noun phrases. Reversible passives like (47), which are widely used in clinical resources, are particularly challenging for young, typically developing children and for children and adults with sentence processing difficulties, and the source of their difficulty is first, the fact that contrary to expectations, the subject and the agent are different entities, and second, that there are no semantic cues to aid their interpretation, because both noun phrases refer to entities that are animate and are thus equally capable of being the agent.

7.5.4   Elements of the clause: object

Subject function is straightforward: there are well-defined criteria for identifying subjects, and a given noun phrase either functions as subject or does not. Object function is more complex, because there are different kinds of object: direct object and indirect object.

Let us first consider the **direct object**. Look at (48) and (49), which are similar to target items in many clinical resources.

48   The girls push the boy.

49   The goat follows the crocodile.

The number agreement and pronoun substitution criteria that were presented in Section 7.5.3 indicate that the subject of (48) is *The girls* and the subject of (49) is *The goat*. But what about the other noun phrases in (48) and (49) – *the boy* and *the crocodile*? These are direct objects.

Although we generally try to avoid or at least de-prioritise semantic criteria when we define syntactic concepts like direct object, introductory texts generally resort to a semantic definition when discussing the direct object in English, saying something along the lines of 'the direct object is the noun phrase that undergoes the action expressed in the verb'. We <u>can</u> make some remarks that draw on grammatical concepts, but we will need to refer to concepts that we have not yet covered, so readers will benefit from coming back to this paragraph after reading the rest of the chapter. If a noun phrase is not the subject of the verb and is not part of a prepositional phrase, then there are several possible classifications in terms of elements of the clause. It could be a direct object. Alternatively, it could be an indirect object, which we will cover later in this section; it could be a complement, which we will cover in Section 7.5.5; or it could be an adverbial in a small number of phrases such as *last year* or *this week*. The indirect object, complement and adverbial functions are constrained by rather specific criteria, which we will explore when we come to them. For the moment, the simplest approach is for us to confine ourselves to examples that contain only two noun phrases until we start to discuss indirect objects, and to promise that, for these examples, the noun phrase that is not the subject (which we can identify using our number agreement and pronoun substitution criteria) is the direct object.

In (50a) and (51a) the underlined noun phrases function as direct objects.

50   a   The storm destroyed <u>those trees</u>.
     b   The storm destroyed <u>them</u>.
51   a   She immediately noticed <u>her brother</u>.
     b   She immediately noticed <u>him</u>.

In the pronoun substitution test the underlined words are replaced by *them* in (50b) and *him* in (51b), not by *they* or *he* (at least, not in standard English). Unfortunately, this is not a conclusive criterion, because, as we will see, the indirect object will also be replaced by the objective form. But at least we know that if a noun phrase is being replaced by a subjective form, it <u>cannot</u> be the direct object.

At this point it is useful to introduce a distinction that is relevant to the concept of the direct object, between **transitive** and **intransitive** uses of verbs. Consider (52).

52   a   He is cooking.
     b   He is cooking the pancakes.

We can see that in both examples, *He* is the subject, because this word is singular as is the verb, and it is in the subjective form. The verbal element is *is cooking*. We promised above that for the moment the only clausal function that would be carried by a non-subject noun phrase would be direct object; so *the pancakes* is the direct object of *is cooking* in (52b). We say that the verb in a clause that contains a direct object is transitive, or is being used **transitively**; so (52b) illustrates the transitive use of the verb COOK. In (52a), the direct object is omitted, and we would say that in this sentence the verb is being used **intransitively**. Verbs vary in the extent to which they are likely to be used transitively or intransitively. Consider the following examples.

53 a Audrey giggled.
    b *Audrey giggled a laugh.
54 a Audrey shouted.
    b Audrey shouted a warning.
55 a Audrey compiled a list.
    b *Audrey compiled.

As we see from these examples, GIGGLE is quite difficult to use transitively, while COMPILE is difficult to use intransitively, but it seems equally easy to use SHOUT transitively or intransitively.

'Transitive' and 'intransitive' are such similar-looking words that it can be easy to confuse them. One way of remembering which is which is to bear in mind that sentences in which the verb is used transitively can usually be translated into the passive. So we could translate (55a) into the passive and say *A list was compiled by Audrey*, but we could not translate (53a) into the passive very easily (*Something was giggled by Audrey*).

Exercise 7.5

You may be familiar with the book by Lynne Truss, *Eats, Shoots and Leaves*, which is about the importance of punctuation (this sounds like a rather dry topic, but it is an entertaining book!). The title is based on the following joke:

'A panda walks into a bar, sits down and orders a beer. He drinks the beer, pulls out a gun, shoots the barman and walks towards the door. "Just a minute!" shouts the manager. "What do you think you're doing? You shot the barman – and you didn't pay for the beer!"

The panda stares icily at the manager and says "I'm a panda; google it" and walks out of the door.

The manager sits down at the computer and googles "panda". The entry reads *Tree-dwelling marsupial of Asian origin, with distinctive black and white appearance. Eats shoots and leaves*'.

Explain the joke using the concepts that have been covered so far in this section (you will need to refer to other concepts that you have encountered in earlier chapters as well).

Let us now turn to **indirect objects**. If a clause contains only a single object, it is a direct object. However, some clauses contain two objects. Consider (56).

56 a Martin baked a cake.
    b He baked a cake.
    c Martin baked Chloe a cake.
    d He baked her a cake.

e   Martin baked a cake for Chloe.
f   He baked a cake for her.

Consistent with our discussion so far, in (56a) we can identify *Martin* as the subject of *baked*, because in (56b) we replace it with the subjective form *He*. As there is only one other noun phrase, *a cake*, in (56a) and (56b), we can, consistent with our earlier promise, assume that this is the direct object. (Don't forget, though, that we also said that later we would see examples where a second noun phrase has other functions). Now what about (56c) and (56d)? Here we have two noun phrases in addition to the subject. In the approach that is usually adopted in clinical resources, *a cake* would still be considered the direct object in (56c) and (56d). *Chloe* must also be some sort of object, because the pronoun that replaces this word in (56d) is in the objective form. According to the approach that is usually adopted in clinical resources, *Chloe* in (56c) and *her* in (56d) would be called the indirect object.[5] The indirect object function is used when referring to the entity that could be loosely said to 'benefit' from the action in the verb. In the alternative forms of (56c) and (56d) that are given in (56e) and (56f), in which the indirect object is expressed as a prepositional phrase, this 'beneficiary' role of the indirect object is perhaps more obvious. You will sometimes find the term **dative** used to refer to the indirect object, especially in its prepositional phrase form (see, for example, the CLIP syntax workbook).

There are many verbs in English that can take two objects. Examples include *buy, bring, lend, make, pour, send, show* and *throw*. In the prepositional phrase form of the indirect object, the preposition can be *for*, as in the earlier examples, but is often *to*, as in *Clark sent a gift to Lois*.

Exercise 7.6

In the following examples, identify direct and indirect objects. If an indirect object is expressed as a prepositional phrase, restructure the example so that the indirect object is a noun phrase and vice versa (for example, *Clark sent a gift to Lois* ↔ *Clark sent Lois a gift*).

1. Catriona lent Angus the car.
2. The chef made a special meal for his favourite client.
3. My mum bought me a bracelet.
4. Don poured a drink.
5. Norman brought flowers for Rosie.
6. Alison showed her holiday photos to her friends at work.

---

[5] We have presented here the approach to direct and indirect object that is most commonly encountered in clinical assessments, but unfortunately there is an alternative approach that you will see in linguistics textbooks. To take the first example in Exercise 6, some grammars of English consider *the car* the direct object and treat *Angus* as 'indirect object', as we have done above; others consider *Angus* the direct object.

In the LARSP, direct and indirect objects are differentiated using subscripts (see Section 7.5.8). In the STASS and the DASS, which are based on the LARSP, the subscripts are abandoned and clinicians only credit 'two objects' rather than identifying each one separately.

We have already seen, in our discussions of active and passive, that the same situation can be conveyed using different constructions. In this section, we have been discussing another such example. Consider (57).

57   a   Catriona lent the car to Angus.
       b   Catriona lent Angus the car.

Sentences (57a) and (57b) denote the same situation but have different syntax. There is no prepositional phrase in (57b), but in (57a) *Angus* is inside a prepositional phrase, *to Angus*, and is at the end of the clause. Sentences (57a) and (57b) differ subtly in meaning. Sentence (57a) presents the car as central to the event, and Angus denoted by a noun inside a prepositional phrase at the end of the clause, is presented as a peripheral participant affected only indirectly. Sentence (57b) presents Angus as central to the event and the participant directly affected by the action.

7.5.5   Elements of the clause: complement

We turn now to the construction illustrated in (58) and (59).

58   Catriona is the new manager.

59   Angus is extremely reckless.

Sentences (58) and (59) are examples of the classic **copula construction,** and *be* is the classic copula. The label comes from the Latin *copula* 'a rope, connection', and the idea behind the metaphor is that *be* does not denote an action or a state but merely links two phrases. The first phrase is usually a noun phrase, as in both examples, while the second can be a noun phrase, such as in *the new manager* (58), or an adjective phrase, such as *extremely reckless* in (59). The second phrase is said to function as the complement of *be*. 'Complement' is from the Latin *com* 'with' and *pleo* 'to fill'. The idea is that complements fill out both the syntax and the meaning of clauses that contain the verb *be*. *Catriona is,* without the complement, is incomplete in syntax and meaning and requires phrases such as *the new manager* to make the clause complete.

Notice that in (58), *Catriona* and *the new manager* refer to one and the same entity. Compare (58) with the superficially similar example (60).

60   Catriona hates the new manager.

In (60), *the new manager* would not normally refer to the same entity as *Catriona*. Here, *the new manager* is not a complement but a direct object.

Following current practice, we also treat *become, appear, feel, seem* and *sound* (and a number of other verbs) as copulas; so they too take complements rather than direct objects. The examples in (61) and (62) all connect a subject noun phrase with another noun phrase or an adjective phrase, and the second phrase refers to or specifies a property of the entity referred to in the subject noun phrase.

61 a Fiona became a lawyer.
    b Kirsty seemed a reliable person.
    c Amelia proved an excellent doctor.
    d Jean remains the best candidate.
62 a Kirsty appeared downcast.
    b Catriona felt/was feeling hungry.
    c The children were becoming restless.
    d Ishbel sounded very tired.
    e Jean ended up miserable.

In a clause with a copula, a prepositional phrase that does not denote a concrete location can also be a complement. See (63) and (64).

63 Kirsty sounded in a panic.

64 Jessie seemed in denial.

As (58), (59) and (61) to (64) show, the complement can be realised by a variety of phrase types, not just noun phrases. Note that in the LARSP, STASS and DASS, the expansion statement for complements only explicitly mentions NPs, but this is not the only phrase type that can appear.

As we pointed out earlier, in the examples that we have used so far in this section, the phrase following the copula refers to or specifies a property of whoever or whatever the subject noun phrase refers to. In (61c) it is the person named Amelia who is an excellent doctor, or in (62e) it is the person named Jean who is miserable. We refer to this kind of complement as a **subject complement**. To reiterate, we can identify a phrase as a subject complement if the verb is a copula, and the phrase refers to the entity denoted by the subject or specifies a property of that entity. Where complements appear in clinical resources, it is usually as part of this construction.

The concept of complement has been extended to another construction called the **object complement**, exemplified in (65). The object complement phrases are underlined.

65 a The painter is going to paint the door dark green.
    b The machine crushed the car flat.
    c The deep-fried Mars bars made me very unwell.
    d The critics consider this novel outstanding.

The verbs in the above examples have direct objects – *the door*, *the car*, *me* and *this novel*. We can tell that these four phrases are not complements because they do not refer to the same entities as the subject noun phrases *The painter*, *The machine*, *The deep-fried Mars bars* and *The critics*. The adjective phrases following the direct objects specify the properties of whoever or whatever is denoted by the direct object noun phrase: the door is to be dark green, the car became flat, the speaker or writer of (65c) became unwell, this novel is outstanding. To see the connection between the adjective phrases in (65) and those in (61), think of (65b), say, as being paraphrased this way: 'The machine affected the car. The car became flat'. That is, the adjective phrase can be thought of as shorthand for a copula clause.

The object complement in this construction can also be a noun phrase, as in (66).

66 a   The committee made Fiona <u>president</u>.
    b   The critics consider this novel <u>the best thriller of the decade</u>.
    c   The voters unexpectedly elected Truman <u>President</u>.
    d   The manager called the players <u>idiots</u>.

The underlined phrases in 65 and 66, then, are object complements, because the entity that they refer to is also the referent of the direct object. As we know from our earlier discussion, when we have a passive construction, the referent of the subject is the same entity that is expressed as the direct object in the corresponding active construction. So in 67 and 68, which use the passive construction, the underlined phrases are subject complements, because they refer to or express a property of the entity that is represented by the subject.

67 a   The door is going to be painted <u>dark green</u> by the painter.
    b   The car was crushed <u>flat</u> by the machine.
    c   I was made <u>very unwell</u> by the deep-fried Mars bars.
    d   This novel is considered <u>outstanding</u> by the critics.
68 a   Fiona was made <u>president</u> by the committee.
    b   This novel is considered <u>the best thriller of the decade</u> by the critics.
    c   Truman was unexpectedly elected <u>President</u> by the voters.
    d   The players were called <u>idiots</u> by the manager.

7.5.6   Elements of the clause: adverbial

The fourth and last function available to phrases in clauses is that of adverbial. An adverbial element supplies information about the place, direction, time or manner of the action expressed by the verbal element. It is crucial to distinguish clearly between the terms 'adverbial' and 'adverb'. 'Adverb' is the label for a word class whose typical members consist of an adjective stem + -ly: *quickly, beautifully, alarmingly, amazingly, indubitably* and thousands of others. 'Adverbial' is the label for a function that can be assigned to adverbs, prepositional phrases and even noun phrases. 'Adverbial' is used for any phrase that has the adverbial function.

How do we recognise when a phrase has the adverbial function? The easiest tests are whether a clause answers a question containing *where, where to, where from, how* or *when*. Consider the examples in (69).

69   a   The dog was sleeping <u>on the armchair</u>.
     b   She was reading her e-mail <u>in her study</u>.
     c   My brother left his briefcase <u>in the train</u>.

Sentence (69a) answers the question *Where was the dog sleeping?* The natural answer would be simply *on the armchair*. We can make similar remarks about (69b,c). (70a–c) answer the question *Where to?* That is, they have to do with direction or movement rather than location.

70   a   We're driving <u>to Granada</u>.
     b   We took the children <u>to the museum</u>.
     c   The locksmith inserted the wire <u>into the lock</u>.

Sentences (71a,b) answer the question *Where from*, as in *Where does he send a box of apples from?* The natural answer would be simply *Canada*.

71   a   My uncle always sends a box of apples <u>from Canada</u>.
     b   The doctor came <u>out of his consulting room</u>.

Sentences (72a–d) answer *how* questions: *How does he speak?*, *How does she write her personal letters?*, *How did the striker put the ball into the empty goal?*. Even if the answer to *How does she write her personal letters?* In the jokey *She writes them with great reluctance*, *with great reluctance* has an adverbial function.

72   a   He speaks <u>very softly</u>.
     b   He speaks <u>with a Welsh accent</u>.
     c   She writes personal letters <u>with a very expensive fountain pen</u>.
     d   The striker <u>casually</u> put the ball <u>into the empty goal</u>.

Sentences (73a–c) answer *when* questions: *When is your cousin arriving?*, *When did you visit the grandchildren?*, *When did the students sit the exam?*

73   a   My cousin is arriving <u>around four o'clock</u>.
     b   We visited the grandchildren <u>in June</u>.
     c   The students sat the exam <u>last week</u>.

Note that the adverbial function is assigned to different types of phrase: the adverb *softly* in (72a), the prepositional phrase *with a Welsh accent* in (72b) and the noun phrase *last week* in (73c). In *See you Tuesday*, a form common in US English though less so in the UK, *Tuesday* is a noun phrase with adverbial function.

Note too that a clause can contain more than one phrase with an adverbial function. An example is (72d), in which the adverb *casually* and the prepositional phrase *into the empty goal* both have an adverbial function. An example such as (74) has three phrases with adverbial function, the adverb *foolishly* and the two prepositional phrases, *in his study* and *on his laptop*.

74   He <u>foolishly</u> left the letter <u>in his study</u> <u>on his laptop</u>.

Exercise 7.7

What function does each underlined phrase have in the examples below: subject, object, complement or adverbial?

1. Jennifer was <u>enthusiastically</u> chopping <u>logs</u>.
2. She was <u>amazed at his lack of concern</u>.
3. Susan was appointed <u>president of the golf club</u>.
4. <u>My aunt</u> left Louise <u>her entire fortune</u>.
5. The lawyer sent <u>Louise</u> a copy of the will.
6. Having forgotten to have lunch, she became <u>very irritable</u>.
7. We sent all the documents <u>to London</u>.
8. <u>Through the window</u> she could see people queuing.

7.5.7 Phrases and grammatical functions

It should be clear from the previous sections that there is not a one-to-one relationship between phrases and functions. In particular, prepositional phrases and noun phrases can each take on a variety of functions. Noun phrases are complements when they follow the copula in the copula construction. They are objects when they come immediately after a verb, can be replaced by *him* or *them*, etc. and can be made the subject of a passive clause. They are adverbials if they answer a question with *when*, *where* and so on. Prepositional phrases can function as complements or adverbials. You can work out which function a given prepositional phrase has by looking at the clause construction. In the copula construction, a prepositional phrase is a complement as long as it does not refer to a concrete location, otherwise it is an adverbial.

Finally, note that complements are typically obligatory, whereas many adverbials are optional. Obligatory adverbials typically have to do with direction, as in *The children ran into the kitchen*.

7.5.8 Notation for clauses

When analysing utterances produced by clients, it is useful to have brief labels for the different clause patterns. One notation is based on the central role played by the verb in a clause and the functions that different classes of verb require or allow. Since it is the notation used in LARSP, we use it here, but readers should be aware that much work on syntax uses representations that focus on the types of phrases that occur in clauses, the types of words that occur inside phrases and the way in which words and phrases are arranged to build up clauses.

For our purposes we need symbols for verbs and for the functions described above.

V: verb
S: subject

O$_d$: direct object
O$_i$: indirect object
C: complement
A: adverbial

These abbreviated labels have the advantage that they can be used to summarise the client's encoding of functions in particular clauses. The patterns that have been discussed in this chapter include the following:

SV: The wall collapsed.
SVO: The car hit the wall.
SVO$_i$O$_d$: Catriona gave her brother the keys.[6]
SVC: Fiona is a lawyer; The children seem restless; Ishbel sounded very tired; The car was crushed flat; She was over the moon.
SVOC: The painter painted the door dark-green; The critics consider this novel outstanding; The committee made Fiona president.
SVA: The car is at the garage; She is working in her garden; The roof was destroyed by the storm; We're driving to Granada; The dog barked furiously.
SVOA: We took the children to the museum; The locksmith inserted the wire into the lock.
SVCA: David Cameron became Prime Minister in 2010; I am busy every evening; The car was crushed flat by the machine; I was made very unwell by the deep-fried Mars bars.

In addition to these elements, the STASS, DASS and LARSP note the presence of question elements with the symbol Q and negative elements with Neg. These are relevant to constructions that we will cover in later chapters (See the account of interrogative clauses in Sections 8.3.3–8.3.5, and of negation in Section 8.5.). These resources use 'wild card' symbols X and Y with these elements – for example, QXY indicates that a client has produced something that contains a question element plus any two other elements – such as QSV in the child utterance *Where Thomas going?* or QSC in *Why Thomas smile?*

The notation can be extended to capture many other distinctions. For example, V can be supplied with subscripts as follows.

V$_{cop}$: a copula verb: *be, become, sound, feel*
V$_{pass}$: a passive verb: *was (destroyed), will be (elected)*, etc.
V$_{mid}$: middle verbs, as in *(The children) photographed (well), (The books) are selling (quickly)*

C and A can be given subscripts to indicate what kind of phrase is functioning as complement or adverbial.

C$_{NP}$: Fiona is the captain.
C$_{AP}$: Fiona is very skilful.

---

[6]Note that the Object element only appears with subscripts when it is necessary to distinguish between direct and indirect object; if the symbol O appears without a subscript, it should be assumed that it is a direct object.

C_{PP}: Fiona is at home.
A_{NP}: Fiona left last week.
A_{ADV}: Fiona replied very grumpily.
A_{PP}: Fiona packed the glasses with great care.

Chapter summary

- There are close connections between syntax and morphology and between syntax and the lexicon.
- One level of description focuses on the way that words combine to form phrases.
- We learned to use the criteria of transposition and substitution to identify a range of phrase types (noun phrase; prepositional phrase; adjective phrase; adverb phrase; verb phrase).
- Every phrase consists of a head word plus optional modifiers. The head word controls the type of modifiers and determines the type of the phrase. The head of a noun phrase is a noun, of a prepositional phrase a preposition and so on. Modifiers may precede the head (premodifiers) or follow it (postmodifiers).
- This chapter used a simplified definition of the clause – a sequence of words that can stand alone as simple sentence.
- The verbal element is the central element of the clause. It may consist of a lexical verb alone or a lexical verb with one or more auxiliary verbs.
- We can identify several major functions that phrases have in clauses:

Subject	(S)	Our new neighbours are keen gardeners.
Direct object	(O_d)	Our new neighbours planted a thick hedge.
Indirect object	(O_i)	Our new neighbours lent us their mower.
Complement	(C)	Our new neighbours are keen gardeners.
Adverbial	(A)	Our new neighbours keep their car in their garage.

Exercises using clinical resources

7.8. At the Phrase level the STASS and DASS Rapid Assessment Score Sheets specify combinations of part-of-speech items to record in clients' speech. Which of these combinations can function as the following at the clause level?
   a. Subject
   b. Direct object
   c. Indirect object
   d. Complement
   e. Adverbial

7.9. Look at the CELF-Preschool; identify the items that explicitly target structures a–d below. Now create at least two more examples of each

that could be used in the same section of the CELF-Preschool. In your new items, underline the target structure.
   a. Verb phrase
   b. Prepositional phrase
   c. Indirect object
   d. Passive

7.10. Section Q in the TROG-2 is called 'post-modified subject'. In items Q2 and Q4, how would you label the group of words that modifies the subject? Think of two more examples that you could use in the same task.

7.11. Look at the Recalling Sentence sub-test of the CELF-4. Identify any passive sentences.

7.12. Look at the items from Sentence Structure subtask in the CELF-4 (it is easiest to look in the manual). Identify items that contain the following:
   a. Indirect object
   b. Complement
   c. Adverbial
   d. Two conjoined clauses

7.13. Identify the elements of the clause in items 1, 3, 9, 10, 16, 17, 19, 21, 24 and 26 of the Sentence Comprehension sub-test of the ACE.

7.14. Here are some sentences that might be elicited by the Cookie Theft Picture in the Boston Diagnostic Aphasia Examination. Identify the elements of the clause in each sentence:
   a. The Mum is washing dishes at the sink.
   b. The Mum is thinking.
   c. The floor is getting wet.
   d. The boy is getting his sister a cookie.
   e. He is falling off the stool.

Further reading

Search for the individual technical terms in Hurford (1994).

'Introduction', 'Chapter 1: Heads and Modifiers' and 'Chapter 2: Constituent Structure' in Miller (2008).

'Chapter 3: Nouns and noun phrases' and 'Chapter 4: Verbs and verb phrases' in Collins and Hollo (2000).

'Chapter 2: LARSP' in Crystal (1992).

8 Sentence Structure 2: Constructions and Main Clauses

> **Clinical resources that will be referenced in this chapter:**
>
> ACE – Assessment of Comprehension and Expression 6–11
> CELF-4, CELF-Preschool – Clinical Evaluation of Language Fundamentals
> ERB – Early Repetition Battery
> PALPA – Psycholinguistic Assessment of Language Processing in Aphasia
> RDLS – Reynell Developmental Language Scales
> TAPS-R – Test of Active and Passive Sentences
> VATT – Verb Agreement and Tense Tests

8.0 Introduction

In this chapter we continue with clause constructions, which were introduced in Chapter 7. There we discussed the central basic clause constructions of English, focusing on main clauses and on full (lexical or main) verbs as central. Many constructions occur in main clauses and in any given clause, depending on the construction, the main verb may be modified by one, two or three noun phrases, by an adjective phrase, by an adverb phrase or by a prepositional phrase.

These modifying phrases stand in different relationships to the main verb (or to put it slightly differently, the modifying phrases have different functions: subject, object, complement and adverbial). The description of each construction specifies the kinds of phrases in the construction, the order of the phrases and, crucially, the function of each phrase. We are now going to examine various other important constructions: in Section 8.3, the constructions that are crucial for allowing speakers and writers to signal whether they are making statements, asking questions or giving commands; in Section 8.4, the constructions that allow speakers and writers to present situations from different perspectives.

For convenience, this discussion of finite clauses is spread over two chapters. Subordinate clauses are important because they allow speakers and writers to build

Introductory Linguistics for Speech and Language Therapy Practice, First Edition. Jan McAllister and Jim Miller.
© 2013 John Wiley & Sons, Ltd. Published 2013 by John Wiley & Sons, Ltd.

up complex sentences and to transmit a complex message. We deal with them in Chapter 9. You may be surprised to find sentences are not mentioned until the final section of Chapter 9. This approach to syntax reflects a particular view: that the important unit of syntax is the clause. All the different syntactic constructions are contained in clauses. Agreement in number and person occurs in clauses; it is clauses that are active, passive or middle, clauses that are main or subordinate and clauses that are declarative, interrogative or imperative. All these different properties of clauses, all the different constructions, allow speakers and writers to produce longer texts such as narratives, which (ideally) set out events, arguments or ideas coherently, in which the links between different chunks of text are clearly signalled, and which hold the listeners' or readers' attention. We will suggest in Section 9.7 that sentences are low-level units of text/discourse that allow clauses to be combined.

8.1   Why do SLTs need this knowledge?

As declared in Chapter 7, syntax – the organisation of words into phrases, phrases into bigger phrases, phrases into clauses and clauses into sentences – is at the core of language. The speaker who wants to transmit a complex message needs at least enough syntax to compose a main clause, and much everyday spoken communication between adults uses some subordinate clauses. Written communication, a central component of modern life at work and home, regularly attains a much higher level of syntactic complexity. Understanding all sorts of texts, from narratives to tax demands, from newspapers to children's stories, requires a command of syntax.

That is why many clinical SLT test materials include instruments for measuring, however roughly, a person's ability to understand and produce syntactic constructions. For instance, the CELF-4 has a section on recalling sentences in which the examples range from passive clauses of the sort *The alpaca was pushed by the llama* to more complicated sentences along the lines of *If we don't get caught up in rush-hour traffic, we should reach Norwich by five o'clock* and *When the students finished their exams, they decided to have a holiday together before returning home.*

The ACE contains a test of 'Syntactic Formulation'. Clients are tested to see if they can use 'Past plus auxiliary' (otherwise known as Perfect auxiliary plus past participle, as in *He's lost the book*), a 'Postmodifying clause' (otherwise known as a relative clause), as in *The boys who are playing football should be in school.* (See the comments on relative clauses in Section 9.4.1.) Clients are also tested to see if they can use subordinate adverbial clauses, such as the *because* clause in *I'm not wearing those shoes because they hurt my feet.* (See the discussion of adverbial clauses in Section 9.4.2.)

The PALPA requires clients to understand different main clause constructions in order to correctly match sentences and pictures. Their sentences are along the lines of *The thief is scaring the Rottweiler, The thief is being scared by the Rottweiler,*

The Rottweiler is hard to scare and *The test is puzzling the client*, *The client is being puzzled by the test*, *The patient is easy to puzzle*.

In the comprehension of narratives clients again have to deal with complicated syntax such as the following paragraph from 'The runaway tractor' in Chapter 16.4.1. Many of the sentences in this narrative consist of a main clause and one or more subordinate clauses. (Subordinate clauses will be dealt with in Chapter 9.) The subordinate clauses are underlined, but note that there is even a subordinate clause, *there was water at the bottom*, inside another subordinate clause, *As soon as he saw there was water at the bottom*.

The tractor raced down the steep field. As soon as he saw there was water at the bottom, he tried to stop. But he didn't know how to put on his brakes. So he fell in the pond with a splash and got stuck in the mud. When the driver found where the tractor was, he phoned for another tractor to pull him out and put him back on the grass.

8.2   Learning objectives

After reading this chapter and doing the exercises, you should be able to:

- Recognise declarative, interrogative and imperative clauses;
- Recognise active, passive and middle clauses;
- Understand the syntactic constructions that are tested in clinical materials;
- Analyse individual examples from clinical materials and appreciate their significance;
- Explain the way that negation is indicated in clauses.

8.3   Declarative, interrogative and imperative clauses

A clause is a construction. We have already met the intransitive, transitive and copula constructions in Chapter 7. The copula construction contains a copula and a complement, as in *Jacob is interested in football* or *Barnabas seemed unwell*. (The construction is represented by the formula SVC or $SV_{cop}C$) The intransitive construction, as in *Katarina is working*, is represented by the formula SV and the transitive construction, as in *Freya read her new book*, is represented by the formula SVO.[1]

In Section 7.5.1, we met examples such as *Catriona gave her brother the keys*. The construction in this example was not given a label but we are now going to give it one – the **ditransitive** construction. It is represented by the formula SVO_iO_d. 'Ditransitive' simply means 'doubly transitive'; that is, the construction contains two objects. One of the objects is called the indirect object, represented by the notation O_i. The other object is called the direct object, represented by the notation O_d.

---

[1] 'Transitive' is from the Latin *trans* 'across' and *ire* 'to go'. The metaphor behind the label is of an action crossing from an agent to a patient. In the intransitive construction there is no patient for an action to cross to. The classic intransitive verbs denote actions or processes that do not involve a patient.

A clause, then, is a very general construction; a phrase is another type of general construction; and a word is a third type – many words consist of stems and affixes that are combined. As we have already said, there are many different types of constructions to be found in clauses. Above we looked briefly at the copula construction, the transitive construction, the intransitive construction and the ditransitive construction. Instead of using a long phrase such as 'a clause containing an example of the transitive construction', people working on syntax say simply 'a transitive clause' (and 'a copula clause', 'a ditransitive clause' and so on). From now on we will use interchangeably phrases such as 'transitive clause', 'transitive construction' and even 'clause containing an example of the transitive construction'.

Most of the examples in Chapter 7 are **declarative**. That is, they represent the construction that speakers and writers use when they make a statement or declaration. Clauses that are used to ask questions are **interrogative**. That is, they are used to interrogate someone (in the general sense of asking questions, not just in police stations or military barracks). **Imperative** clauses are typically used for issuing commands, though commands can be issued using interrogative and declarative clauses. (See the discussion of speech acts in Chapter 13 on language in use.)

8.3.1   Basic constructions: declarative clauses

All work on syntax recognises a set of central basic constructions with which all syntactic analysis begins. These basic constructions are all declarative and neutral, in the sense that none of the words or phrases is emphasised or focused on. ('Focus' is a technical term that you will meet in Chapter 15 on narrative.) For example, *James likes this music* is neutral. *James* and *this music* are not highlighted and are not emphasised or contrasted with other people or things, and similarly for *likes*. (In speech, intonation could obviously be used to highlight items without changing the word order. Here we are focusing on syntax.) The clause *This music James likes* has an unusual word order that highlights the phrase *This music*, in contrast with other pieces of music. It is not a basic construction.

An important reason for taking declarative clauses as basic is that we can think of interrogative and imperative clauses as built up out of them. Declarative clauses allow the widest range of structures; for instance, adverbials can occur at the front of declarative clauses, as in *This morning Jacob played football*, but not in interrogative or imperative clauses: *This morning did Jacob play football?* is not absolutely incorrect but it is highly unusual. A second reason why declarative clauses are taken as basic is that the meaning of interrogative and imperative clauses depends on the meaning of declarative clauses. The speaker who understands an interrogative clause such as (1a) must first be able to understand the declarative clause in (1b).

1   a   Did Jacob play football this morning?
    b   Jacob played football this morning.

Basic declarative clauses are also positive, that is, they do not contain negation. As with interrogative and declarative clauses, a major reason is that the speaker who understands the negative clauses in (2a) and (2b) must first be able to understand the positive clauses in (3a) and (3b).

2   a   Jacob didn't play football this morning.
    b   Pavel doesn't eat broccoli.

3   a   Jacob played football this morning.
    b   Pavel eats broccoli.

A third reason for taking the declarative clause/construction as basic is that it is less complex. Sentence (1a) contains *did*, (1b) does not. Sentences (2a) and (2b) contain the verb *do* as well as the negative *n't*. It is generally accepted in syntactic analysis that simpler constructions be treated as more basic than more complicated constructions.

A fourth reason for taking the declarative clause/construction as basic is that it is more flexible, allowing words and phrases to occur in a different order. Sentences (4a) and (4b) are the most basic of declarative clauses but the underlined prepositional phrases can be moved to the front of the clause as in (5a) and (5b).

4   a   The children ran <u>into the kitchen</u>.
    b   A desk stood in <u>a corner of the room</u>.

5   a   <u>Into the kitchen</u> ran the children.
    b   <u>In a corner of the room</u> stood a desk.

The prepositional phrases cannot be moved to the front of interrogative and imperative clauses. The interrogative clauses in (6a), (6b) and (6c) are peculiar, as is the imperative clause in (7).

6   a   *Into the kitchen did the children run?
    b   *Into the kitchen who ran?
    c   *In the corner did a desk stand?

7   *Into the kitchen run!

Note that the examples in (4)–(7) contain a verb of location, *stand*, and a verb of movement, *run*. The first requires a prepositional phrase denoting a place in which something is located, while the second requires a prepositional phrase denoting a place to which something moves. The link between the verb and the prepositional phrase is strong; the prepositional phrase is a complement of the verb. Where the link is looser, prepositional phrases can occur at the front of interrogative clauses. Thus *He prefers red wine with his meal* can be converted to *Does he prefer red wine with his meal* and *With his meal he prefers red wine* can be converted to *With his meal does he prefer red wine?*

8.3.2   Imperative clauses

Imperative clauses, that is, clauses containing an imperative construction, typically have no subject noun phrase, as in (8).

8   a   Return the book immediately! [transitive]
    b   Come back here! [intransitive]
    c   Give your brother the keys. [ditransitive]

What (8) also shows is that a clause can (indeed, typically does) consist of several constructions. Sentence (8a) is imperative, as opposed to a declarative clause such as *She returned the book immediately* and an interrogative clause such as *Did she return the book immediately?* Sentence (8a) is transitive, as opposed to the intransitive clause in (8b) and the ditransitive clause in (8c). Furthermore, (8a) is positive, as opposed to the negative clause *Don't return the book immediately!* All this is summed up by saying that (8a) is an imperative, transitive, positive clause.

Another imperative construction does contain the subject noun *you*, as in (9).

9   a   You just stay there!
    b   You put that down immediately!

The two imperative constructions in (8) and (9) are used when speakers issue a command to a specific individual. Situations arise in which speakers issue commands to a group in general, hoping that some individual will respond. The imperative construction for use in this situation has *somebody* as the subject noun, as in (10).

10   a   Somebody phone for an ambulance!
     b   Somebody open the door before I drop this pile of books!

8.3.3   Interrogative clauses: yes–no interrogatives

There are various interrogative clauses/constructions. The **yes–no interrogative** construction is used for asking questions about whole situations: did some event take place or did it not? The construction gets its name from the fact that such interrogative clauses can be answered by *yes* or *no*. (Another name for the construction is 'polar interrogative'. The idea behind this label is that the answer *yes* is at the positive pole while the answer *no* is at the negative pole.)

Let us return to the idea that declarative clauses are basic. Suppose we have a declarative clause that we want to turn into a yes–no interrogative clause. If the declarative clause has the construction with BE, BE (*is, are, am, was, were*) is moved to the front of the interrogative clause, as in (11). If the declarative clause contains an auxiliary verb such as *have, will* or *can*, that auxiliary verb likewise moves to the front of the clause, as in (12).

11   a   Katarina <u>was</u> unhappy? ⇒ <u>Was</u> Katarina unhappy?
     b   Freya <u>is</u> at home? ⇒ <u>Is</u> Freya at home?
12   a   James <u>will</u> be at the party. ⇒ Will James be at the party?
     b   Philippa <u>has</u> been in Liverpool. ⇒ <u>Has</u> Philippa been in Liverpool?

The declarative clause may of course not have the BE construction nor contain an auxiliary verb. In that case, the auxiliary verb *do* is brought in to carry tense and number, as in the conversion of (13a) into (13b) and (14a) into (14b).

13   a   Jacob plays football on Saturdays.
     b   <u>Does</u> Jacob play football on Saturdays?
14   a   Barnabas learnt to swim.
     b   <u>Did</u> Barnabas learn to swim?

If the copula is *become* or *seem*, *do* is also required: *She seemed happy* → *Did she seem happy?*; *She became determined to win* → *Did she become determined to win?*

8.3.4   Interrogative clauses: wh interrogatives

Another type of interrogative construction enables speakers

- to ask questions about a particular participant in an event or state, as in (15a) and (15b);
- to ask questions about where and when a situation happened, as in (16a) and (16b);
- to ask questions about the manner in which something happened, as in (17).

15   a   Who lost the keys? [Someone lost the keys.]
    b   What did Rene lose? [Rene lost something.]

16   a   Where did Rene lose the keys? [Rene lost the keys somewhere.]
    b   When did Rene lose the keys? [Rene lost the keys (at) some time.]

17   How did Rene (manage to) lose the keys? [Rene lost the keys somehow.]

This interrogative construction is called the **wh-interrogative** because clauses containing the construction begin with one of the wh-words *who, what, which, where, when* and *how*. (*How* is counted as a wh-word.) We can think of these clauses as being constructed from the declarative clauses in square brackets in (15)–(17). If the <u>some</u>-word being questioned is the subject of the verb, as in (15a), it is simply replaced by the corresponding wh-word:

<u>Someone</u> lost. ⇒ <u>Who</u> lost?

<u>Something</u> frightened the dog. ⇒ <u>What</u> frightened the dog?

If the <u>some</u>-word is not the subject, as in (15b), it is moved to the front of the clause. If the declarative clause contains an auxiliary verb such as *can, will, do, have* or the copula *be*, it too moves to the front of the clause, into second position following the wh-word, as in (18).

18   a   Rene has lost something. ⇒ <u>What has</u> Rene lost?
    b   James will go somewhere. ⇒ <u>Where will</u> James go?
    c   Jennifer is somewhere. ⇒ <u>Where is</u> Jennifer?

If the declarative clause simply contains a main verb, the auxiliary verb *do* is brought into the interrogative clause to carry tense and number, as in the yes–no interrogative. See (19).

19   a   Katarina found something. ⇒ <u>What did</u> Katarina find?
    b   Sabrina fixed the lock somehow. ⇒ <u>How did</u> Sabrina fix the lock?

8.3.5   Interrogative clauses: tag questions

English has a third type of interrogative construction. It is usually treated as one construction or clause but is actually a combination of two clauses and two constructions. One is a declarative clause and the other is a cut-down interrogative clause, as in (20).

20   Kenneth is older than Donald, isn't he?

The declarative clause is *Kenneth is older than Donald*. The interrogative clause is *isn't he*. This can be thought of as a reduced version of *Isn't he older than Donald?* The bit that is left after the reduction is tagged on to the declarative clause, hence the label '**tag question**'. (They are not usually called 'tag interrogatives'.) Tag questions are used when the speaker, having made a statement, decides that they are not completely confident that the statement is accurate and appeals to the listener for confirmation. (The speaker may be quite confident in the accuracy of the statement but wish to appear less confident or to make the listener help decide what is to be taken as fact.)

In (20) the declarative clause is positive and the tag question is negative. In (21) the declarative clause is negative and the tag question is positive.

21   Kenneth isn't older than Donald, is he?

Sentences (20) and (21) show by far the most frequent patterns, but you will come across examples with both clauses positive or both clauses negative. We leave these for later chapters on language in use but point out that speakers who utter examples such as (20), positive declarative clause + negative tag, expect the answer 'yes' ('Kenneth is older'), whereas speakers who utter examples such as (21), negative declarative clause + positive tag, expect the answer 'no' ('Kenneth isn't older').

Exercise 8.1

For each of the examples below, say whether it is a declarative, interrogative or imperative clause.

1. The incessant rain has finally stopped.
2. Isn't anybody going to help.
3. Barnabas doesn't feel like going to school today.
4. Just leave the parcel in the porch.
5. Could I just borrow your scissors for a minute.

Exercise 8.2

Convert each of the following examples into a tag question.

1. You like oysters.
2. Susan didn't leave a message.
3. We will go to the cinema.
4. Your brother can read German.

8.4   The active, passive and middle constructions

In this section we look at three other central constructions, the **active**, the **passive** and the **middle**. These are central constructions for the organisation of narrative, allowing narrators to present situations from different perspectives, focusing on different participants and backgrounding or excluding others. At the risk of becoming wearisome, we repeat the point that any given clause represents or realises several constructions: a given clause can be active or passive or middle plus declarative or interrogative or imperative. Active clauses can be transitive or ditransitive or intransitive. Passive and middle clauses are always intransitive, since there is no direct object. Examples are given in (22).

22 a James fell off his bike. [active, declarative, intransitive]
    b Jennifer cleaned her room. [active, declarative, transitive]
    c Jennifer cleaned something. [active, declarative, transitive]
23 a The room was cleaned by Jennifer.
       [passive, declarative, intransitive]
    b Was the room cleaned by Jennifer?
       [passive, yes-no interrogative, intransitive]
    c What was cleaned by Jennifer?
       [passive, wh interrogative. intransitive]
24 a This material cleans easily. [declarative, middle, intransitive]
    b Does this material clean easily? [middle, interrogative (yes–no), intransitive]

8.4.1   Active clauses/constructions

The prototypical active transitive clause presents a situation and its principal participants. Situations include actions such as cutting and concocting or states such as knowing and believing. Actions involve agents carrying out actions and patients affected by actions. Agents are typically animate (and often human), as in (25), but may be inanimate, as in (26). 'A' is for 'agent' and 'P' is for 'patient'.

25 The children [A] painted the shed [P].
26 This stone [A] is supporting the whole wall [P].

The prototypical patient is inanimate, as in (27), but many are of course animate, as in (28).

27 Freya [A] rewrote the rules [P].
28 The noise [A] deafened her [P].

Sentence (29) is an example of a clause in which both agent and patient are inanimate.

29 The flood [A] destroyed many houses [P].

Active intransitive clauses denote situations involving one major participant, either an agent or a patient depending on the type of situation. Thus, *Katarina shouted* denotes a situation in which Katarina is an agent (*What did Katarina do? – She shouted*) and *Katarina tripped* denotes a situation in which Katarina is a patient (*What happened to Katarina? – She tripped*). Anticipating the chapter on narrative, we simply note here that basic active transitive clauses highlight agents, which occupy the first slot (after any adverbs): *Freya rewrote the rules* and *Yesterday Freya rewrote the rules*. Active intransitive clauses highlight the single participant (*Sabrina fell*, *Sabrina ran up the stairs*) or what is presented as a single participant (*The book sold out in a day*).

8.4.2   Passive clauses/constructions

The passive constructions – there are several – allow speakers and writers to present situations in such a way that patients are highlighted but agents are either pushed into the background or not mentioned at all. Some examples of passive clauses are given in (30).

30   a   The toddler was knocked over by the dog.
      b   The toddler was knocked over.
31   a   The toddler got knocked over by the dog.
      b   The toddler got knocked over.
32   The mahogany table was polished.

Sentence (30a) is an example of the passive construction most frequently found in written English. The subject *The toddler* denotes an animate patient who is affected by an action of knocking over. The agent that carries out the action is denoted by *the dog*. This phrase comes at the end of the clause and has an adverbial function – (30a) can be thought of as answering the question *How was the toddler knocked over?* The syntax of the construction puts the patient phrase, *the toddler*, at the front of the clause and makes it prominent, while demoting the agent to the end of the clause. The whole prepositional phrase containing the agent phrase can be omitted, as shown by (30b). This construction is called the **short passive**, in contrast with the construction in (30a), which is called the **long passive**.

(31a) is the same as (30a) and (31b) is the same as (30b) apart from the fact that the auxiliary verb is *got* and not *was*. The construction is called the ***get* passive**. *Get* passives are dynamic, that is, they denote situations involving events. *Be* passives can be dynamic or static, denoting states. Sentence (32) is ambiguous between a dynamic interpretation, as in *The table was polished by the staff once a week*, and a static interpretation, as in *(As soon as we entered the room) we saw that the table was polished*. The addition of the adverb *highly* makes the static interpretation unmistakable: *As soon as we entered the room we saw that the table was highly polished*.

Get passives are frequent in spoken English, especially in informal circumstances. Short passives, whether with *be* or *get*, are far more frequent than long passives. Various counts have found that typically more than 90% of the passives in a given text are short passives – 'typically', because long passives are more frequent in formal written texts such as academic monographs and official documents than in other types. Most clinical resources use long passives, though the TAPS-R contrasts long and short passives.

The typical long passive can be interpreted by children because the subject is an inanimate noun and the adverbial is an animate noun. In picture tests, children can associate the correct picture with *The car is pushed by the boy* or *The ball Is thrown by the girl*. Trickier to interpret are clauses in which both the subject and the adverbial are animate, as in (33).

33   a   The boy is called by his father.
     b   The girl is helped by the boy.

What makes these passive clauses tricky for young children to interpret is that if the subject and the adverbial phrases swap places, the clauses still make sense, as in (34).

34   a   His father is called by the boy.
     b   The boy is helped by the girl.

Passives in which the subject and the adverbial phrases can swap places are called reversible passives (see Chapter 4).

8.4.3   Middle clauses/constructions

The third construction we need to discuss at this point is the middle. Examples are given in (35). They are all genuine examples or based on genuine examples.

35   a   The book <u>reads</u> well.
     b   These cars <u>sell</u> quickly.
     c   It was claimed that the nano <u>scratches</u> excessively during normal usage.
         [New Zealand Herald, 2005]
     d   The Checking Requirement: Uninterpretable features must be checked, and once checked they <u>delete</u>.
         [David Adger (2003) Core Syntax. A Minimalist Approach. OUP. p. 91]
     e   'Sunset' [type of apple] is well named, striped with red on a golden, slightly russety skin. ... It's ready to pick by late September and **will** <u>store</u> until the end of the year.
         [*The Independent Magazine,* 20th October 2007, article by Anna Pavord]

Sentences (35a,b) are the type of example cited in grammars of English. They have a subject noun phrase, *The book* and *These cars* but no object noun phrase; in fact, the construction excludes direct objects. Adverbials are possible, as in (36).

36   a   These cars sell quickly <u>in France</u>.
     b   The book reads well <u>in my view</u>.

The middle is like the passive in excluding direct objects, but otherwise is very different. The verb is active – *reads* and *sells* as opposed to *is read* and *are sold* in passives. See (37).

37   a   **Passive** The cars were sold quickly. (That is, the salesmen were efficient. The quality of the cars is not relevant.)
         versus
     b   **Middle** The cars sold quickly. (That is, the cars had certain qualities that appealed to customers. The skill of the salesmen is not relevant.)

The middle construction excludes Agent *by* phrases. Sentences (38a,b) are ungrammatical.

38 a *The book reads well by my students.
    b *These cars sold quickly by this salesman.

Moreover, middles and passives have different interpretations. *These cars are sold quickly by this salesman* presents the cars as patients, undergoing the action of selling carried out by the agent, the salesman. It is a comment on the abilities of the salesman. In contrast, *These cars sell well* is a comment on the qualities of the cars. The cars are presented, not quite as agents, but not as patients either. It is the cars that control the situation and they are called '**controllers**'.

The other examples in (35) show that the middle construction is not confined to simple examples such as (35a,b) but extends to other verbs and is found in different types of text. In fact, the middle construction, which is quite frequent in eighteenth century literature, did seem in the early twentieth century to be confined to a handful of verbs but is now undergoing a revival.

Exercise 8.3

For each underlined chunk in the examples below, decide whether it is an example of the active, passive or middle construction.

1. There was torrential rain that afternoon. Six or seven people were waiting at a bus stop for a bus that <u>had been delayed</u>.
   <u>They got soaked by a lorry</u> that drove right through a huge puddle.
2. The driver <u>had driven his lorry</u> from Manchester to Glasgow
3. These apples <u>will be stored</u> in a cold room all winter.
4. 'Sunset' is well named, striped with red on a golden, slightly russety skin. ... It's ready to pick by late September and <u>you can store them until the end of the year</u>.
   [*The Independent Magazine*, 20 October 2007, p. 99, Anna Pavord *Be Amazed*.]
5. Celia <u>tells very interesting stories</u> about her time in Africa.
6. Her stories <u>tell very well</u>.
7. My assistant <u>is always being interviewed</u> for other jobs. I don't think she's happy with her job.
8. Well how else am I supposed to get him out of the way so I can slip out and <u>interview for other jobs</u>? [Not 'interview other people']
   [New Zealand Herald, Alex cartoon 23.XI.05]
9. Our new teapot <u>actually pours without spilling</u>.
10. Beef had remained strong because of the artificial trading conditions caused by the bans, a situation that was always going <u>to correct</u>.
11. Several slates <u>were blown off the roof by the storm</u>.
12. The dog <u>has scratched our new door</u>.

13. The lawsuit ... claims that the nano <u>scratches 'excessively during normal usage'</u>.
    [New Zealand Herald]
14. The PC version of Skype is a 7.6 MB download and it <u>installs painlessly</u>.
    [NZH]
15. The napkin ring <u>polishes up very nicely</u>.
16. Her books <u>translate</u> easily.
17. After the outbreak of c-difficile these two wards have been closed and <u>are being thoroughly cleansed and disinfected</u>.
18. All the moving parts have <u>to be lubricated with special oil</u> once a year.
19. If untreated, the eyes gradually become more and more inflamed as they are unable <u>to cleanse and lubricate properly</u>.
    [*Esk Valley Veterinary Surgery News*, Spring 2011, p. 2. 'Eyes: taking the long view!']

8.5 Negation

We have twice mentioned negation in this chapter: once when remarking in passing that a particular clause was positive as opposed to negative and once in the previous section on notation. LARSP uses 'Neg' to represent negation. Before closing the chapter we need to discuss, even if briefly, the structure of negative clauses. We begin with (39).

39 a The dog isn't fierce.
    b The dog is not fierce.

In (39a) negation is signalled by *n't*, which is part of the word form *isn't*. In (39b) negation is signalled by *not*, which is an independent word. *Isn't* can be considered as deriving from *is* + *not*, with *not* being reduced to *n't* and being attached to *is*. Sentences (39a) and (39b) are identical in meaning – as logicians might put it, 'It is not the case that the dog is fierce'. The logicians' paraphrase neatly brings out the fact that the negation applies to the remainder of the clause. We can show this thus: NEG (The dog is fierce).

Apart from showing that the negation applies to whole clauses, the logicians' approach is interesting in another respect. Very young children often produce utterances in which a negative item precedes the clause, as in the real examples in (40).

40 a No the sun shining
    b No fall
    c No Mommy do that

What the children appear to be doing is using the negative particle *no* (which should probably be followed by an exclamation mark given the energy with which small children utter it). When they first start to use it, it is a response to a request (*Put the worm down.*) or an offer of food and so on. At a later stage they tack *no* onto a clause. Eventually, they arrive at the constructions in (39), and at the other negative constructions of English.

We begin our review of negative constructions with (39). Sentences (39a) and (39b) are negative versions of *The dog is fierce*. To produce the corresponding negative clause you simply insert the independent word *not* into the clause to give (39b) or add *n't* to *is* to give (39a). The negative declarative clause is turned into a negative interrogative clause by moving *isn't* or *is* to the front of the clause, as in (41a) and (41b).

41   a   Isn't the dog fierce?
    b   Is the dog not fierce?

Be is one of the primary auxiliaries, the other one being *have*. The primary auxiliary *have* follows the same patterns as *be*, as shown by (42). (Note that *have* also functions as a main verb, as in *She has a flat in Glasgow*. The main verb *have* follows a different set of patterns.)

42   a   Juliet has bought an alpaca.
    b   Juliet hasn't bought an alpaca.
    c   Juliet has not bought an alpaca.

These negative declarative clauses yield negative interrogative clauses by *hasn't* or *have* being moved to the front of the clause, as in (43) and similarly to (41).

43   a   Hasn't Juliet bought an alpaca?
    b   Has Juliet not bought an alpaca?

The primary auxiliary *have* follows the same pattern, as in the declarative clause in (44), the negative declarative clauses in (45) and the negative interrogative clauses in (46).

44   The engineer has repaired the boiler.

45   a   The engineer hasn't repaired the boiler.
    b   The engineer has not repaired the boiler.

46   a   Hasn't the engineer repaired the boiler?
    b   Has the engineer not repaired boiler?

The pattern is also followed by the modal auxiliary verbs, *can* as in (47).

47   a   Freya can come to the party.
    b   Freya can't come to the party.
    c   Freya can not come to the party.
    d   Can't Freya come to the party?
    e   Can Freya not come to the party?

The construction with the independent word *not* is the one that is typical of written English, particularly formal written English. But the construction with *isn't*, *hasn't*, *can't*, etc., is used in informal writing and is making an appearance in more formal texts – but is probably not yet acceptable in university essays. SLTs need to be aware that their clients will present various usages in speech. The construction with the independent word *not* is common in Scotland and the north of England, especially with BE. Note too that some of your clients, especially in Scotland and North East England will have the negative *no*, as in *They're no leaving*, and a range of forms such as *dinnae* 'don't', *cannae* 'can't'.

The second author's spoken usage is exemplified in (48).

48 a   I'm not coming to the party.
    b   Is she not leaving tomorrow? (= Isn't she leaving tomorrow?)
    c   Can you not get the box open?

Not can be stressed or unstressed. Sentences (48a–c) are to be interpreted as neutral statements and questions.

Verbs that are not auxiliaries have various negative and interrogative constructions. One is the construction you have seen above for the primary auxiliaries BE and HAVE, because they occur in the Progressive and the Perfect, as in (49).

49 a   The dog is barking.
    b   The dog has lost her ball.

The negative construction is shown in (50) and the interrogative one in (51).

50 a   The dog isn't barking.
    b   The dog is not barking.
    c   The dog hasn't lost her ball.
    d   The dog has not lost her ball.

51 a   Is the dog barking?
    b   Isn't the dog barking?

Where there is a modal auxiliary, as in the Future Tense, the construction shown in (47) is used. Thus, the clause *We shall complete the book next week* has as its negative and interrogative the examples in (52), and (53) shows the negative and interrogative versions of the clause *Katarina will help*.

52 a   We shan't complete the book next week.
    b   We shall not complete the book next week.
    c   Shall we complete the book next week?

53 a   Katarina won't help.
    b   Katarina will not help.
    c   Will Katarina help?

Many, probably most, of your clients will not use *shall*. It was noted long ago that it was disappearing from English, though it survives in formal English and in the speech of a small but influential number of speakers.

Where there is no primary or modal auxiliary, the dummy auxiliary DO is brought into play. This happens with the Simple Past tense and the Simple Present tense, exemplified in (54) and (55).

54 a   Sabrina bought a blue pashmina.
    b   Sabrina didn't buy a blue pashmina.

  c   Sabrina <u>did not</u> buy a blue pashmina.
  d   <u>Did</u> Sabrina buy a blue pashmina?

55 a   Jennifer <u>plays</u> cricket.
    b   Jennifer <u>doesn't</u> play cricket.
    c   Jennifer <u>does not</u> play cricket.
    d   <u>Does</u> Jennifer play cricket?

Semi-auxiliaries follow two patterns. In Chapter 6, you met the semi-auxiliary *be going to* as in *She's going to sell her car*. This particular semi-auxiliary contains the primary auxiliary *be* and the negative and interrogative patterns are those shown in (50) and (51): *She's not going to sell her car* and *Is she going to sell her car?* Another semi-auxiliary is *need*, which follows complex patterns. In the positive, declarative construction, shown in (56), *need* is followed by the infinitive. (See the account of the infinitive in Section 10.3.)

56   We need to buy a new washing machine.

Need has two negative patterns. One is the pattern for primary and modal auxiliaries in which *n't* is attached to the verb, as in (57a), and the other is the pattern for ordinary verbs using the dummy auxiliary *do*, as in (57b).

57 a   We <u>needn't</u> buy a new washing machine.
    b   We <u>don't need to</u> buy a new washing machine.

Likewise it has two interrogative patterns, as in <u>*Need we buy a new washing machine?*</u> and <u>*Do</u> we <u>need to buy a new washing machine?*</u> The auxiliary pattern in (57a) is confined to written English and the speech of a few (but again, influential) speakers. Most of your clients will have the pattern in (57b).

Negative clauses typically contain the determiner *any* and not the determiner *some*. (Note the word 'typically'; the patterns of usage are actually quite intricate but need not concern us here. [Note 'need not']) Sentence (58) shows the construction with the count noun *dog* and (59a,b) have the mass noun *sugar*. Sentences (58a) and (59a) are positive (or non-negative) and contain *some*; (58b) and (59b) are negative and contain *any*.

58 a   Pavel saw <u>some</u> dogs in the garden.
    b   Pavel didn't see <u>any</u> dogs in the garden.
59 a   Rene bought <u>some</u> sugar.
    b   Rene didn't buy <u>any</u> sugar.

There are clauses that are covertly negative. What we mean by that is they do not contain an overt negative like *n't* or *not* but they have *any* and not *some*. The key words are *seldom* and *hardly*, as shown in (60) and (61).

60 a   She <u>seldom</u> buys books.
    b   She <u>seldom</u> buys <u>any</u> books.
61 a   He <u>hardly</u> reads novels.
    b   He <u>hardly</u> reads <u>any</u> novels.

She seldom buys some books and *He hardly reads some novels* are at the very least unusual, and at best might be given an interpretation requiring some unusual context. In some varieties of English an overt negative turns up: there is a well-known rockabilly song entitled 'Can't hardly stand it'.

Chapter summary

Section 8.3.1 deals with some of the frequent clause constructions in English.

Basic clause constructions

Declarative	Pavel drives a Porsche.
Imperative	Drive carefully!
	You drive carefully!
	Someone open the gate!
Interrogative	
Yes-no	Does Pavel drive a Porsche?
Wh	Who drives a Porsche?
	What does Pavel drive?
Tag-question	Pavel drives a Porsche, doesn't he?
	Pavel doesn't drive a Porsche, does he?

The most basic construction is the declarative.

Section 8.4 introduces the active, passive and middle constructions. Any one clause represents a number of different constructions simultaneously. A declarative or interrogative clause can represent the active, passive or middle constructions. Imperative clauses could in principle be active, passive or middle but the vast majority are active. An active clause can be transitive and intransitive. Passive and middle clauses are always intransitive.

Declarative	Active	Intransitive	The wall collapsed.
Declarative	Active	Transitive	The workmen demolished the wall.
Declarative	Passive	Long	The wall was demolished by the workmen.
Declarative	Passive	Short	The wall was demolished.
Declarative	Get passive		The wall got demolished (by the workmen).
Declarative	Middle		The book sold out in two days.

Long passives with an inanimate subject as in *The wall was demolished by the workmen* are easily interpreted by children but not so easy are passives in which the subject is animate or human and the noun in the *by* phrase is also animate or human. An example is *The man was blamed by the boy*. These are called reversible passives.

Section 8.5 discussed negation.

Exercises using clinical resources

8.4. In the Complex Sentences section of the New RDLS, which items have the passive structure?

8.5. In the Recalling Sentences sub-test of the CELF-4, which items illustrate the following structures?
    a. Passive interrogative
    b. Active interrogative
    c. Negative

8.6. In the VATT, which items illustrate the ditransitive construction?

8.7. In the TAPS-R, which items illustrate the short passive?

8.8. In the Sentence Imitation Test of the ERB, which items illustrate the following:
    a. Negative
    b. Yes–no interrogative
    c. Imperative
    d. Ditransitive

8.9. In the Sentence Structure sub-test of the CELF-Preschool, which items illustrate the following:
    a. Imperative
    b. Wh-interrogative

Further reading

'Chapter 3: Constructions' in Miller (2008).

Search for the individual technical terms in Hurford (1994).

9 Sentence Structure 3: Subordinate Clauses and Sentences

Clinical resources that will be referenced in this chapter:
ACE – Assessment of Comprehension and Expression 6–11
CELF-4, CELF-Preschool – Clinical Evaluation of Language Fundamentals
Renfrew Bus Story
RAPT – Renfrew Action Picture Test

9.0 Introduction

In the previous chapter, we discussed the finite clauses and some of the major constructions that occur in them. In this chapter, we turn our attention to subordinate clauses. Speakers and writers combine subordinate clauses with main clauses to build sentences. In traditional terms, main clauses can stand on their own as the first contribution to narrative but subordinate clauses cannot. *Sabrina sat down at the piano* might not provide much information but it is a good beginning and the listener or reader would not be surprised by a continuation such as *She loved practising in the spacious music room*. In contrast, *When Sabrina got home* and *which she didn't like at all* and *whether Jennifer wanted to play duets* are not good beginnings on their own. The traditional definition has to be supplemented with other properties, and this we do in Section 9.2.

9.1 Why do SLTs need this knowledge?

The ability of SLT clients to process subordinate clauses is targeted explicitly in many clinical resources, including the Renfrew Bus Story, RAPT, CELF-Preschool, CELF-4 and ACE. As we noted in Chapter 8, and will explore further in later chapters, successful expression and reception of narrative depends on accurate processing of a wide range of subordinate clause types.

Introductory Linguistics for Speech and Language Therapy Practice, First Edition. Jan McAllister and Jim Miller.
© 2013 John Wiley & Sons, Ltd. Published 2013 by John Wiley & Sons, Ltd.

9.2   Learning objectives

When you have studied the chapter and done the exercises, you should be able to:

- Discuss the differences between main and subordinate clauses;
- Understand and apply the criteria distinguishing relative clauses, complement clauses and adverbial clauses;
- Recognise the different types of subordinate clause in clinical assessment materials;
- Recognise some of the constructions used by clients that are not accepted in formal written English but are nonetheless in regular use in spoken English.

9.3   Main and subordinate clauses

We turn now to the major distinction between main and subordinate clauses. They can be regarded as different major types of construction. We can recognise main clauses as a type that, among other things, allows a large range of constructions such as interrogatives and imperatives. It also allows clauses such as those in (1).

1   a   Into the kitchen ran the children.
     b   Never have buildings rented so cheaply.

Sentences (1a) and (1b) illustrate a syntactic process called **fronting.** In (1a), the adverbial/prepositional phrase *Into the kitchen* is at the front of the clause; in (1b) the negative *never* is at the front of the clause. In (1a), the main verb *ran* is followed by the subject *the children* (cf. *The children ran into the kitchen.*). In (1b), the auxiliary verb *have* follows the negative and is in turn followed by the subject, *buildings*.

We recognise three major types of subordinate clause construction: relative clauses, complement clauses and adverbial clauses. They all exclude interrogatives and imperatives. Sentences (2a–c) are unacceptable.

2   a   *Since do you have a driving licence, you can borrow my car.
          (*Since you have a driving licence,* . . . is OK)
     b   *My friend, who does she have a driving licence, can borrow my car.
          (*who does have a driving licence* is OK with emphasis on *does*)
     c   *I suspect that do they not have a plan B.
          (*that they do not have a plan B* is OK)

The fronting of adverbials and negatives, as in (1) is not allowed either, as shown by (3).

3   RELATIVE CLAUSE   The animal that into the room came was our dog.
                            (*that came into the room* is OK)

     ADVERBIAL CLAUSE   *When into the room came our dog, our guest screamed.
                            (*When our dog came into the room* is OK)

Main and subordinate clauses play different roles in the unfolding of narratives; indeed the traditional definition of main clauses relates to texts. They are said to be able to stand on their own but this can usefully be rephrased as 'A main clause is one that can stand alone as the first sentence in a text, or as a whole text, and is syntactically complete.'

Thus, the subordinate clause in (4) is not complete but requires some other clause to complete it, as in (5).

4   If she visits them next week [incomplete: what will happen if the visit takes place?]

5   If she visits them next week, we might find out who her fiancé is.

In contrast, if the narrative begins with *We might find out who her fiancé is*, no other clause is required, though listeners or readers might feel happier with more clauses conveying information about when and where, and why the speaker thinks they will learn the identity of the fiancé.

9.4   Recognising different types of subordinate clause

Three types of subordinate clause are recognised: relative clauses, adverbial clauses and complement clauses. How do we recognise one type of subordinate clause from another? To decide what type a given subordinate clause is we need to ask two questions. One is: does it modify a clause? If the answer is 'yes', the clause is an adverbial clause. If the answer is 'no', the next question is: what kind of word does it modify? If it modifies a verb or an adjective, it is a complement clause. If it modifies a noun, it could be a relative clause or a complement clause, but the two types are distinguished by another criterion, as discussed in Section 9.5 on complements.

9.4.1   Relative clauses

In *the castles that King Edward built* the relative clause *that King Edward built* modifies *castles*; that is, it provides information about the castles and helps to identify them. Suppose we have the main clause in (6) and the relative clause in (7).

6   The guest will not be invited here again.

7   who stole my book
    The two clauses can be combined as in (8).

8   The guest will not be invited here again
    + who stole my book

The guest who stole my book will not be invited here again.

As the first chunk in a narrative or piece of conversation, *who stole my book* – not uttered as a question! – will not do. Likely responses from listeners would be *What do you mean?* or *Who are you talking about?* It is worthwhile commenting that some SLT clinical work seems to suggest that relative clauses are different from subordinate clauses. Relative clauses are certainly different in their syntax from adverbial and complement clauses but the criteria mentioned in Section 9.2 apply to all three types of clause. Relative clauses will be discussed in more detail in Section 9.6.

9.4.2 Adverbial clauses

We begin with the underlined adverbial clauses in (9).

9 a <u>When the snow fell</u>, the major roads were blocked.
  b The road will be empty <u>if we leave before seven o'clock</u>.
  c <u>Since/because you've spent all your money</u>, you won't be able to buy more time on your mobile.
  d <u>Although my brother is going,</u> I'm staying at home.

The label 'adverbial' suggests that adverbial clauses modify verbs, but they modify whole clauses. In (9a), *when the snow fell* denotes one situation and *the major roads were blocked* denotes another situation. The clause *when the snow fell* specifies the time at which the second situation came about. It does not just modify *were blocked* but *the major roads were blocked*. Such adverbial clauses are called **adverbial clauses of time**.

In (9b), *if we leave before seven o'clock* denotes one situation, the speaker and other(s) leaving before seven. The other clause, *the road will be empty*, denotes another situation. This other situation will come about if the first situation comes about. The clause *if we leave before seven o'clock* sets out the conditions or circumstances in which they will find the road empty. It is known as an **adverbial clause of condition**.

In (9c), the clause *Since/because you've spent all your money* describes one situation: the person spoken to has spent all their money. The second clause, *you won't be able to buy more time on your mobile*, denotes another situation: the person addressed is unable to buy time for their mobile phone. The first clause provides the reason for the second situation and is called an **adverbial clause of reason**.

Sentence (9d) is slightly trickier than the others. As before, one clause denotes one situation and the other clause denotes another situation. The speaker uses the clause *I'm staying at home* to state one situation. The speaker uses the first clause to concede a point in the discussion. The clause *although my brother is going* can be glossed 'OK, I'll concede one point: it is true that my brother is going'. Such clauses are called **adverbial clauses of concession**.

It is worthwhile mentioning that, life being short, linguists often just talk of time clauses, conditional clauses or conditionals, reason clauses and concessive clauses or concession clauses. The sentences in (10) are based on sentences that are used in various clinical SLT materials on the understanding of paragraphs and demonstrate the kind of adverbial clauses that SLT practitioners will come across. The adverbial clauses are underlined.

10 a As they got out of the car, they could see the crowds of people.
       [Adverbial clause of time]
    b When they switched on the computer, they didn't notice the e-mail.
       [Adverbial clause of time]
    c The driver swerved to avoid the dog, even though his front tyres were bald.
       [Adverbial clause of concession]
    d Juliet was annoyed because the electrician did not turn up.
       [Adverbial clause of reason]
    e That all happened before he went to work in Paris.
       [Adverbial clause of time]
    f As soon as he saw his card had been stolen, he alerted the bank.
       [Adverbial clause of time]

An example similar to (10f) occurs in the Renfrew Bus Story. The adverbial clause of time is introduced by *as soon as*, that is, by three words, whereas the time clauses in (10a, b, e) are introduced by one word: *as*, *when* and *before*. These single words are subordinating conjunctions; that is, they conjoin one clause with another, and make the conjoined clause subordinate. The simplest analysis is to treat the three words as one complex conjunction (following the practice whereby, e.g. analysts treat *in front of* as a complex preposition).

9.4.3 Complement clauses

We move on to complement clauses, as exemplified and underlined in (11) and (12).

11 a The Government declared that they had no Plan B.
    b Nobody knew that the match had been rigged.
    c The witness admitted that she had been threatened.
    d She found out who had started the rumour.
    e The fans asked if the referee was blind.

12 a It is clear that they haven't a clue.
    b It is surprising that anybody can pay that kind of money.
    c It is regrettable that she resigned.
    d It is incredible that the driver survived.

The underlined clauses in (11a–e) modify verbs: *declared* in (11a) – *that they had no Plan B* answers the question *What did the Government declare?*; *found out* in (11d) – *who had started the rumour* answers the question *What did she find out?*; *asked* in (11e) – *if the referee was blind* answers the question *What did the fans ask?*.

In some syntactic work such clauses are called **subordinate noun clauses**, since in sentences such as those in (11) they occur where noun phrases can occur, as demonstrated in (13) and (14).

13 a   Nobody knew [that the match had been rigged].
    b   Nobody knew [her address].

14 a   [That she decided to resign surprised everyone].
    b   [Her sudden death] surprised everyone].

In much contemporary syntactic theory the label used is 'complement clause'. The account of the complement function in Section 7.5.5 began with the examples in (15) and moved on to the examples in (16) and (17). The complement phrases are underlined.

15 a   Catriona is a good driver.
    b   Angus is extremely reckless.

16 a   Kirsty appeared downcast.
    b   Catriona felt/was feeling hungry.
    c   The children seem restless.
    d   Ishbel sounded very tired.

17 a   Kirsty seemed a reliable person.
    b   Jean remains the best candidate.
    c   Amelia proved an excellent doctor.

Phrases that function as complements are obligatory, since they fill out and complete the syntax of the clause and its meaning. *Kirsty appeared, Angus is, Ishbel sounded* and *Amelia proved* have incomplete syntax and meaning. (*Appear* in (16a) means 'have a certain appearance', not 'come into sight'.) The clauses in (11) that we are calling complement clauses are also obligatory, filling out and completing the syntax and the meaning of the bigger clause. *The Government declared* and *The witness admitted* are unacceptable in any circumstances. (Cricket teams declare but not Governments.) *Nobody knew, She found out* and *The fans asked* are only acceptable if some piece of syntax has been ellipted (omitted), as in *He didn't tell her where he had been but she found out [where he had been].*

Each example in (12) contains the copula *is*, but the complement clauses modify the adjectives *clear, surprising, regrettable* and *incredible*. A clause such as *It is regrettable* is syntactically complete but something more is needed to specify what *it* refers to – here, *that she has resigned*. Note that the complement clauses can function as subject, as in (18). Sentence (18a) can be thought of as answering the question *What is surprising?* and (18b) as answering the question *What is incredible?*

18 a   That anybody can pay that kind of money is surprising.
    b   That the driver survived is incredible.

Sentences such as (18a,b) occur regularly in written texts but are rare in spontaneous speech such as informal conversation. Speakers prefer the construction *It is surprising that anybody can pay that kind of* money and *It is incredible that the driver survived.*

Exercise 9.1

The subordinate clauses in each of the following examples are underlined. For each one say whether it is a relative, complement or adverbial clause. For each adverbial clause, say what kind it is – time, condition, reason, manner, etc.

1. I did tell you that Sabrina doesn't like camping.
2. The book she took so long to write has been a big success.
3. Once they had a good night's sleep the children decided they liked our idea of going sailing.
4. Did you ask when they would arrive?
5. The house my grandparents lived in was demolished last year.
6. He listened carefully as she explained the route.
7. Torquil sighed when he heard that Alice was leaving.
8. Harriet grimaced as though she had tasted something sharp.
9. It's a shame that our friends had to sell the house they'd just bought.
10. Charles wasn't listening, although his sister tried several times to talk to him about his decision.

9.5 Clauses that modify nouns

Clauses that modify nouns are either relative clauses, as in (19), or complement clauses, as in (20).

19 a I prefer the books which you chose.
    b I prefer the books that you chose.
    c I prefer the books you chose.

20 a I can't accept the idea that the house will be demolished.
    b The theory that the earth is flat has been discredited.
    c They abandoned the plan that they would hold an election.

The underlined clauses in (19) are relative clauses and those in (20) are noun complement clauses. Both types modify nouns but there are major differences between them. Relative clauses can be introduced by wh words such as *which*, as in (19a), or *who* as in *The policeman who spoke to us*, or by *that* as in (19b). Complement clauses can only be introduced by *that*. The examples in (21) are all ungrammatical.

21 a *I can't accept the idea which the house will be demolished.
    b *The theory which the earth is flat has been discredited.
    c *They abandoned the plan which they would hold an election.

There are some complement clauses that, contrary to (21), are introduced by a wh word, as in (22).

22 a the question why the house is to be demolished
    b the reason why they want to hold an election
    c the problem where to store the books

These apparent counter-examples can be handled by treating *the question why* and so on as fixed phrases. That is, there is a small set of nouns such as *question*, *reason* and *problem* that require or allow complement clauses introduced by a wh word.

Noun complement clauses present the content of some plan, idea, intention, suggestion, theory, hypothesis and so on and typically modify a noun such as *plan*, etc. Relative clauses present the property of some entity but not the content of a plan, project and so on.

A third difference is that if the wh word in relative clauses is deleted, what is left is often an incomplete clause, as in (23).

23   a   We're going to visit the town <u>where I was born</u>.
           →*We're going to visit the town [ ] I was born.
      b   I'll lend you the book in which I found the data.
           →*I'll lend you the book in [ ] I found the data.

In contrast, when *that* is deleted from a noun complement clause, what is left is a complete clause. The construction may be informal in style but is grammatical, as shown by (24a–c).

24   a   I can't accept the idea [ ] <u>the house will be demolished</u>.
      b   The theory [ ] <u>the earth is flat</u> has been discredited.
      c   They abandoned the plan [ ] <u>they would hold an election</u>.

That can also be deleted from complement clauses modifying verbs, as in (25).

25   I knew that he was up to no good.
      →I knew [ ] he was up to no good.

In spoken English such complement clauses are typically not introduced by *that*. The fact that *that* can be removed but leaves behind a complete complement clause suggests that it is not part of the clause at all. In adverbial clauses too, the initial word can be removed without making the clause incomplete. Thus, *When we were on holiday in Granada, we visited the Alhambra* becomes *We were on holiday in Granada, we visited the Alhambra*. The clause *We were on holiday in Granada* is no longer an adverbial clause but it is complete and could be a good main clause.

(A more recent term for *that* is 'complementiser'. It was first applied in the analysis of complement clauses but has been extended to adverbial clauses. We will use the term 'subordinating conjunction'.)

Exercise 9.2

For each underlined clause in the following examples, say whether it is a relative clause or a complement clause.

1. The idea <u>that she might borrow our flat</u> is ridiculous.
2. The idea <u>that she describes in her book</u> is brilliant.

3. She's not ready to publish the theory <u>that she has been working on</u>.
4. He doesn't accept the theory <u>that plants and animals evolved over millions of years</u>.

9.6 Optional extra on relative clauses

We return to relative clauses because they occur frequently in narrative and because English has several relative clause constructions. Sentences (26a) and (27b) are examples of the classic **wh relative clause**.

26 a   the person <u>who phoned</u>
    b   the person <u>who/whom you phoned</u>

In order to explain the relative clauses we start from an 'ideal' structure showing the function of the wh word in the relative clause. The ideal structures for (26) are in (27a,b).

27 a   the person [the person phoned]
    b   the person [you phoned the person]

One of the nouns in the relative clause, here *person*, is identical with the noun modified by the relative clause. In the relative clause, the phrase containing that noun is replaced by *who* (if the noun is human) or by *which*. If the noun in the relative clause functions as the object, it may be replaced by *whom*. (But *whom* is pretty well confined to formal writing and for many speakers is archaic.) These operations give the structures in (28).

28 a   the person [who phoned]
    b   the person [you phoned who]

If the wh word is not already at the front of the relative clause, it is moved there. Sentence (28b) becomes (26b). If there is a preposition, as in *the person to whom you gave the book*, there is a choice of moves. We start with the ideal structure in (29), and replace *the person* with *who* or *whom*, to give (30).

29   the person [you gave the book to the person]

30   the person [you gave the book to whom/who]

The wh word can be moved to the front of the sentence on its own, leaving behind the preposition *to*, to give (31a). Alternatively, the whole prepositional phrase can be moved to the front to give (31b).

31 a   the person who you gave the book to.
    b   the person to whom you gave the book.

The wh relative clause is found mainly in formal writing. Two other relative clause constructions are the ones typical of spoken language, the th construction as in *the person that you phoned* and the contact relative construction as in *the person you phoned*. We go back to our ideal structures, repeated in (32).

32   a   the person [the person phoned]
      b   the person [you phoned the person]
      c   the person [you gave the book to the person]

To get to the **th relative clause** we insert *that* and delete *the person* (in this particular example) from the relative clause. The bold brackets in (33) show the gap where the phrase has been deleted.

33   a   the person [that [ ] phoned]
      b   the person [that you phoned [ ]]
      c   the person [that you gave the book to [ ]]

Note that the wh words are pronouns: there is the contrast between *who* and *whom*, which is parallel to the contrast between *he* and *him*, *she* and *her*, *I* and *me*, *we* and *us*, *they* and *them*; and the wh words can be preceded by a preposition, as in *to whom you gave the book*, *from whom I received the award*. In contrast, *that* is not a pronoun but a conjunction. It is invariable; that is, it always has the same form, *that*. It cannot be preceded by a preposition: *the person to that you gave the book* is unacceptable.

The third construction is the **contact relative clause**, so called because the relative clause is right next to the noun it modifies, with no wh word or *that* to act as a buffer. Examples are in (34).

34   a   the person you phoned.
      b   the person you gave the book to.

To get to the contact relatives you take the ideal structures in (35) and simply delete the relevant phrase as for the th construction. The results are shown in (36a) and (36b).

35   a   the person [you phoned the person]
      b   the person [you gave the book to the person]
36   a   the person [you phoned []]
      b   the person [you gave the book to []]

But suppose the ideal structure is the one in (37), where *the person* functions as the subject of the relative clause.

37   the person [the person phoned]

In this case, you have to insert *who* or *that*. *The person [that phoned] spoke unclearly* is fine; *the person [phoned] spoke unclearly* is unacceptable (at least in written English and for many speakers of standard English). But, a construction called the **existential** allows just this sort of relative clause. The existential is used to introduce entities into conversations or narratives. An example is (38).

38   There's a strange dog in the garden.

If there is more than one dog, the construction typical of spoken English is *There's strange dogs in the garden*, with *there's* and not *there are*. *There are strange dogs in the garden* is typical of formal written English. Suppose our ideal relative clause structure is that shown in (39).

39 There's a guy here [the guy speaks Turkish].

It is possible, in spoken English, to simply delete the phrase *the guy* to give (40).

40 There's a guy here [speaks Turkish].

Many native speakers deny, almost with oaths, ever having heard examples like (40), far less using them. Nonetheless, the construction is the norm for informal spoken English and is to be heard in not-so-informal contexts too.

Some speakers do not like to use *that* relative clauses for human nouns. For example, the CELF-Preschool UK record form has a list of questions to be asked with respect to pictures. The sample questions are shown in (41) and (42). The questions to do with humans all have *who* and the questions to with non-humans all have *that*.

41 the one who is pointing up
    the one who is first
    the one who is tall
    the one who is alone

42 the one that is inside
    the one that is empty
    the one that is cold
    the one that is long
    the one that is full

In spoken English, the *that* and contact relative constructions are used, regardless of what sort of noun is modified by a given relative clause. The same usage is found in written English.

Another factor affecting the use of the wh, th or contact relatives is the relationship between the relative clause and the noun it modifies. Consider (43).

43 a We found the house that Fiona is selling.
    b It took us about ten minutes to find the house, which Fiona is selling (by the way).

In (43a), the relative clause *that Fiona is selling* is an integral part of the description of the house and helps the listener or reader to pick out the correct house. In (43b), the relative clause *which Fiona is selling (by the way)* merely adds some information. Sentence (43a) contains what is called a **restrictive** (or **defining**) **relative clause**: it restricts or defines the set of houses to be identified by the listener. Sentence (43b) contains a **non-restrictive** or **non-defining relative clause**. In writing it is separated by a comma from the noun it modifies and in speech it may be separated from the noun by a short pause.

The practice among users of British English has been to use *wh* pronouns with either restrictive or non-restrictive relatives but to use *that* only with restrictive relatives. The practice recommended by style guides for American English is for *wh* pronouns to be used with non-restrictive relatives and *that* with restrictive relatives. The latter practice seems to be gaining ground in Britain.

The final comment to be made on relative clauses has to do with their use in subject and object noun phrases. Two of the criteria listed in TROG-2 are 'Relative clause in subject' and 'Relative clause in object'. Examples analogous to those in TROG-2 are in (44) and of the latter in (45). The whole noun phrases are underlined and the relative clauses are in bold brackets. Note that all the relative clauses are restrictive and all have *that*.

44   **Relative clause in subject**
    a   The girl [that is reading] is sitting at the table.
    b   The car [that is all rusty] is outside our house.
    c   The boy [that is swimming] waves to his friend.
    d   The flower [that is white] is in the vase.

45   **Relative clause in object**
    a   The girl helps the toddler [that is walking].
    b   The farmer shouts at the sheep [that are grazing].
    c   The plates are in the cupboard [that is grey].
    d   The laptop is on the desk [that is tidy].

A number of analysts working with corpus data of different sorts have demonstrated clearly that in informal spoken English, subject noun phrases are kept simple. The typical subject noun phrase consists of a single noun, such as *dogs*, *Fiona* or *she*, or a determiner + noun, as in *a snake*, *the children*, *those books*, *two cars*. In spoken English, subject noun phrases are typically first in clauses. More complex noun phrases, such as those in (44) and (45) are used in object, complement or adverbial noun phrases, which come towards the end of clauses.

Exercise 9.3

In the following sentences say whether the relative clauses (underlined) are wh, th or contact relative clauses and whether they are restrictive or non-restrictive.

1. I really like the coat you bought the other day.
2. Did you recognise the girl who waved to us?
3. This is the house that Jack built.
4. Show me the book you found this example in.
5. The computer on which I keep the exam questions is password-protected.
6. This computer, which our son persuaded us to buy, is not all that good.
7. We received 67 applications, many of which were not relevant.

9.7 Sentences

Why put the section on sentences at the end of the two chapters on finite clauses? Usually introductions to syntax begin with some definition of sentence, and you come across the term 'sentence' much more often than the term 'clause'. Moreover, the concept of 'sentence' plays a large part in schooling. Early in their school careers, pupils start learning to write in sentences and to read written texts aloud with pauses at the end of sentences. Written texts are set out in sentences (though many sentences to be found in novels and newspapers do not match the 'ideal' sentences taught in the school classroom) and speakers who produce disjointed language are said to be unable to talk in sentences.

In spite of these facts, the sentence is not the best large unit for analysing syntax. Constructions go with clauses, phrases are held together in clauses and the controlling role of main verbs typically stretches over one clause. Analysts of spontaneous spoken language have found it impossible to work out criteria for recognising a chunk of syntax as a sentence; in contrast, clauses can be recognised by the presence of a main verb and the phrases that modify it. Certainly, sentences are recognisable in written texts, but only because writers, or at least competent writers, mark the beginning of sentences with capital letters and the end of sentences with full stops. In speech, there are no sounds corresponding to capital letters and full stops. (If you google 'Victor Borge', you will find a link to a comedy routine called 'Phonetic Punctuation'.) Readers might be surprised to learn that in many spoken texts, especially in spontaneous spoken language, intonation and pauses give no reliable or consistent clues as to where one sentence might end and another begin. Many scholars specialising in the analysis of spoken language simply talk about clause combinations; we will follow their example.

Even the written sentence has proved very hard to define. There are many definitions, none of which is accepted by all linguists working on English, not to mention linguists working on other languages. The view taken here is that sentences are best thought of as units of discourse (see chapters on narrative), created by speakers or writers either presenting a single clause as a piece of text to be processed as a unit or combining two or more clauses and presenting the combination to be processed as a unit. (These remarks on sentences have a bearing on clinical practice. It would be unhelpful to worry about patients who are perceived as not speaking in sentences. But patients who cannot produce clauses do not have a normal degree of competence.)

A speaker or writer may choose to present a single clause as a sentence; such sentences are known as simple sentences. (The term **'simplex sentence'** has also come into use; it appears to have been coined by analogy with 'complex sentence', defined in the next paragraph). For the idealist, the single clause is a main clause containing a finite verb. In practice, many writers, including the great nineteenth-century novelists such as Dickens, produce, for good stylistic reasons, text sentences that do not contain a finite verb or even a verb. The text sentences in (46) and (47) are from a detective novel (Mark Billingham 2005, *Lifeless*. Sphere, p. 80). The underlined text sentences in (46) are adjective phrases and those in (47) are noun phrases.

46   . . . you could catch the whiff of desperation almost everywhere.
Pungent and unmistakeable. Classless and clinging, and far stronger than anything being rubbed on to wrists, or rolled across armpits, or sprayed over shoppers by those grotesquely made-up hags in Harrods and Selfridges.

47   Where he was walking, the desperation was of the common or garden variety. A need for warmth, food or a fix. A need for comfort.

A writer may choose to combine two main clauses with a conjunction such as *and*, *or* and *but*; thus, the clauses *It will rain today* and *tomorrow will be sunny* can be linked by *but* and presented as the single sentence *It will rain today but tomorrow will be sunny*. Such sentences are said to be **compound**. A writer may choose to combine a main clause with one or more subordinate clauses. For instance, the main clause *She took the dog for a walk* can be combined with the clause *the rain stopped* to yield *When the rain stopped she took the dog for a walk*. The main clause *it surprised us all* can be combined with the subordinate clause *she married Angus* to yield *It surprised us all that she married Angus*. Such sentences are said to be **complex**. (Our fictitious writers could have written *The rain stopped. She took the dog for a walk* with two sentences, and *She married Angus. It surprised us all*, also with two sentences.)

Exercise 9.4

For each of the following sentences, decide whether it is simple, complex or compound.

1. Margaret drives and Jim navigates.
2. It'll be chilly, so don't forget to bring warm clothes.
3. Peter remembered that he had not walked the dog.
4. After he was elected, new facts came to light.
5. Can you send me a copy of the document you received?
6. Rain is forecast for tomorrow but apparently it is to be sunny for the rest of the week.
7. The house is easy to run, plus it has excellent insulation and eco- friendly heating.
8. Angus has to sit the exam whether he wants to or not.
9. I'll give you five pounds to cut the grass.
10. Remind me who was at the meeting.

Chapter summary

Section 9.3 deals with subordinate clauses, which are special constructions. Main clauses can stand on their own as the beginning of a narrative but subordinate clauses cannot. Main clauses allow a wide range of constructions but subordinate clauses allow a narrower range.

MAIN TYPES OF SUBORDINATE CLAUSE		
Section 9.4.1	Relative	Modifies a noun
	The book that you wrote sent me to sleep.	
	That you wrote modifies *book.*	
Section 9.4.2	Adverbial	Modifies a whole clause
	When he arrived, he got a surprise.	
	When he arrived modifies *he got a surprise.*	
Section 9.4.3	Complement	May modify a verb
	Freya declared that the example was rubbish.	
	That the example was rubbish modifies *declared.*	
		May modify a noun
	They rejected the proposal that the traffic flow be changed.	
	That the traffic flow be changed modifies *proposal.*	

Section 9.5 deals with clauses that modify nouns: complement clauses and relative clauses. Nouns modified by complement clauses include *plan, proposal, theory, hypothesis, belief* and so on and the complement clause specifies the content of the plan, theory or belief. Such complement clauses cannot be introduced by a wh word: **They rejected the proposal which the traffic flow be changed.*

Section 9.6 deals in more detail with relative clauses. There are three types in English.

wh relative clause	the flat *which they rent*
th relative clause	the flat *that they rent*
contact relative clause	the flat *they rent*

A major distinction is between restrictive and non-restrictive relative clauses. Restrictive relative clauses help the listener or reader to identify what is referred to, as in *the car you were driving*. Non-restrictive relative clauses merely provide incidental information, as in *The new houses, which cost a bomb, are an eyesore*.

Section 9.7 gives an account of sentences. A sentence is a low-level discourse unit. Various types of sentence are recognised.

Simple/simplex sentence	just one main clause
Compound sentence	two or more main clauses
Complex sentence	one main clause and one or more subordinate clauses

Exercises using clinical resources

9.5. According to the CELF-Preschool, item 7 of the Sentence Structure subtest targets subordinate clauses. Give a more explicit label for the type of subordinate clause in this item.

9.6. Which items in the Sentence Structure subtest of the CELF-4 assess subordinate clauses? Using the terminology introduced in this chapter, give more precise labels to the examples.

9.7. In the Narrative Syntax section of the ACE, one item is labelled 'subordinate clause'. Give it a more precise label based on the information in this chapter.

9.8. In the Recalling Sentences section of the CELF-4, identify items that target the following structures:
   a. relative clause
   b. adverbial clause of condition
   c. adverbial clause of reason
   d. adverbial clause of concession
   e. adverbial clause of time

Further reading

Search for the individual technical terms in Hurford (1994).

'Chapter 6: Clauses 1 (clauses and sentences, main and subordinate clauses, different types of subordinate clause)' and 'Chapter 7: Clauses 2 (subordinate clauses)' in Miller (2008).

'Chapter 7: Subordination and coordination' in Collins and Hollo (2000).

10 Sentence Structure 4: Non-finite Clauses

Clinical resources that will be referenced in this chapter:

Boston Diagnostic Aphasia Examination
CELF-4 – Clinical Evaluation of Language Fundamentals
LIST – Listening Skills Test
PALPA – Psycholinguistic Assessment of Language Processing in Aphasia
TROG-2 – Test for the Reception of Grammar

10.0 Introduction

The clauses examined in Chapter 8 and 9 are all finite clauses; that is, clauses consisting of words and phrases held together by a main verb that is finite. For the moment, we will simply say that a finite verb is one that has tense (and person): *wrote* and *writes* are finite forms of the verb *write* while *writing* and *to write* are non-finite forms. There are several types of clause built around **non-finite verbs**; some examples are underlined in (1).

1 a The boys wanted <u>to play football</u>.
   b She likes <u>playing chess</u>.
   c Ken likes to read <u>sitting in his armchair</u>.
   d We had to throw out the books <u>chewed by the dog</u>.

Some types of **non-finite clause** are very common in both speech and writing but others are typical of writing and occur frequently in narrative. (Written narrative can be, and often is, read aloud, but that does not make such clauses typical of speech.) Non-finite clauses enable speakers and writers, but especially writers, to condense their syntax so that a small chunk of syntax carries a lot of information.

Introductory Linguistics for Speech and Language Therapy Practice, First Edition. Jan McAllister and Jim Miller.
© 2013 John Wiley & Sons, Ltd. Published 2013 by John Wiley & Sons, Ltd.

10.1 Why do SLTs need this knowledge?

In Section 8.1, we stated the general point about the central, indispensable role of syntax in communication by means of language. It does not need to be restated here. But we need to supplement the general point with a particular point about non-finite clauses: they look like very simple pieces of sentence structure, but interpreting some of the constructions is far from simple and causes difficulties for children whose language skills are developing slowly. Clinical assessment materials focus on examples such as those in (2) and (3).

2 a My sister was thinking what to do about the mark on the carpet.
  b We suggested (to her) what to do about the mark on the carpet.

3 a She was anxious to clean the carpet.
  b She was easy to spot in her yellow track suit.

The crucial points for anyone interpreting (2), especially as part of a narrative, are who was going to do something about the mark, *My sister* in both cases, but *my sister* is the subject of *was thinking* but not of *suggested*. In (3a), *she* is the one who will do the cleaning, but in (3b), *she* is the one who will be spotted, not the one who is going to do the spotting.

10.2 Learning outcomes

When you have read the chapter and done the exercises, you should be able to:

- Recognise different types of non-finite clause;
- Explain why we talk of non-finite clauses and not just of phrases;
- Understand the difficulty some of your clients will have in interpreting non-finite clauses;
- Use non-finite clauses in summarising texts.

10.3 Infinitives and (Type 1) gerunds

We need to begin with a brief look at the concept of a finite verb. The traditional definition is 'one that is marked for tense and person, and also for number'. It applies very neatly to languages such as Latin, Russian, Italian and Turkish but does not apply all that straightforwardly to English. The best examples are forms of the verb BE: *am*, *is*, *was* and *were*. *Am* (present tense, first person, singular number, combining with *I*) contrasts with *is* (third person), *are* (plural number, combining with *we* and *they*), *was* (past tense) and *were* (past tense and plural number). *Was* contrasts with *were* (singular vs. plural), and so on.

Verb forms such as *runs* and *stands* are present tense, third person and singular number; they combine with *he*, *she* and *it*. *Run* and *stand* in combination with *they*, *we*, *you* are simply present tense and not third person. *Ran*, *stood*, *struggled* and so on are past tense but any person and any number. ('Finite' comes from the Latin term 'finitus' 'having a boundary or limit'. *Run*, without the ending *-s* and not part of any construction, denotes a kind of movement. The form *runs* brings limits to that movement: it denotes a movement in present time and carried out by a single person who is not the speaker 'I' or the hearer 'you'.)

One last point before embarking on non-finite clauses: remember that, as we noted in Chapter 7, the definition of 'clause' applies to structures containing a verbal element, but that the verbal element may consist of either a main verb alone, or a main verb supported by one or more auxiliaries. It applies to examples such as *The dog chewed its bone* but it has to apply also to examples such as *The dog was chewing its bone*. This contains two verbs, *was* and *chewing*. We will say that a clause is a collection of words and phrases held together by a main verb that is finite (*chewed*), or by a finite auxiliary verb and a main verb (*was chewing*).

What are non-finite clauses? The examples in (1) illustrate the most basic types of non-finite clause: infinitives and gerunds. Infinitives are preceded by *to*, as in (1a). Gerunds end in *-ing*, but while this distinguishes them from infinitives it does not distinguish them from other non-finite forms in *-ing*, as we will see later. What turns out to be crucial is what the non-finite clauses modify.

4   a   The boys decided <u>to visit their grandparents</u>. [**infinitive**]
   b   The dog loves <u>chasing pheasants</u>. [**gerund**]

In traditional grammar, chunks like the underlined ones in (4) were treated as phrases; <u>to visit their grandparents</u> was called an infinitive phrase and <u>chasing pheasants</u> was called a gerund phrase. This treatment ignored the fact that such 'phrases' are like finite clauses in many respects. They allow objects – *their grand-parents* and *pheasants* in (4); complements – *They want <u>to paint their room yellow</u>, I want <u>to be a lawyer</u>*; adverbials – *They enjoy <u>sitting in the garden</u>* answering the question *Where did she enjoy sitting?* and *She wanted <u>to visit Australia in July</u>* answering the question *When did she want to visit Australia?*

Infinitives allow the Progressive and the Perfect, as in (5). Note the two adverbials in (5a), *in Nice* and *right now*, and the adverbial in (5b), *by Easter*.

5   a   I'd like <u>to be working in Nice right now</u>.
   b   Our goal is <u>to have completed the hotel by Easter</u>.

Infinitives differ from finite clauses in that they do not allow tense: *to work* is tenseless compared with *works*, *worked* and *will work*. Neither do they allow modal verbs forms such as *to can* or *to must* do not exist.

Like infinitives, gerunds allow objects, complements and adverbials, as in (6).

6   a   Rene enjoys <u>chopping logs</u>.
   b   James hates <u>being unemployed</u>.
   c   We prefer <u>going to France</u>.

Unlike infinitives, gerunds do not allow the Perfect or Progressive, and they also do not allow modal verbs; there are no forms **musting*, **maying* and so on.

What about subjects? There is a type of gerund that occurs in formal writing but not in informal speech. An example is (7).

7   We enjoyed John's spending the whole summer with us.

The word *John's* is a possessive – of which more below – but it can be regarded as the equivalent of an agent. (Although it is found in formal writing, this type of gerund is unfamiliar to many speakers of English. Recently, the second author had to persuade a class of mature postgraduates that he was not just making up the construction to baffle them.)

There is a special infinitive construction with what looks like the equivalent of a subject noun, with *for to* as in (8).

8   For Jennifer to miss a game is unheard of.

The parallel between infinitives and gerunds on the one hand and finite clauses on the other has long been recognised in the traditional concept of the 'understood subject'. Consider sentences (9a–c).

9   a   John wants to breed alpacas.
     b   John wants Juliet to feed the alpacas.
     c   Jennifer loves grooming the alpacas.

10.3.1   Understood subject and control

The infinitive in (9a) is traditionally interpreted as having an **understood subject**. That is, it is interpreted as denoting a situation in which there is an action of breeding and patients that undergo the action. The patients are denoted by the object *alpacas*. There is a missing subject that would denote the agent. It is as though the structure of the infinitive is [ ] *to breed alpacas* and it is up to the listener or reader to find a suitable subject to put inside the square brackets. In (9a), the subject to be inserted is *John*, the subject of *wants*. In (9b), the suitable subject is *Juliet*, the object of *wants*. And in (9c), the suitable subject is *Jennifer*, the subject of *loves*. *John* is the understood subject of *to breed*, *Juliet* is the understood subject of *to feed* and *Jennifer* is the understood subject of *grooming*. The nouns *John*, *Juliet* and *Jennifer* are said to control the understood subject.

The concept of understood subject is relevant to examples that turn up in SLT clinical test materials. Consider the following examples similar to those in the auditory PALPA Sentence–Picture Matching test, with the infinitives underlined.

10   a   The tourist is wondering who to ask.
      b   The woman is considering where to fly to on holiday.

11   a   The salesman is demonstrating what to buy.
      b   The waiter is suggesting what to eat.

In (10a), *who* is the object of the verb *ask*. In (10b), *where* is an adverbial. What listeners have to do is work out the understood subject, *the woman*. In (10a), the understood subject is *the tourist*, in (10b), it is *the woman*. That is, the understood subject is the same as the subject of the main verb *'s wondering* or *'s considering*. In

(11a,b) the understood subject is NOT the same as the subject of the main verb. It is not the salesman who is going to do something but whoever he is demonstrating to; it is not the waiter who is going to eat but whoever he is making the suggestions to. The understood subjects can be identified from the pictures in the test form.

The standard analysis of (10) and (11) shows this **subject gap** thus: *[ ] to ask who*, *[ ] to fly where*, *[ ] to buy what* and *[ ] to eat*. That is, they all have gaps where there should be a subject. The PALPA materials label (10a,b) 'GS' for 'Gap as subject', and (11a,b) 'GO' for 'Gap as non-subject'. The PALPA labels presumably reflect the fact that the understood subject in (10a,b) is controlled by the subject of the main verb, whereas the understood subject in (11a,b) is controlled by the object or complement of the main verb, or indeed by an adverbial, since you demonstrate *to someone*. The word 'gap' is very misleading in a syntactic context: 'subject control' and 'non-subject control' would be more accurate labels.

Other examples from the PALPA materials demonstrate how important it is to apply the term 'gap' consistently. Consider (12).

12   a   My sister is eager to see (the rugby match).
     b   The tiger is difficult to see. (in the jungle)

In (12a), the understood subject of *to see* is *my sister*. A representation showing that it is the subject that is missing and that *my sister* controls it is in (13). The non-finite clause is enclosed in large square brackets.

13   My sister₁ is keen [[ ]₁ to see].

The subscript '1' indicates that the items to go in the square brackets are *my sister*. In (12b), *the tiger* is the object of *see* and the understood subject of *to see* is not controlled by anything. It could be the speaker who finds it difficult or a group of tourists on safari, say, being addressed by the speaker. We can capture the lack of control in our representation of the syntax of these examples. We will use 'pro' (for 'pronoun') to represent this uncontrolled subject and a subscript '1' as in (13) to show that the understood object of *see* is *the tiger*. Sentence (14) contains a sample representation.

14   The tiger₁ is difficult [pro to see [ ]₁].

Other examples similar to the PALPA materials that can be handled in the same way are *The snake is ready to strike* (analogous to (12a)) and *The snake is easy to kill* (analogous to (12b)).

10.4   Type 2 gerunds

Two other types of non-finite clause appear in SLT materials. The first is from the CELF-4, illustrated by the examples in (15), analogous to examples in tests of paragraph understanding.

15   a   They could still see the lava <u>flowing down the mountainside</u>.
     b   Instead, they heard a car <u>tooting at the front gate</u>.
     c   [He] saw yellowish smoke <u>pouring from the chimney</u>.

Let us briefly return to infinitives and gerunds. Infinitive chunks contain *to* or *for to*; gerunds have *-ing* added to a verb: *I like <u>swimming</u>*. Infinitives and gerunds function as subjects, objects or complements.

16   Subject
   a   <u>To catch moles</u> is very difficult.
       (cf. <u>Japanese</u> is very difficult.)
   b   <u>Catching moles</u> is very difficult.

17   Object
   a   Fiona loves <u>to go cycling</u>.
       (cf. Fiona loves <u>dogs</u>.)
   b   Freya loves <u>weeding the garden</u>.
       Freya loves <u>ice-cream</u>.

18   Complement
   a   His technique is <u>to use a heavy hammer</u>.
       (cf. His technique is <u>very advanced</u>.)
   b   The secret is <u>using enough sugar</u>.
       (cf. The secret is <u>widely known</u>.)

Instead of calling *catching moles* and *weeding the garden* simply gerunds, we will call them Type 1 gerunds in order to distinguish them from the underlined chunks in (15), which we call Type 2 gerunds. Type 1 gerunds and Type 2 gerunds differ in two respects: Type 1 gerunds function as subjects, as in (16b), or objects, as in (17b). Type 2 gerunds do not function as subjects or objects. They are found in examples such as (15b) in which there is a verb, here *heard*, followed by a direct object, here *a car*, followed by the Type 2 gerund, here *tooting at the front gate*. The verb is often a verb of perception such as *hear*, *see* as in (15) and *feel* or *notice* as in (19), but also verbs such as *catch* or *draw*, as in (20).

Type 1 gerunds, functioning as subjects, objects or complements, modify verbs. Type 2 gerunds modify nouns; the above examples tell us more about the rain, the birds, the tail, the spider, the cyclist, the dog and the horse.

19   a   Catriona felt the spider <u>moving over her hand</u>.
     b   We noticed the cyclist <u>going through the red light</u>.

20   a   Sabrina caught the dog <u>eating the cake</u>.
     b   Katarina drew the horse <u>jumping over the hedge</u>.

Type 1 gerunds also occur inside prepositional phrases. In (21), the prepositions are in bold and the gerunds are underlined.

21   a   **On** <u>hearing the news</u>, everyone cheered.
     b   **Before** <u>leaving the room</u>, make sure the lights are switched off.
     c   **After** <u>watching the appeal on TV</u>, Barnabas decided to make a large donation.
     d   **By** <u>adopting this policy</u>, the government damaged the economy.

10.5   Bare-verb clauses

Another simple type of non-finite clause consists of just a verb stem, possibly accompanied by an object, complement or adverbial. The verb is said to be bare, and the clause can be called a **bare-verb (non-finite) clause**. The clause in (22a) only contains a verb stem but the clause in (22b) contains a verb stem, an object – *their cases* and an adverbial – *into the house*.

22   a   Katarina watched the building <u>collapse</u>.
    b   Sabrina helped them <u>carry their cases into the house</u>.
    c   Freya made James <u>do his homework</u>.

The bare-verb non-finite clause is a central component of another construction, to be discussed in Chapter 15 on narrative. The construction is known as the WH cleft and it has important functions in narrative. Here we merely give the example in (23), with the bare-verb clause underlined.

23   What they do is <u>dismantle the ships</u>.

10.6   Free participle clauses

A fourth type of non-finite clause occurs in SLT materials. Sentence (24) is analogous to an example in tests of paragraph understanding in the CELF-4.

24   The little red squirrel hopped through the grass, sniffing the air.

Here is yet another word ending in *-ing*, *sniffing*. The traditional name for it is '**free participle**', and we will call the whole chunk a **free participle clause**. Ending in *-ing*, it looks like a Type 2 gerund but there are two crucial differences. Type 2 gerunds, as in (20a), come after a verb and a direct object: *(Sabrina) caught + the dog + eating the cake*. The chunks that we call 'free participles' occur at the end of a sentence, as in (24), or at the beginning, as in (25), or in the middle, as in (26).

25   <u>Sniffing the air</u>, the little red squirrel hopped through the grass.

26   The little red squirrel, <u>sniffing the air</u>, hopped through the grass.

In addition, we saw that Type 2 gerunds modify nouns. In contrast, free participles modify whole clauses. In (24)–(26), *sniffing the air* modifies *the little red squirrel hopped through the grass*. In this respect, free participles are very like finite adverbial clauses, and sometimes free participles can be paraphrased by means of adverbial clauses, as in (27) and (28).

27   a   <u>Knowing the area well</u>, Kirsty was able to take a shortcut.
    b   <u>As/because she knew the area well</u>, Kirsty was able to take a shortcut.

28   a   <u>Going down the stairs</u>, Jean smelled gas.
    b   <u>As/when she was going down the stairs</u>, Jean smelled gas.

One very important point must be made here. We have just said that free participles can be paraphrased by adverbial clauses. This does not mean that you get a free participle clause by taking an adverbial clause and cutting it down to size. You could cut down (28b) to get (28a) by deleting *As she was*, but (27b) cannot be cut down in the same way to get (27a). This process is blocked by the fact that *know* does not occur in the progressive: **Kirsty was knowing the area well* is not a correct sentence of English and there is no adverbial clause **Because she was knowing the area well*. *Know* is not alone, as demonstrated by (29) and (30).

29 a   Believing that Torquil had already left, Jean drove home.
    b   *As she was believing that Torquil had already left, Jean drove home.

30 a   Seeing that the track petered out, we turned back.
    b   *Since we were seeing that the track petered out, we turned back.

10.7   Reduced clauses

There are two final types of non-finite clause to be mentioned. One, known as a reduced relative clause, turns up in SLT materials such as the TROG-2. The other one, known as a reduced adverbial clause, does not but is very common in written narrative. The reduced relative clauses in (31) are analogous to examples in the TROG-2. The reduced relative clauses are the underlined chunks.

31 a   The men <u>pushing the car out of the snow</u> are strong.
    b   The hounds <u>chasing the fox</u> are too slow.

The reduced relative clauses, *pushing the car out of the snow* and *chasing the fox*, contain the present participles *pushing* and *chasing*. They convert straightforwardly into the relative clauses in (32) and (33) with the addition of a wh word or *that* (see Section 9.6) and some form of *be*.

32 a   The men <u>who are pushing the car out of the snow</u> are strong.
    b   The men <u>that are pushing the car out of the snow</u> are strong.

33 a   The hounds <u>which are chasing the fox</u> are too slow.
    b   The hounds <u>that are chasing the fox</u> are too slow.

Chunks containing passive participles, such as those underlined in (34), also convert into relative clauses.

34 a   The car <u>driven by Fiona</u> went off the road.
    b   We all admire the dogs <u>trained by Kirsty</u>.

The passive participles are *driven* and *trained*. *Driven by Fiona* expands into the full relative clauses in (35) and *trained by Kirsty* expands into the full relative clauses in (36).

35 a   The car <u>that was driven by Fiona</u> went off the road.
    b   The car <u>that was being driven by Fiona</u> went off the road.
    c   The car <u>which was driven by Fiona</u> went off the road.
    d   The car <u>which was being driven by Fiona</u> went off the road.

36 a   We all admire the dogs <u>that have been trained by Kirsty</u>.
    b   We all admire the dogs <u>that are trained by Kirsty</u>.
    c   We all admire the dogs <u>which have been trained by Kirsty</u>.
    d   We all admire the dogs <u>which are trained by Kirsty</u>.

Reduced adverbial clauses are chunks introduced by subordinating conjunctions but containing either a finite verb or no verb at all. Examples of clauses with no verbs are in (37) while (38) and (39) have examples containing non-finite verbs. The ones in (38) are present participles, while those in (39) are passive participles.

37 a If in doubt, consult your doctor.
   b When in Rome, do as the Romans do.
   c Although not the sharpest tool in the toolbox, he never misses a day's work.

38 a While waiting for his appointment, he read all the notices.
   b When giving lectures, Harold always wears a suit.

39 a Although impressed by the car, Jane didn't buy it.
   b When delayed in traffic, Roger checks his e-mails.

The reduced adverbial clauses expand into full adverbial clauses with the addition of a subject noun and some form of *be*, as in (40), (41) and (42).

40 a If you are in doubt, consult your doctor.
   b When you are in Rome, do as the Romans do.

41 a While he was waiting for his appointment, he read all the notices.
   b When he is giving lectures, Harold always wears a suit.

42 a Although she was impressed by the car, Jane didn't buy it.
   b When he is delayed in traffic, Roger checks his e-mails.

A full adverbial clause as in (40)–(42) is reduced to a non-finite clause by the deletion of the subject and whatever form of *be* it contains. This means that reduced adverbial clauses consist of a subordinating conjunction followed by a phrase which can be one of a number of different types, as shown by (43).

43 a Although Head of Department, he relies on the Departmental Secretary. [Noun Phrase]
   b Although seriously ill, he came to the meeting. [Adjective Phrase]
   c Although on holiday, Susan responded to the request for help. [Prepositional Phrase]
   d Although waiting in a long queue, Catriona stayed calm. [Participial Phrase]

Non-finite clauses are important constructions. Infinitives and gerunds, Type 1 and Type 2, and bare-verb clauses occur frequently in spoken and written English. Free participle clauses and reduced relative and adverbial clauses are typical of written English and play a central role in the construction of narrative texts.

Exercise 10.1

Identify the types of underlined non-finite clauses in the examples below.

1. Sailing in shark-infested waters is not my idea of fun.
2. Freya was reluctant to lend her laptop to James.

   3. Look at the monkey <u>sitting up in the tree, watching us</u>. [2 clauses]
   4. You'll find the information in the book <u>lying on my desk</u>.
   5. <u>Although not very tall</u>, he's quite powerful.
   6. You have to be very careful <u>when using electric carving knives</u>.
   7. You can't learn about birds without <u>spending hours sitting quietly and watching</u>.
   8. You can't learn about birds without spending hours <u>sitting quietly and watching</u>.
   9. <u>Seeing that the youngster was in difficulty</u>, the lifeguard dived into the pool.
  10. Nowadays he spends a lot of time in his library, <u>working on his memoirs</u>.
  11. It was an education <u>watching the team outplay their opponents</u>.
  12. They would just hate <u>for us to win the competition</u>.

Exercise 10.2

Pick out and identify the non-finite clauses in the following piece of narrative from a label on a bottle of wine.

Made in the classic Médocaine style, it was aged in French oak barriques to marry the blend and imbue the wine with subtle oak flavours... Though drinking well now, it will reward cellaring for a year or two and should be decanted before drinking.

Exercise 10.3

Pick out and identify the non-finite clauses in the following real piece of narrative.

I give every student a balloon, and ask them to blow it up and then slowly let out the air such that the balloon emits a rather annoying squeaky noise. They seem to have to do this at least once or twice to get over the apparent humour involved in the chorus of a classroom of 40 students emptying balloons simultaneously.

Jennifer Hay (2007) A toolbox for teaching phonetics. *Te Reo* 50, 7–16.

Exercise 10.4

Here again is a longer paragraph of real narrative, from Terry Pratchett's novel *Snuff* (London: Doubleday, 2011, pp. 106–107). This time, identify and label all the non-finite clauses.

And he woke again to hear the sound of heavy cartwheels rumbling over stones. Half-asleep as Vimes was, suspicion woke him the rest of the way. Stones? It was all bloody gravel around the Hall. He opened a window and stared out into the moonlight. It was an echo bouncing off the hills. A few brain cells doing the night shift wondered what kind of agriculture had to be done at night. Did they grow mushrooms? Did turnips have to be brought in from the cold? Was that what they called crop rotation? These thoughts melted into his somnolent brain like little grains of sugar in a cup of tea, slithering and dripping from cell to synapse to neuro-transmitter until they arrived in the receptor marked 'suspicion', which if you saw a medical diagram of a policeman's brain would probably be quite a visible lump, slightly larger than the lump marked 'ability to understand long words'. He thought, Ah yes, contraband! And, feeling cheerful, and hopeful for the future, he gently closed the window and went back to bed.

Chapter summary

Finite and non-finite verbs.

Finite verb: one marked for tense (and, for some verb forms, for person). A non-finite verb is not marked for tense or person.

A clause: a collection of words and phrases held together by a finite main verb or by a finite auxiliary verb and a main verb (*was chewing*).

Reasons for recognising non-finite clauses: they contain phrases that can function as object, complement or adverbial, just as in finite clauses. Understood subjects can be identified.

Role of non-finite clauses in narrative text.

Different types of non-finite clauses:

Infinitive

The boys decided <u>to visit their grandparents</u>.

<u>For Jennifer to miss a game</u> is unheard of.

Type 1 gerund

The dog loves <u>chasing pheasants</u>. (These can function as subject, object or complement.)

Bare-verb clause

Freya made James <u>do his homework</u>.

Type 2 gerund

Sabrina caught the dog eating the cake. (Does not function as subject, object or complement. Occurs in the construction V O Type 2 gerund, where V is typically, but not necessarily, a verb of perception.)

Free participle clause

The big, black bear walked slowly through the burned-out forest, sniffing the ground. (Functions like an adverbial clause to modify the whole clause it is attached to.)

Reduced relative clause

The elephant pushing the boy is big.

The car driven by Fiona went off the road.

Reduced adverbial clause

If in doubt, consult your doctor.

While waiting for his appointment, he read all the notices.

Although impressed by the car, Jane didn't buy it.

Exercises using clinical resources

10.5. Page 5 of the LIST shows 20 test items. Which ones contain a reduced relative clause?

10.6. Look at Section D3 of the Boston Diagnostic Aphasia Examination Auditory Comprehension block. Which items contain a reduced relative clause?

10.7. Examine the Test Paragraphs in the Understanding Spoken Paragraphs section of the CELF-4. Identify instances of the following:
a. Infinitive
b. Gerund
c. Free participle

10.8. Look at the short stories in the Boston Diagnostic Aphasia Examination record booklet, pages 14–15 (Complex Ideational Material) and identify instances of the following:
a. Infinitive
b. Free participle
c. Reduced relative

Further reading

Search for individual technical terms in Hurford (1994).

'Chapter 8: Clauses III (non-finite clauses)' in Miller (2008).

11 Language in Use 1: Deixis and Reference

Clinical resources that will be referenced in this chapter:

ACE – Assessment of Comprehension and Reception 6–11
Boston Diagnostic Aphasia Examination
CAPPA – Conversation Analysis Profile for People with Aphasia
CCC-2 – Children's Communication Checklist
CELF-4, CELF-Preschool – Clinical Evaluation of Language Fundamentals
ERRNI – Expression, Reception and Recall of Narrative Instrument
The Squirrel Story
The Renfrew Bus Story
Western Aphasia Battery

11.0 Introduction

In the previous chapters, we have been looking at the meaning of lexical items; at how words are constructed (morphology); at how phrases, clauses and sentences are constructed (syntax, or sentence structure); and at the different types of clause. That is, we have been looking at the code used by speakers and writers of English. In this chapter, we begin to think about speakers and writers of English using the code in particular situations. We are not abandoning the code, since we will be discussing the system of **deictic** items such as *this* and *that*, *here* and *there*, *now* and *then*. In order to discuss reference, we have to consider not only deictic items but **definite noun phrases** and **indefinite noun phrases**.

11.1 Why do SLTs need this knowledge?

Language users would be unable to communicate successfully if they were unable to identify what speakers are talking about in a given situation or to follow who is doing what in a narrative. The CELF-Preschool assessment involves asking children to point in sequence at animals in pictures. To do this, children have to understand the deictic word *then* in instructions such as 'Point at X and then at Y' and they have to understand the difference between *a pangolin* and *the pangolin* and between *the pangolin in the middle* and *the pangolin at the end*. The set of tests in the CELF-4 includes one that allows SLTs to assess children's ability to understand spoken paragraphs. And the ERRNI assessment manual has one test in which children have to compose a narrative relating the events shown in a series of pictures. For children to perform successfully in these tests and for SLTs to analyse what might have gone wrong, concepts such as deixis and reference are essential.

11.2   Learning objectives

After reading the chapter and doing the exercises, you should be able to:

* understand the central concepts of deixis;
* understand the extended uses of deictic items;
* recognise deictic items in narrative;
* explain the use of a particular deictic item in narrative;
* understand the central concept of reference;
* explain the use of definite and indefinite noun phrases in narrative;
* be ready to start applying the concepts in your clinical work.

11.3   Reference and deixis

One of the most frequent acts performed by speakers is **reference**, which is the act of drawing a listener's attention to something. In order to do this successfully, speakers must assess, in a particular situation, how easily listeners will identify the referent. If the referent is judged to be easily identifiable, it is said to be **given**. The referent may have been mentioned before in which case it is enough to use a simple noun phrase such as *the ball* or *your crayon*. If it has not been mentioned before, the speaker may have to supply a more detailed description, such as *the ball you were throwing for the dog* or *the crayon that James was chewing*. If the referent stands out in what is called the **context of utterance** or **situation of utterance**, that is, if it is salient in the immediate surroundings of the speaker and the hearer, a pronoun such as *it* or *that* will suffice. If the referent is something that is judged to be central to the culture and world-knowledge shared by the speaker and the hearer, it may be possible to use a pronoun such as *she* or *I*, a simple noun phrase such as *the boss*, or a proper name such as *Dot* or *Barry*.

If the referent is judged not to be easily identifiable, it is said to be **new**. Thus, if the referent has not been mentioned before, or is not salient in the context of utterance, or is judged unlikely to belong to the culture and world-knowledge of the listener, pronouns will not do. A particular referent may require a long noun phrase such as *The guy I was meeting in Leeds the other day*, or may even need to be specifically introduced into the conversation and established as a topic of discussion: e.g. *You remember I was meeting a guy in Leeds the other day? It turns out he would like to visit our research group.*

11.3.1   Deixis: introduction

Many acts of reference are much simpler to perform, because typically the speaker and the listener(s) are in the same place and face to face. In such situations, speakers can draw attention to something by physically pointing at it or by using linguistic pointing words such as *that* or *this*, or by doing both. Pointing words provide no description of a thing but they are extremely frequent in speech because in conversation and in spoken narrative much can be understood with reference to only four factors:

- the speaker and the addressee;
- where they are in the location;
- where other things in the location are relative to them;
- the moment of speech (time of utterance).

Pointing words and phrases are known as **deictic words** (*Deixis* derives from the Classical Greek verb *deiknumi* 'to show, point out'. The root *deik-* is connected with *dig-* in *digit* (= finger), the body part that is used for pointing.). They fall into various deictic categories: personal pronouns, demonstratives, **spatial expressions**, **temporal phrases**, **verbs of movement** and tense. A convenient term for what is pointed at is '**deictic target**'. The demonstratives, but also the personal pronouns, have basic uses that can be analysed by means of the four factors in the above list. The deictic targets associated with these basic uses may appear obvious but, as we will see below, even a very basic use may have a shifting deictic target. As we will see in Section 11.3.8, deictics also have extended uses, especially in connection with social relationships and the organisation of narrative.

In order to analyse how deictic words are used in context, two more concepts are required: **construal** and **perspective**. Human beings do not (or should not!) just look at a landscape blankly. They **construe** or interpret it; that is, they assign a structure to it and base any linguistic description of the landscape on that structure. A farmer will construe a landscape in a different way from an office worker who has spent all her life in a big city, and the latter office worker will construe a city street scene differently from her country cousins visiting a big city for the first time.

Consider a scene in a film showing two young men turning from a sunlit street into a dark passageway. One viewer might construe the action as unremarkable; perhaps the young men are returning to their flat. Another viewer might construe the scene as sinister: who knows who is lurking in the passageway. Filmmakers guide the viewers' construal by adding music to encourage the reaction they want.

Construal involves perspective, that is, particular viewpoint. Consider two towns, say Shrewsbury and Telford. A speaker might say *This road lies between Shrewsbury and Telford*, adopting a perspective in which the two towns are locations and the road is located between them – just like the representation on a map. The speaker can adopt a different perspective, imagining themselves in Shrewsbury and saying *This road goes from Shrewsbury to Telford*. They might instead imagine themselves in Telford and say *This road comes to Telford from Shrewsbury*. Looking at a path lying on a hill between a car park and a monument, they can say *A path goes up to the monument from the car park* or *A path goes down from the monument to the car park*. The two descriptions correspond to different perspectives.

Perspectives apply to relations that are not spatial. The second author was once sitting next to a woman at a social gathering. She gave her name as (the name has been changed) Patricia Greig. The second author, knowing that a colleague of his called Angus Greig had a sister Patricia, said *Oh, are you Angus Greig's sister?* Clearly taking offence, the woman replied *No, Angus Greig is my brother*.

11.3.2   Deixis: personal pronouns

The interpretation of the personal pronouns (*I, you, he, she, it, we, they*) is governed by who is playing the role of the speaker and who is playing the role of the addressee at a given moment. Consider the following dialogue.

 1   A1:   Did you know that Freya has a job in Brussels?

 B1:   No, I didn't. How did you hear about it?

 A2:   I had an e-mail from her. They're very pleased, her parents I mean.

You in A1 refers to the addressee, B. In B1, *you* also refers to the addressee, who is A. *I* refers to speaker B, but in A2 *I* refers to speaker A. The speaker and the addressee are roles in a dialogue and the participants in a dialogue take it in turn to play each role. *I* refers to whoever is speaking and *you* refers to whoever is the addressee. The speaker is central to each act of speaking, as is recognised by the traditional term 'first person'. The addressee is slightly less central, as is recognised by the term 'second person'. Anyone or anything other than the speaker and the addressee is a third person; hence the label 'third person pronoun' for *he, she, it* and *they*. The shifting reference of personal pronouns makes them tricky for small children. Many parents realise this and address infants by their first name and refer to themselves as *Mummy* or *Daddy* or whatever label they use. An example is *Will Daddy make orange juice for James?* (spoken to James by James' father).

The interpretation of plural pronouns is different from that of plural nouns. The deictic target of *we* always includes the speaker plus one or more other people, but not necessarily the addressee. In English, the reference can be made clear by the construction in (2).

 2   a   Him and me, we're going to Glasgow on Friday.
   b   You and me, we're going to find out what's going on right now.

In (2a), the phrase *him and me* excludes the addressee, whereas in (2b) *you and me* includes the addressee. *We* in (2a) is known as the **exclusive *we***: the addressee is excluded. *We* in (2b) is the **inclusive *we***: the addressee is included. Some languages have two forms of the first person plural pronoun, an exclusive one and an inclusive one. English signals the difference via its syntax.

Personal pronouns are also used in writing, where their usage is to be explained with reference to their use in speech (This is not surprising, as spoken language evolved before written language and individuals typically acquire spoken language before they learn to read and write.). *I* in a letter or e-mail refers to the writer of the letter or e-mail and *you* refers to the person addressed by the writer (who is not necessarily the person reading the letter or e-mail). Narratives can contain layers of reference. A narrative may begin with *I* referring to the author. Suppose the author includes the text of a letter written by a character in the narrative. In that letter, *I* refers to the author of the letter, not to the author of the major narrative. Analogously, *you* refers to the person the letter is addressed to, not to a reader of the narrative.

Such layering of reference is not confined to written narratives, as shown by the piece of (fictitious) conversation in (3).

3   Well, when I heard that I thought I would have it out with him — he just said 'You just mind your own business — I'm not going to discuss anything with you'.

In (3), the first three occurrences of *I* (not underlined) refer to the speaker of (3). The underlined occurrences of *you*, inside the inverted commas, also refer to the speaker of (3), but are in a chunk that is signalled as being spoken by whoever *him* and *he* refers to and addressed to the person producing the narrative in (3). In that chunk in inverted commas, the *I* refers to the same person as *he* and *him*. This shifting of reference is complex, as is made clear by attempts to spell it out in writing. Some clinical resources recognise that processing texts (written or spoken) containing shifting reference is something that clients may find difficult. See, for example, the ACE Narrative Syntax section, 'Direct Speech' item, or the use of quoted speech in various narrative resources such as the Squirrel Story or the Renfrew Bus Story.

They is described in grammars of English as being used to point to two or more persons other than the speaker or the addressee. Another usage has become more and more prominent over the past 40 or 50 years, namely to point to one person whose gender is not known, as in (4).

4   a   Somebody is coming to help but they don't know the house number.
    b   Somebody is coming to help but he or she doesn't know the house number.
    c   We always tell the author beforehand that they must submit a pdf document.

5   A   Somebody phoned while you were out.
    B   Oh. What did they want?

They is used in instead of *he or she*. The usage is still controversial and is unacceptable to many, possibly most, educated users of written English over the age of 40. Nonetheless, the usage is the norm in spoken English and its penetration into written English is unstoppable, even if it takes many years to become accepted in formal writing. Note that speaker B in (5) would hardly ask *Oh, what did he or she want?*

A final comment on personal pronouns: their reference is not always clear. In this textbook, for instance, *we* and *you* are used. Does *we* refer to the two authors or to the two authors and the readers? The latter is in many cases the intended reference, in such sentences as 'In Chapter 9 we looked at finite clauses'. And does *you* refer to any individual reader, although unknown to the authors, or to all the readers collectively?

11.3.3   Deixis: demonstratives

The set of demonstratives contains *this*, *that*, *these* and *those*. They can be used as demonstrative pronouns, as in (6) or as demonstrative determiners, as in (7).

6   a   This is going to cause trouble.
   b   That was delicious.
   c   These are too dear.
   d   Those won't fit you.

7   a   This car is uneconomical.
   b   That programme was absolute rubbish.
   c   These trainers are too dear.
   d   Those trousers won't fit you.

The interpretation of *this* and *that* depends on where the speaker and the addressee are in a given location and where things or people are relative to them. *This* is used for things that are relatively near the speaker or the speaker and the addressee, as in (8).

8   a   I'll give you this book as soon as I've finished it.
     (The speaker indicates a book on the desk beside her.)
   b   Can you guess what's in this parcel?
     (The speaker has come in holding a parcel.)
   c   These animals are very dangerous.
     (The speaker and the addressee at the zoo watching a pack of African wild dogs.)

That is used to refer to things that are relatively far from the speaker or the speaker and the addressee, as in (9).

9   a   Could you pass me that dictionary please?
     (The speaker points to a dictionary on the other side of the table, next to the addressee.)
   b   Oh, what's in that parcel you've got?
     (The speaker referring to a parcel just brought in by the addressee.)
   c   Those dogs are frightening the children.
     (The speaker is referring to dogs held by the addressee, who is standing some distance away.
   d   Do you see those houses on the other side of the square?
     (The speaker and the addressee are on the opposite side of the square from the houses.)

Sentence (9d) has been included because it is the sort of example in which some, possibly many, speakers of Scottish English and other Northern English varieties would use *yon* (And literary, especially poetic, texts offer examples of *yonder*, now archaic.).

10   Do you see <u>yon</u> houses on the other side of the square?

These varieties of English have *this* for things near the speaker, *that* for things near the addressee but not near the speaker and *yon* for things that are far from both the speaker and the addressee.

The addressee may be unable to build an enriched interpretation of *this* or *that*, as in the following dialogue from a novel.

11   'Well, my dear, I am heartily glad we've done with that,' Miss
       Dunstable said to her, as she sat herself down to her desk in the drawing-room
       on the first morning after her arrival at Boxall Hill.
       'What does "**that**" mean?' said Mrs Gresham.
       'Why, London and smoke and late hours, and standing on one's legs for four
       hours at a stretch on the top of one's own staircase, to be bowed at by anyone
       who chooses to come . . . '
       Trollope, A. (1996) *Framley Parsonage*. London: Folio Society, 383.
       Text based on the Penguin edition, 1984. First published 1860–1861.

Sentence (11) is useful in another respect: it shows that the apparently simple demonstratives have complex extended uses, not just pointing at tables and chairs but at different aspects of a situation considered collectively. We pick up this point in the discussion of extended uses at the end of this account of deixis.

The following piece of (real) dialogue illustrates the difficulty in understanding pointing words without being present in a situation or being able to see the interlocutors. In the dialogue below, the speaker has been talking about his experiences when he was working in Nigeria, and in particular the day he and his companions came across a lion-hunter caught in one of his own traps. The speaker is asked how a lion trap works.

12   A: So how do these things work?
      B:
      i   The trap has two bits, like <u>this</u>.
      ii   <u>This</u> bit has teeth like <u>these</u>.
      iii   It's pulled back and propped open like <u>so</u>.
      iv   A chunk of meat is placed <u>here</u>.
      v   When an animal tries to take the meat, it knocks out <u>this</u> prop.
      vi   <u>This</u> bit slams shut.

The video recording of the dialogue shows the speaker using his hands to demonstrate the working of the trap. *These things* in A's utterance refers to animal traps, which had just been brought into the conversation. *This* in Bi refers to B's two hands used to represent the two parts of an animal trap. *These* in Bii refers to the fingers on B's right hand, which was being used to represent the teeth. *So* in Biii refers to the alignment of B's hands representing the open trap. *Here* in Biv points to the hollow of B's left hand, representing the part of the trap in contact with the ground. *This bit* in Bvi points to B's right hand, which B brought down in contact with his left hand to imitate the trap snapping shut. The pointing words make perfect sense when the conversation can be both heard and seen.

11.3.4   Deixis: spatial expressions

The classic **spatial deictics** are *here* and *there*. *Here* is prototypically used to point to the location of the speaker or to a location near the speaker and *there* to a location distant from the speaker (Distance is relative. A location referred to by means of *there* might be five feet away from the speaker or many miles.). Consider the examples below.

13   a   Jacob isn't here at the moment.
         (The speaker refers to the house in which they are answering the phone.)
     b   The memory stick is there on the table.
         (The speaker points to the object on a table at the other side of the room. The addressee may be next to the speaker or sitting at the table.)

14   a   She's coming here to give a lecture this autumn.
         (The speaker refers to the town or institution where the conversation is taking place.)
     b   Have you been in Brittany? We're going there for two weeks in July.
         (The speaker refers to a location at some distance from where they are.)

15   a   Here's the book you were looking for.
         (The speaker hands the book to the addressee. Alternatively, the speaker is going along the library shelves looking for the book and produces the above utterance when they reach the book. In either case the speaker and the book are in the same location.)
     b   There's the book you were looking for.
         (The speaker catches sight of the book lying on a chair. The book is distant from the speaker.)

The words 'near' and 'distant' are used above to describe the relation between an object or location and the speaker. 'Distant' can be defined as 'not near', and what counts as near depends on the context and perspective, as discussed in Section 11.3.1. If James is standing near the vase when it falls to the floor, 'near' is interpreted as a foot or less. When we say of two towns in Britain that one is near the other, we mean five or ten miles but not fifty miles. Looking at the map we think of New Zealand as being near Australia, and on a global scale that judgment is sensible. From the perspective of someone actually in New Zealand, Australia is not near; it takes three and half hours to fly from Auckland to Melbourne.

Other spatial terms are deictic in that they are interpreted with respect to the speaker's and/or the addressee's location. The speaker's and the addressee's location is the **landmark**. Thus, given two buildings, either can be taken as the landmark or reference point for describing the location of the other. If we say *Sheffield is east of Manchester*, we take Manchester as the landmark; if we say *Manchester is west of Sheffield*, we take Sheffield as the landmark. A landmark can be left unmentioned. If Freya says *My friend lives opposite* or *My friend lives across the road*, she means *My friend lives opposite my house* or *My friend lives across the road from my house*. 'My house' is the unspoken landmark.

11.3.5 Deixis: verbs of movement

The classic deictic verbs of movement are *come* and *go*. Prototypical examples are in (16).

16 a   Rene went to Edinburgh yesterday.
        (The speaker is not in Edinburgh.)
    b   Rene came to Edinburgh yesterday.
        (The speaker is in Edinburgh.)
    c   *Rene went here yesterday.
        (The deictic target of *here* is the location of the speaker.)
    d   *Rene came there yesterday.
        (The deictic target of *there* is some place that is not the location of the speaker.)

In these basic examples the use of *come* or *go* is governed by whether somebody moved towards the speaker or away from the speaker. This regularity is brought out even more clearly in imperative clauses, as in (17).

17 a   Come over here and tell me what's wrong.
        (The speaker summons the child to move closer to them.)
    b   Go over there and sit quietly for two minutes!
        (The speaker orders the child to move away from them.)

Sentences (16) and (17) are examples produced by a speaker talking about someone else moving from one location to another. Speakers can talk about themselves moving and when they do slightly different patterns of usage prevail (depending on which perspective they adopt, as discussed in Section 11.3.1). Consider (18).

18 a   I'm going to Glasgow tomorrow to meet Elspeth and see the exhibition.
    b   I'm coming to Glasgow tomorrow to go to the exhibition with you.

When uttering (18a), the speaker is not in Glasgow and the addressee is not in Glasgow either. *I'm going* is appropriate because the speaker is referring to movement away from their current location. When uttering (18b) the speaker is talking to an addressee who is in Glasgow. The use of *I'm coming* can be explained as the speaker mentally placing themselves in Glasgow with the addressee and talking as though they were moving towards themselves. The speaker will certainly be moving towards the addressee.

Bring and *take* are another pair of verbs whose use is governed by whether something or somebody is moved towards the speaker or away from the speaker. This is particularly clear in imperative clauses, as in (19).

19 a   Bring me the scissors please.

    b *Take me the scissors please.
       (The speaker asks the addressee to pick up the scissors and move to where
       he or she is.)

20 a Take the book over to Dad.
    b *Bring the book over to Dad.
       (Assume that the speaker is not Dad and is not addressing a very small
       child as discussed after (1) in Section 11.3.2. The addressee is asked to
       pick up the book and move away from the speaker towards Dad.)
    c Bring the book over to Dad.
       (The speaker is not Dad but is standing next to Dad. This means that in
       picking up the book and moving towards Dad the addressee also moves
       towards the speaker.)

In commands such as those in (19) and (20) *bring* must be used for movement
towards the speaker and *take* for movement away from the speaker. Variation on
this pattern is possible when the speaker makes the sort of mental adjustments
mentioned in connection with (18).

21 a Hi. Is that Katarina? Just phoning to say that I'm bringing you the CDs
       this afternoon.
    b * Hi. Is that Katarina? Just phoning to say that I'm taking you the CDs this
       afternoon.

22 a Hi. Is that Freya? Just phoning to say that I'm taking Katarina the CDs
       this morning. Are you going round to her flat for lunch?
    b *Hi. Is that Freya? Just phoning to say that I'm bringing Katarina the CDs
       this morning. Are you going round to her flat for lunch?

Sentence (21a) can be explained if we assume that the speaker mentally places
himself or herself in the place where Katarina is. Sentence (22b) would only be
possible if Freya were at Katarina's flat. This would allow the speaker to mentally
place themselves with Freya at Katarina's flat and to talk as though they were
going to move towards themselves. Sentence (22a) makes it clear that Freya is not
at Katarina's flat, and such mental adjustments are excluded.

Exercise 11.1

Point out all the instances of deixis in the following examples. What type of
deixis is involved in each instance (personal pronoun, demonstrative, spatial,
temporal, verb of movement)?

1. I understood that there would be an opportunity to meet her there later that
   week, and that I would be responsible for bringing the documents. At least,
   that's what John said.
2. Come out from behind there at once!
3. I met this guy at the concert, and we got talking. He said that this Christmas
   had been the worst he had ever had. I'm meeting him again and taking him
   a copy of that new CD you recommended.

Exercise 11.2

The following examples are from a draft of a film script. What difference will the choice of version A or version B make to what the cinema audience see?

Version A

Leonardo locks the door of the staffroom, sits in the furthest corner of the room and opens a copy of a subversive linguistic tract. Suddenly the door is kicked open and four members of the linguistics thought police come in.

Version B

Leonardo locks the door of the staffroom, sits in the furthest corner of the room and opens a copy of a subversive linguistic tract. Suddenly the door is kicked open and four members of the linguistics thought police go in.

11.3.6   Deixis: temporal expressions

Words and phrases such as *today, tomorrow, yesterday* and *next week* are also deictic. *Today* points to the day on which the speaker is speaking or the writer is writing. To interpret correctly utterances such as *Granny and Grandpa are coming today,* small children have to grasp the conventional concept of a day and then understand that the referent of *today* shifts as time passes, as do the referents of *tomorrow* and *yesterday*. An utterance such as *We're leaving tomorrow* cannot be given a full interpretation unless the person who hears it or reads it knows the date on which it was produced. If it was uttered on Wednesday 11 January 2012, *tomorrow* points to Thursday 12 January 2012. This is difficult for small children to get to grips with, but situations arise in which even adults have difficulties. Some years ago, the second author, living in New Zealand, regularly phoned friends and family living in the United Kingdom. Depending on the time of year, New Zealand is either 11 hours or 13 hours ahead of the United Kingdom. If he phoned at 9 am on 10th July, the recipient of the call in the United Kingdom would answer the phone at 8 pm on 9th July. If the second author said *She arrived yesterday,* he would be referring to 9th July but the person in the United Kingdom would initially interpret this as referring to 8th July. Analogous problems affect the interpretation of *yesterday* and *tomorrow.*

Expressions such as *next week* or *the next three months* also pose problems of interpretation: you need to know the date on which the expression was used. That is, you need to know which date to take as the landmark (see Section 11.3.4). Sitting in a dentist's waiting room, the second author read a notice saying *Anyone who signs up with the practice in the next three months will be entitled to a free dental examination.* The notice was undated, and from the dust and the texture of the paper looked as though it had been pinned up in the waiting room for some time. Perhaps the dentist intended the temporal landmark to be vague in order to bring in as many patients as possible. At any rate, he sold his practice not long afterwards.

Sentences (23a,b) exemplify another pair of deictic temporal adverbs, *now* and *then*.

23   a   Barnabas is walking the dog just now.
    b   Pavel will be playing rugby then (so come round a bit later).

The deictic target of *now* in (23a) is a period of time that includes the time at which the speaker is speaking (Note the phrase *even as we speak* (*such and such is happening*).). *Now* can also point to a moment of time. The exasperated parent who utters (24) does not expect the child to respond at some point or other in the period including the moment of speech but right at or right after the moment of speech.

24   I'm not telling you again. Come to the table (right) now.

Then in (25b) denotes a period of time that is not now. It can point to the past, as in (25a,b) or to the future, as in (25c).

25   a   By then everybody was ready to go home.
    b   Very few people had a car then.
    c   Good weather is forecast for Tuesday. We'll go for a picnic then.

The deictic target of *then* is determined by the context. It might involve a date, say the 1930s for a low level of car ownership, or a sequence of events, as in (26).

26   The children built sandcastles, dug enormous holes, swam in the sea and ran up and down the beach. They had a picnic, and by then everybody was ready to go home.

The interpretation of *now* is actually more complex than indicated by (23a) and (24). It always has as its deictic target a period of time including the moment of speech. The extra component in the interpretation is the perspective from which the period of time is viewed. In (27), the phrase *just now* points to a period of time including the moment of speech but beginning earlier and going on after the moment of speech.

27   James is at school just now (but he'll be back around half-past three).

Now in (28a,b) targets the same period of time but presents it as a change in a sequence of periods of time. James was not attending school before *now* but is *now*, and for the foreseeable future will be, attending school.

28   a   James is at school now (and is away all day).
    b   James is now at school (and is away all day).

To take another pair of examples, in uttering (29a) the speaker simply points to the period of time including the moment of speech and says what Pavel is doing in that period of time. In uttering (29b) the speaker refers to a change of occupation.

29   a   Pavel is working at the bank just now. (He's working late this week to help install a new IT system.)

b Pavel is working at the bank <u>now</u>. (Previously he was working for an insurance company.)

c Pavel is <u>now</u> working at the bank. (Previously he was working for an insurance company.)

Note that the straightforward deictic *now* as in (23a), (24) and (27) can be modified by *just* or *right*. The sequential *now*, as in (28a,b) and (29b,c) cannot be modified by these adverbs but can occur after the verb *be* or after an auxiliary verb, *is now at school* and *is now working*. It can occur at the beginning of a clause, as in (30), and in the stage magician's formula *Now you see it, now you don't*.

30 <u>Now</u> Pavel is working at the bank. (He left the insurance company last week.)

It is worth mentioning that many speakers of Scottish English, and perhaps other varieties of Northern English, have a distinction between *the now* and *now*. *The now* is the straightforward deictic and *now* is the sequential. Some years ago a colleague of the second author at Edinburgh University, not a Scot, was telling another non-Scot the old story of the severe Scottish Presbyterian who arrives at the gates of heaven fully expecting to be admitted but is turned away by St Peter. The latter informs the Presbyterian that he had committed some serious sin. The Presbyterian exclaims *But I didnae ken* (= But I didn't know), to which St Peter replies *Weel, ye ken noo* (= Well, you know now). The speaker got it wrong and produced the punch line *Weel, ye ken the noo*. Unfortunately, the punch line sounded very wrong both in syntax and meaning.

11.3.7 Deixis: tense

In their basic, primary use of present and past tense are interpreted in relation to the moment of speech, as shown in (31).

31 Dad   Jennifer, what <u>are</u> you doing?

Jennifer   I'<u>m</u> doing my homework.

The present-tense verb *are you doing* includes the moment at which A speaks and *'m doing* includes the moment at which Dad speaks. Past tense is interpreted as pointing to a period or moment of time preceding the moment of speech, as in (32).

32 a Moira <u>phoned</u> Margaret to tell her about Alastair.

b Moira <u>phoned</u> Margaret just a couple of minutes ago.

c Moira <u>phoned</u> Margaret several months ago.

The past tense verb *phoned* in (32a) has a very general interpretation, just some moment or period of time earlier than the moment of speech. Moira might have phoned in the very recent past, as described in (32b), or in the more remote past, as in (32c). To specify such details speakers have to use adverbs of time such as *a couple of minutes ago* or *several months ago* or even *many years ago*. A particular moment or period of past time can be pinned down very exactly by means of phrases such as *at 11.25 on the morning of the 25th January 2012* (a moment of time) or *during July and August 2011* (a period of time).

In narrative, the interpretation of present and past tense is more complex. Suppose that (33) is part of an e-mail from Lucie to Margaret.

33   I'm planting annuals in the border. What are you doing in your garden?

The present tense *'m planting* is to be interpreted in relation to the period of time at which Lucie is writing her e-mail message. Suppose Lucie writes her message on 15th May and Margaret reads it on 17th May. The deictic target of *'m planting* is different from the deictic target of *are you doing*. Margaret's reply may be as in (34), that is, she interprets the present tense *are you doing* in relation to the period of time at which <u>she</u> is writing <u>her</u> reply to Lucie.

34   I'll plant my annuals next week. Still too cold. But I'm cutting the lawn today.

The present tense *'m cutting* points to 17th May, not to 15th.

In stories the interpretation of tense is even more complex. Sentence (35) is an example of a narrative technique by which the writer uses the present tense although narrating events that took place in the past.

35   On a sunny day in May 1881 Henry Grant is admiring his garden, unaware that his life is about to be rudely interrupted.

The deictic target of the present tense *is admiring* is neither the time at which the writer is writing the words nor the time at which some reader might be reading the words. Rather, the narrator places himself or herself in an imagined world at an imagined time and invites readers to follow. The deictic target of *is admiring* is a moment or period of this imagined time.

11.3.8   Deixis: extended uses

Pointing words are frequently extended beyond the space and time in which a speaker is speaking, as shown by the dialogue in (36). The dialogue comes from *The Wellington Corpus of Spoken New Zealand English* (1998), created by the Department of Linguistics at the Victoria University of Wellington, New Zealand. The dialogue is an excerpt from a radio phone-in programme. In the corpus it is labelled DGB 005. Annotations have been removed to make the dialogue easier to read and em-dashes have been inserted to mark pauses. The transcription contains no capitals or punctuation. *These* and *that* have been underlined by the authors.

36   A1   now the — <u>these</u> persons I would like to a — you to ask them if you can — if you EVER get on to them um

    B1   flush them out you mean

    A2   \<laughs>yes\<laughs> — is for them to do a budget for a — um — ONE person — one adult and two teenagers

    B2   but that's not his argument you see

    A3   <u>this</u> is the scary thing

In A1, *these* signals that the persons are near to the speaker and the addressee, near in the sense that they have been under discussion and are going to be central in the next chunk of dialogue. In B2, *that* points to the argument that A is putting forward but B uses *that* to signal that the argument (budgeting on a small income for a family consisting of a parent and two teenagers) remains distant from B because B is not accepting it. *This* in A3 signals the proximity of the topic: the refusal of the third person (mentioned earlier in the programme) to consider family budgeting. It is mentioned in A3 and, together with that person's views on the problem, is about to be discussed in the next chunk of dialogue.

Another example of *this* being used to signal that a person or thing is to be made the topic of conversation is in (37). The participants are speakers of Scottish English recorded in Edinburgh. B and C are students at a secondary school and A is the researcher. The transcription has no capital letters or punctuation apart from em-dashes to indicate pauses. The relevant phrases are *that technician* in B3 and *this technician* in A4. *That* is used in B3 because the speaker is referring to a person who is remote from the location where the conversation is taking place and remote from the conversation, since he has not been mentioned. *This technician* is used in A4 because the speaker wants to bring the technician, metaphorically speaking, towards B and C and into the conversation and to stay in the conversation as someone to be talked about. In this sense, the technician ceases to be remote and becomes close.

37   B2   it was great fun — I didn't have any appetite so I existed on oranges and I lost about three pounds

A3   goodness me

C1   you'll have put it back on by now

B3   I know — start putting it back on again — eating a bit more yeah it's unfair — that technician — I think he ought to be shot

C2   yeah cause we're getting these films at

B4   very interesting films with any luck

C3   sex education

B5   they're boring at the beginning

C4   and he must have slept in or something

B6   and the roads were icy — we were late — I was late in — the car was all over the place

C5   my Mum was going awful slowly

A4   so what's this technician got to do with it?

Sentences (35) and (36) are examples of **discourse deixis**; that is, the use of deictic words to signal that some person or thing is close, in the sense of having been brought into the narrative or conversation, or remote, in the sense of the narrative or conversation having moved on to other topics.

The following incident illustrates **psychological deixis**; that is, the use of deictic words to signal that some entity is psychologically close to or remote from the speaker. Consider this exchange between the second author and a student. The former came across the student looking at the departmental notice board assigned to the second-year Linguistics course. After an exchange of greetings the student asked *Has that essay of yours been marked yet?* The *that* signalled that the student was putting a psychological distance between himself and the essay. The second author found the question slightly offensive (more so since the student had not put much effort into the essay and had obtained a low mark). Fortunately he was able to reply politely *The essays were marked two weeks ago. You can collect yours from the Departmental Office.* (The exchange took place well before the use of e-mail and the Internet for all departmental business.)

A different kind of extension is exemplified in (38).

38   This has suddenly decided Europe is a good thing.
      (The speaker holds up a copy of the *Daily Bulldog*.)

The deictic target of *this* is not the newspaper that the speaker is holding in their hand. It is not the particular issue of the newspaper, realised in many thousands of copies. It is not the journalists who have written the articles. Rather it is the owner, possibly in cooperation with the editor. The copy of the newspaper present in the immediate context acts as a bridge to the other possible targets. Of course, the bridge can only be understood and exploited by speakers and listeners who have the necessary information about how newspapers are produced and who decides what line a particular newspaper follows on social and political issues. (Such information is said to constitute a frame. We discuss frames in the following chapter as they are crucial for successful communication.)

Personal pronouns too have extended uses, which are more obvious in languages other than English. For instance, the second person plural pronoun *vous* in French is certainly used when the speaker addresses more than one person. More importantly (from the point of view of good social relationships), *vous* is also used in certain circumstances when the speaker is talking to just one person. If the speaker is talking to someone older and not a friend, or talking to someone senior in an organisation, or talking to an employee (not a friend) in a bank, at a supermarket check-out, in any type of shop, *vous* must be used. Why the plural? One explanation is that in using *vous* the speaker acts as though they are addressing more than one person. A one-to-one interaction is direct and relatively intense; in a one-to-many interaction, there is no direct contact between the speaker and just one of the addressees and the intensity of the contact is dissipated. The speaker's attention is distributed over the set of speakers. The inverse in English is the use of the 'royal' *we*. A monarch using the 'royal' *we* acts as though several people are addressing a subject. This act makes it appear that there is no direct one-to-one connection. The use of *vous* in French and the 'royal' *we* in English is known as **social deixis**. The deictic words are exploited to signal social relationships and how an individual perceives the social relationship between himself or herself and another person.

Exercise 11.3

Discuss the targets of the underlined deictics in the following examples:

1. The policy may work in your country but I don't think it will work <u>here</u>.
   [The speaker and the addressee are sitting in a pub in York.]
2. We really have quite dry weather <u>here</u> compared with Cumbria.
   [The same speaker and location as for (1)]
3. The traffic police <u>here</u> are very polite compared with the French ones.
   [A Home Secretary talking on a discussion programme.]
4. The major sources of pollution are <u>here</u> and <u>here</u>.
   [The speaker draws imaginary circles on the map.]
5. <u>She</u> clearly understands the topic inside out.
   [The speaker taps the assignment she is holding.]
6. I remember the riots of 1968. We were on holiday in Paris <u>then</u>.

11.4   Reference

Many **acts of reference** require the speaker or writer to use full lexical items to enable the addressee(s) to pick up the referent. Instead of simply saying *She has a good sense of humour* or *I bought this today*, using the underlined deictic words, they could say *The tall, dark-haired girl from Manchester has a good sense of humour* and *I bought this blue woollen jacket today*, using the underlined referring expressions. These referring expressions are noun phrases containing the lexical items *tall*, *dark-haired*, *girl*, *from*, *Manchester* and *blue*, *woollen* and *jacket*. The lexical items are clues to the addressee as to what sort of person or thing the speaker is drawing attention. They are said to have a **denotation**, which influences the sense relations discussed in Section 3.4.5. Denotation is a property of lexical items. Reference is an act performed by speakers, and it is this act that we focus on here. In order to refer, speakers (and writers) use noun phrases (called referring expressions when we are focusing on their function in acts of reference) and the things they refer to are referents.

What is important for speakers is that they refer <u>successfully</u>. In many situations, it does not matter if the speaker comes up with an incorrect referring expression, because the addressee can work out the referent anyway. It may be quite obvious what the speaker is referring to because it is salient in the situation and highly imageable (see Chapter 2). The addressee may have detailed knowledge, stored in a frame or several frames, that enables them to work out who or what the speaker is referring to. Quite frequently, all the participants in a dialogue work together to establish correct interpretations of utterances as intended by the speakers. To take an extreme example, a sympathetic parent will make repeated attempts to interpret utterances from a small child: *Here's Teddy. Oh, you don't want Teddy? Dolly?*

No? Ah, the monkey! That's right, monkey [Child tries the word again.] *Here you are.* Two adults will work together on a more equal basis, as in (39).

39   Husband: Can you pass me that thingummy?

      Wife: What thingummy?

      Husband: The pointy thing. I want to make a hole for the screw to go into.

      Wife: Oh, you mean a bradawl. Will this one do? [picks up one of two]

      Husband   Bradawl. That's the word! But 'pointy thingummy' sounds good.

Well, 'pointy thingummy' sounds good but is not much use for instantly successful reference, although helpful listeners do their best to solve the puzzle. In fact, a speaker may get a referential description hopelessly wrong but still refer success-fully, as in (40).

40   a   Who did you give the file to?

      b   I gave it to the departmental secretary over there

      a   That's not the departmental secretary. That's the Dean's PA.
          Get the file back now!

For successful reference, the speaker must be able to supply enough information to identify the referent and mark it out from other possible referents. The hearer must be able to use the information to pick out the referent. Speakers and hearers usually just assume that these conditions are met, though in real life things can go wrong, as in (39) and (40). Of course it is easier to identify referents that are imageable, that is, that have definite shape, size and colour; tulips, chairs and bottles of wine can be seen and touched, but truth and sincerity cannot. Imageable objects are typically referred to by means of phrases containing familiar and frequently used lexical items. One last point: usually acts of reference are included in larger speech acts (to be discussed in Section 13.4). An act of reference is usually included in a statement (*I'm going to transplant the young bush*) or question (*Are you going to transplant the young bush?*) or command (*Transplant the young bush before the spring growth starts*) or even just an exclamation, as in *What a mess!* (Parent on opening the door of children's bedroom.)

Suppose a speaker uses a definite noun phrase, that is, a noun phrase introduced by the definite article *the*, as in (41a), or a demonstrative, *this* or *that*, as in (41b), or a possessive pronoun, as in (41c).

41   a   They've appointed the applicant from Belgium.

      b   Can you pass me that small blue bowl please?

      c   My laptop is in your office.

The speaker is said to perform an act of **specific reference**. That is, they refer to specific people or things that they consider identifiable or given, to use the technical term from the analysis of narrative (see Section 11.3.1). The speaker might instead use an indefinite noun phrase, that is, a noun phrase introduced by the indefinite article *a*, as in (42).

42   A snake bit him but he survived.

The snake cannot be identified by the listener (and possibly not by the speaker) and has not been mentioned before and is not in the immediate context. In uttering (42), the speaker performs an act of **non-specific reference**. Speakers can also use indefinite noun phrases for specific reference, and the listener usually requires extra information in order to work out whether the reference is specific or non-specific. Consider (43a) and (43b).

43   a   I left a book on first language acquisition on my desk. Have you seen it?
      b   I'm looking for a book on first language acquisition. Can you recommend one?

In (43a), the underlined indefinite noun phrase is used for an act of specific reference, as is made clear by the pronoun *it*. In (43b), the same indefinite noun phrase is used for an act of non-specific reference, as is made clear by the pronoun *one*. A humorous line from a TV series of the mid-90s turns on the distinction between specific and non-specific reference and on the range of meanings expressed by idiomatic expressions containing the verb *feel*. Sentence (44) is uttered by a middle-aged woman whose doctor (also a woman) has successfully diagnosed a chronic ailment and cured it.

44   I feel like a new woman — and like a new man. [The em-dash signals a long pause.]

A new woman has specific reference, at least for the speaker, whereas *a new man* has non-specific reference. Non-specific reference is typical for words such as *sometime* and *somewhere*, as in (45).

45   a   Come and have a meal with us sometime.
      b   I know I've seen your glasses somewhere in the house.

Sentence (45a) is highly non-specific and commits the speaker to nothing. Sentence (45b) may be nothing more than an encouraging remark, unless the speaker suddenly remembers the particular place they saw the glasses. The pronoun *somebody* allows degrees of specificity, as shown by (46)–(48).

46   Somebody left a parcel for you — but I didn't see who it was. I found the parcel on the doormat.

47   Somebody left a parcel for you — I'd recognise them if I saw them again.

48   Somebody left a parcel for you — I think it was your friend from Exeter.

The speaker who utters (46) performs an act of non-specific reference in that they cannot identify the person. The speaker who utters (47) also performs an act of non-specific reference, but the reference is less non-specific. The speaker does not know their name but could identify the person in the right conditions. The speaker who utters (48) is able to say tentatively who the *somebody* is. Some languages have different pronouns for *somebody* depending on how non-specific the reference is.

Speakers and writers who perform acts of specific reference using deictics or definite noun phrases assume that listeners or readers can pick up what they are referring to. The referents may have already been mentioned, or may be very salient in the immediate context, or may be something or someone so well known that it can safely be assumed that everyone belonging to a particular culture will recognise the referent. Such referents are said to be given, or are assumed to be given. Speakers can make incorrect assumptions.

Speakers and writers who use indefinite referring expressions, even for specific reference, assume that listeners or readers will not be able to pick out the referent. In such cases the referent is not salient in the context, or is assumed not to be well known to the listener or the reader, or has not been mentioned. Such referents are said to be new. The distinction between given and new referents, or between given and new information, is discussed in more detail in Section 15.3.

The final kind of referring act is when speakers refer to a whole set of things. In spoken English, plural indefinite noun phrases are used, as in (49), but singular indefinite noun phrases are also used, as in (50).

49   Tasmanian Devils are frightening animals.

50   A Tasmanian Devil is a frightening animal.

More frequent in written English is the use of definite noun phrases, as in (51).

51   The Tasmanian Devil is a frightening animal.

Out of context, (51) might be interpreted as specific reference to an individual, as in (52), or as a reference to the whole set of Tasmanian Devils, as in (53).

52   The Tasmanian Devil is a frightening animal. Just have a look in its cage.

53   The Tasmanian Devil is a frightening animal. The first settlers were very scared of them.

Reference to a whole set is known as **generic reference**.

We close this section by pointing out that some lexical items have different but very closely related denotations. This allows speakers to refer to different facets of some entity, possibly with humorous intent. *Book*, for example, denotes an imageable physical thing with pages, binding, kind of type and illustrations. It can also denote something less imageable: the plot, the characters, the unfolding of events, the quality and quantity of text. *The book* in (54) denotes the physical object, in (55) the abstract properties.

54   The book is unattractive (The type is ugly, the paper feels wrong and the binding is shoddy.).

55   The book is unattractive (The plot is convoluted, the characters are off-putting and the action unfolds far too slowly.).

In an early Garfield cartoon, the first panel shows Garfield the cat sitting in an armchair looking very full and very satisfied. The second panel carried the caption *That book was pretty good*. The third one carries the punch line *But the bookmark was absolutely delicious.* The punch line leads us to reinterpret the second panel: when Garfield uses the phrase *the book* he is referring to the book as a physical object (which he has just eaten) and not as a story with good plot and characters.

In Section 11.3.8 we looked at an extended use of *this* and *that*. The example involved a speaker holding up a newspaper and commenting *This has just decided that Europe is a good thing.* A frame of information about how newspapers are produced and how the content is decided provides a bridge from the apparent deictic target, the copy of the newspaper the speaker is holding, to the real targets, the editor and the owner. Frames of information and the process of bridging can be crucial for the correct interpretation of definite noun phrases. Consider (56).

56   A1:   The new conductor's enjoying the job.

      B1:   I heard he had some problems.

      A2:   Well, the cellos keep turning up late for rehearsals.

      B2:   Hmm, there's always some people who make life difficult.

            Does he get on with the other members of the orchestra?

A mentions 'the cellos'. Cellos are musical instruments but B understands correctly that A is referring to the people who play the cellos. This may look obvious, but B has to apply a frame relating to orchestras and a subframe relating to the way people can be referred to indirectly via the instruments they play, the clothes they wear and so on. A well-known example in the linguistics literature involves restaurant staff who refer to customers by the food and drink they are consuming. In *The ham sandwich wants another black coffee* the phrase *the ham sandwich* is used to refer to the person eating a ham sandwich.

We have looked at reference, and paid some attention to the connection and distinction between denotation and reference and to the important role played by frames in controlling the identification of referents by listeners and readers. In Chapter 14, on narrative, we look at how different types of noun phrase/referring expression are used at different places in narrative.

Exercise 11.4

BUY, HUNT, DRY, CHASE, WASH, COOK, POLISH, etc., are listed in many dictionaries as verbs that are used transitively (Some are also listed as verbs that are used intransitively.). Which of the following examples are acceptable? How are the acceptable examples to be explained, the ones in which the verbs that are typically used transitively are not accompanied by a direct object NP?

1. They hunt in the Autumn.
2. She's hunting upstairs (= She's hunting for her driving licence.).
3. Barry washes, Jim dries and Dot puts away.
4. I'm cooking just now — I'll phone you back.
5. The accountant is cooking just now — he'll phone you back
   (= The accountant is cooking the books.).
6. Jane buys for John Lewis.

Exercise 11.5

What words and phrases are missing from the following pieces of text? Why is the text quite comprehensible in spite of the missing items?

From a cardboard packet containing a bottle of cough linctus:

Warnings
May cause drowsiness. If affected, do not drive or operate machinery. Avoid alcoholic drink.
Do not use if bottle seal is broken when purchased. Keep bottle tightly closed. Store below 30°C.
Keep out of the reach of children.

Chapter summary

Deixis is a phenomenon of words that are the linguistic equivalent of pointing. Words such as *this* and *that*, *now* and *then*, and I, *you* or *she* provide no information about the properties of entities (animate or inanimate) but are used to point to them. Crucial to the interpretation of deictic words and phrases are the location of the speaker relative to some other entity, whether the entity is the speaker, the addressee or a third person, and the moment at which the speaker is speaking. Deictic items can be used to signal perceived proximity or remoteness with respect to time, the place of an entity in a narrative, social relations and the speaker's attitude.

Reference has to do with the use of noun phrases/referring expressions to draw the attention of listeners or readers to some entity or entities. It is an act, whereas denotation has to do with the information carried by lexical items. Speakers and writers can refer to entities that are given, that is have already been mentioned or are prominent in the immediate context or in the culture shared by speaker or writer and the addressee. Reference may be to entities that are new, that is have not been mentioned or that cannot, in the judgment of the speaker, be (easily) picked up by the addressee. Given entities are specific; new entities may be specific or non-specific. Philosophers focus on whether referring expressions are correct but in ordinary language use many instances of referring are successful without being correct.

The interpretation of both deictics and definite noun phrases may involve bridging. The addressee builds a bridge from an apparent deictic target or referent to the intended target or referent, making use of frames of information about some area of a given culture or world.

Exercises using clinical resources

11.6. In Section 11.3.2 we noted that it can be challenging to process the 'shifting deixis' associated with direct speech in narrative. Consider the Recalling Sentences in Context subtest of the CELF-Preschool, and look at the items that include direct speech (i.e. words in inverted commas). In which items could shifting deixis be an issue?

11.7. The following resources involve the clinician asking questions of the client. Which questions contain deictic expressions?
  a. Boston Diagnostic Aphasia Examination (page 2, section A of the record booklet).
  b. Western Aphasia Battery (Part 1, section A).

11.8. In the following clinical resources, identify any items that specifically target the client's processing of deixis:
  a. CAPPA (Part A, section 1)
  b. CCC-2

Further reading

'Chapter 16: Reference and deixis' in Cruse (2004).

12 Language in Use 2: Frames and Scripts, Metaphor and Irony, Implicature, Explicature

Clinical resources that will be referenced in this chapter:

ACE – Assessment of Comprehension and Expression 6–11
ASDS – Asperger Syndrome Diagnostic Scale
CAPPA – Conversation Analysis Profile for People with Aphasia
CAPPCI – Conversation Analysis Profile For People With Cognitive
  Impairment
CCC-2 – Children's Communication Checklist
CELF-4 – Clinical Evaluation of Language Fundamentals
Don't Take It So Literally!
MCLA – Measure of Cognitive-Linguistic Ability
Narrative Intervention Programme.
TALC – Test of Abstract Language Comprehension
TOPL – Test of Pragmatic Language
Sheffield Screening Test for Acquired Language Disorders
Understanding Ambiguity

12.0 Introduction

Fully competent speakers and writers in any language are those who have mastered the language code: the patterns for creating new lexical items out of stems and derivational affixes; the patterns for building phrases, clauses and sentences; vocabulary, including whatever technical vocabulary is required for professional activities, whether legal language, the language of plumbing or the language of some academic discipline. This knowledge is also important for listeners and readers. Without it they cannot process what is being said or what has been written in order to interpret it. Note that we talk of speakers and writers, listeners and readers as though they were different set of people but being a speaker, listener and so on is to act different roles. To avoid repeating the list of roles, we will talk of 'language users'.

Introductory Linguistics for Speech and Language Therapy Practice, First Edition. Jan McAllister and Jim Miller.
© 2013 John Wiley & Sons, Ltd. Published 2013 by John Wiley & Sons, Ltd.

There are two more sets of skills that language users must control in order to be recognised as competent language users. One is the capacity to construct full and accurate interpretations of utterances on the basis of limited information. Speakers do not spell out all the information that they wish to convey. Information is left unspoken that they think listeners can supply from context, both the immediate situation in which talk is being produced and the cultural knowledge that speakers (sometimes mistakenly) assume is available to their addressees. Cultural knowledge includes knowledge of a particular society and knowledge of the broader world. Language users learn, with varying levels of success, how much information to leave out in a given situation and what information to infer.

The second set of essential skills has to do with the ability to interact with others: to initiate a conversation, to have one's say without interrupting, to finish a conversation, to make assertions, ask questions and issue requests, suggestions, advice and instructions in a manner befitting the type of interaction (domestic conversation, consultation with a doctor, interview for a job and so on) and the relationship between the participants, determined by such characteristics as rank, age, gender and experience.

In this chapter, we look at the first set of skills, leaving core interactional skills for the next chapter.

12.1   Why do SLTs need this knowledge?

Mature speakers acquire and learn not just the structures of words and sentences but a very large number of language practices. These language practices are not innate and some children do not acquire the social skills with which language is used by adults. The topics to be discussed in this chapter relate directly to skills such as constructing interpretations of utterances that contain all the information that speakers and writers convey without expressing it explicitly (see Section 12.5 on implicature and Section 12.6 on explicature). The Pragmatics Profile in CELF-4 includes the following checks on clients' control and use of language in communication. The checks come under the heading of 'Rituals and Conversational Skills' (which we look at in Chapter 13) but require the capacity to make invited inferences (implicatures) and to fill out an interpretation with information that has not been explicitly mentioned because, for most language users, it is obvious in a given situation.

- Makes relevant contributions to a topic during conversation/discussion
- Asks appropriate questions during conversations and discussions
- Avoids use of repetitive/redundant information
- Shows appropriate sense of humour during communication situations.

The last point is important. A central part of language use, at home and in the workplace, is the use of humour. Language users crack jokes but, more subtly, produce ironic utterances and speak or write metaphorically. The importance of using humour in various forms of narrative is emphasised in the Narrative Intervention

Programme. Of course, there are otherwise perfectly average speakers who do not understand the use of humour and take utterances literally. And not every other-wise average language user appreciates or is able to use metaphorical language. The tricky task for the SLT is to establish for a given client whether such characteristics are symptoms of something more serious or whether they are superficial.

12.2   Learning outcomes

After reading this chapter and doing the exercises, you should:

- Understand the concepts of frames and scripts and be ready to learn to apply them in clinical work;
- Understand the concepts of explicature and implicature and be able to recognise failures of understanding in your clients;
- Be aware of the role of jokes and irony;
- Be aware of the prevalence of metaphor in everyday communication.

12.3   Frames and scripts

Two fundamental concepts are essential for any sensible account of how language users convey and construct these rich meanings, how they manage to communicate coherently with one another and even how they manage to refer successfully to people and things. One concept is that of a **frame**. A frame is a representation of some area of experience in a given culture. It is widely used in Artificial Intelligence as a way of organising information that has to be supplied to computers to enable them to understand texts. The concept is also widely used in the analysis of narrative and the area of linguistics known as Discourse Analysis or Text Linguistics. A frame contains schematic information about some area of experience, particularly concerning the main types of actors and the relations between them. Thus, the frame for shopping in a British supermarket contains entities such as rows of tiered shelves (gondolas), a line of checkouts, people stacking the shelves, people operating the checkouts, shoppers, many different items for sale, labels stating the price of individual items and the price by weight or volume. The frame for shopping in a Middle Eastern souk, say in Aleppo, contains small individual shops, not always accessible to the shopper, goods set out on display but with no prices shown, no checkouts. The frame for British supermarkets does not contain people whose job is to persuade shoppers to part with their money – that is done by more subtle methods. The frame for the Middle Eastern souk (at least, the second author's frame) contains people whose goal is precisely to part shoppers from their money.

Frames are constantly updated and are used in reasoning. Over the past few years many people have updated their frame 'British supermarket' to include special 'self-checkouts', where shoppers scan and pay for their purchases using a computerised checkout system. Frames include information about many other aspects of each area of experience, such as different language practices. Informal conversation with family members in domestic settings calls for informal, colloquial language, whereas discussion in school classrooms calls for formal language. Even something as basic as the interpretation of individual lexical items is controlled by frames. For example, in the frame relating to the collection and delivery of mail, *letter* denotes envelopes containing written messages on paper and is in a lexical field with such lexical items as *parcel*, *packet* and *envelope*. In the frame relating to typography *letter* denotes a particular set of marks on paper representing sounds. In the frame 'tennis' *server* is the player serving the ball; in the frame 'IT' *server* is the piece of equipment that distributes mail and other documents to individual PCs.

The second fundamental concept is '**script**'. It was originally developed to enable computers to 'understand' texts such as narratives and conversations and to handle the many inferences that even a single sentence gives rise to. It was soon extended to models of language processing by humans. Scripts differ from frames – like frames, they store knowledge about the roles of the people taking part in some situation and about the inanimate entities involved, but they also store knowledge about stereotypical sequences of events and actions in given situations. Thus, the script for catching a plane involves checking in (finding the check-in desk, queuing, showing ticket and passport, putting luggage on the conveyor belt to be weighed and labelled), going to the departure lounge, the sequence of events that constitute going through security and so on.

Scripts for British supermarkets involve the sequence of events in a visit: picking up a basket or taking a trolley, going round the store, picking the appropriate checkout, the appropriate comments to make to the person operating the checkout, putting the purchases into bags and making the payment. Applying this script in an American supermarket may cause trouble if there is someone who is employed to pack the bags and who expects a tip. (Each major component of the script may consist of sequences of smaller components. The second author's subscript for going round the store differs from his wife's in the order in which different areas of the supermarket are visited and the process of choosing what items to buy.)

The above paragraphs talk about scripts for two types of public actions, checking in at an airport and shopping in a supermarket. We will see in Sections 12.5, 12.6 and 13.4 that frames and scripts govern every area of our lives, down to the most banal domestic exchanges. Children have to acquire and learn not just their first language but the frames and scripts that go with it in the culture they are brought up in. The degree to which clients have mastered such frames and scripts is an important part of clinical appraisal by speech and language therapists. And adults with acquired communication difficulties may not retain full control of the scripts they require in order to take part fully in everyday life.

Frames contain all sorts of information, including information that is so banal that normally nobody bothers to mention it. In one of the Paddington Bear stories, Paddington takes part in a television quiz. He picks mathematics as his subject and is given, one at a time, various problems to solve mentally. One involves two men filling a 50-gallon bath with one tap running. If they fill the bath in x minutes how long will it take another man to fill the same bath with two taps running? The quizmaster wants the answer 'x/2 minutes' but Paddington declares the answer is no time at all. His reasoning is that the quizmaster specified that the one man was filling the same bath and the bath was already full, since the two men had filled it. The quizmaster had not said that anyone pulled out the plug and emptied the bath before the one man started his task. The audience applaud Paddington's reasoning and force the quizmaster to hand over the prize money. Of course, the humans in the culture concerned have a frame 'examinations' containing the information that examination or quiz questions focus on the essential points, are not trick questions and do not mention information that can be taken for granted (by those who know the conventions).

Frames and scripts play an essential role in connection with meanings and interpretations that go far beyond the meanings of the lexical items and grammatical constructions in a particular clause or sentence. Meanwhile here are two more examples to illustrate the phenomenon.

1   A1:   Will you be baking a Christmas cake?
    B1:   My husband doesn't like it.
    A2:   You can have a bit of mine if you like.

B does not say explicitly that she is not going to make a Christmas cake but A infers that she is not. Christmas cakes take a lot of time to mix (and possibly to leave maturing in brandy) and to bake. (Even ready-made mixes require long baking.) The trouble is not worthwhile if the person most likely to eat a large part of the cake is not interested. We can think of A as having all this cultural information at her disposal stored in various frames: a frame related to baking in general, a frame related to the baking of Christmas cakes, a frame related to the provision of food for Christmas and getting all the different foods eaten up when Christmas is over. Speaker A uses these frames to build a complete understanding of B's reply. ('Cultural' is used in its broadest, anthropological sense to cover all the practices and behaviours in a given society, from art, music and literature, through many linguistic and social practices, to cooking and eating, joking and so on.)

The second example shows how listeners have to apply different frames in order to interpret different examples of the same construction, here the Perfect. Consider the small dialogues in (2) and (3).

2   A   Has anybody seen my glasses?
    B   I saw them on the kitchen table just a minute ago.
3   A   Has anybody seen that film?
    B   Freya has seen it, but it was so long ago she doesn't mind seeing it again.

The problem is that the Perfect by itself does not specify whether an event happened very recently or some time ago. To interpret A's question in (2) and give an appropriate answer, B has to apply a frame with the information that somebody who wears glasses typically uses them regularly or even constantly throughout the day and assumes that the question has to do with the recent past. In contrast, a question about who has seen a film may relate to the recent or to the more remote past. What is important is that if Freya has seen the film that may affect the decision about what cinema to go to.

Exercise 12.1

What information goes into a frame and script for

a. using an automatic teller;
b. on landing at an airport, getting from a plane to the exit from the terminal?

Exercise 12.2

How do frames help us to explain the use of the underlined definite noun phrases in the following examples?

1. We're going to my parents for Christmas but I don't know how we'll get the Christmas tree into the car.
2. A train drew into the station and the driver got down onto the platform.
3. We leave St Pancras at 11. The train arrives in Paris at 12.30.

12.4 Metaphor, irony, humour

Mark Haddon's novel *The Curious Incident of the Dog in the Night-Time* (Vintage edition, 2004, first edition Jonathan Cape, 2003) is purportedly written by a 15-year-old boy who has Asperger's syndrome. The novel illustrates the problems that people with Asperger's have in dealing with **metaphor** (and other aspects of language use, as we will see later). Chapter 29 begins with the declaration *I find people confusing*. One reason is given in (4).

4   The second main reason is that people often talk using metaphors. These are examples of metaphors.

I laughed my socks off.
He was the apple of her eye.
They had a skeleton in the cupboard.
We had a real pig of a day.
The dog was stone dead.

The word metaphor means carrying something from one place to another and it comes from the Greek words *meta* (which means 'from one place to another') and *ferein* (which means 'to carry') and it is when you describe something by using a word for something that it isn't. This means that the word metaphor is a metaphor.

I think it should be called a lie because a pig is not like a day and people do not have skeletons in their cupboards. And when I try and make a picture of the phrase in my head it just confuses me because imagining an apple in someone's eye doesn't have anything to do with liking someone a lot and it makes you forget what the person was talking about'.

The narrator in (4) does not mention a problem with **similes,** possibly because similes are straightforward. A simile makes a direct comparison: if you say that a room is like a fridge, the addressee has to figure out in what respect the room and a fridge are alike, but temperature will probably be salient. Metaphors suggest similarities indirectly and demand more complex mental processing in order to relate a **source domain** to a **target domain.** To interpret the assertion *The firm is on the rocks* you have to establish the source domain, an enterprise carrying on a business, and the target domain, voyaging on the ocean. You then have to work out that the firm is being compared to a ship that has been blown off course and driven onto rocks. At the very least, it is difficult to refloat a ship once it has gone onto rocks and often the ship breaks up and sinks. The assertion is to be interpreted as saying that the firm is about to come to an end.

Exercise 12.3

Explain the following metaphors, using the concepts of source domain and target domain.

1. In her new school she blossomed.
2. The proposal turned out to be a lead balloon.
3. In their anger they had a heated argument.
4. He can't get over the death of his wife.

Children have to learn about the use of **irony,** and many adult speakers have difficulty understanding irony, even if they are not affected by Asperger's syndrome. The traditional definition of irony is that it is a property of utterances that have a meaning opposite to the one intended. A speaker seeing a colleague gazing out of the window may remark *I see you're busy today.* Not all ironical utterances say the opposite of what the speaker means but may involve simple understatement. A speaker who produces the apparent question *Isn't the meat a bit underdone?* is not actually asking a question and means that the meat is not slightly underdone but very underdone. As with metaphors, the interpretation of ironic utterances calls for a considerable amount of mental processing. We can think of irony as the speaker pretending to say something positive while intending something negative and the hearer going along with the pretence.

Language users also have to learn to distinguish irony from **sarcasm.** Ironic comments are not intended to hurt other people's feelings, but may simply be intended to start a conversation or to shake up someone who is feeling down, as when a speaker, coming in out of wind and sleet, comments *Wonderful weather this morning!* or *Nothing like a bit of healthy sleet to set you up for the day!* Sarcastic comments, in contrast, are intended to affect others negatively, as when a lecturer says to a student handing in a very short essay several days late *I see you're really excited by this topic*, or when a parent comments to a son wearing some garish outfit *Couldn't you have bought something brighter?*

Jokes are utterances that are intended to make the recipients laugh or chuckle and are not to be taken seriously. They may take the form of extended stories, such as the one cited by Lynn Truss about the panda that eats shoots and leaves (see Chapter 7). They may simply consist of one-liners produced off the cuff. The daughter of a friend of the second author was talking about her success at a game of Scrabble, when she had scored 30 points with the word *sex*. Quick as a flash her father said *Nobody's ever given me 30 points for sex* – much laughter, followed by a comment from his wife. Jokes can enliven lectures, especially impromptu one-liners. Sadly, it is said that 30 years on a group of students will remember none of the content of a lecture series but will remember any good jokes.

In many clinical resources, this aspect of language is targeted in items that refer to 'literal' versus 'indirect' meaning. Such resources include the CAPPCI, Don't Take It So Literally!, the TOPL and Understanding Ambiguity.

12.5 Implicature

The other major property of daily communication that children have to learn about is that much of the information conveyed by speakers to listeners is not stated overtly but must be inferred. Dealing with this sort of inference requires sophisticated skills that are sometimes targeted in resources; see, for example, the Inferential Communication sub-test of the ACE, or level 4 of the TALC.

Consider the following (not so) imaginary dialogue:

5   Child: Can I go round to Freya's house after lunch?
    Mother: Granny and Grandpa are coming. They'll be here by half past two.
    Child: But I'll take my watch and come back before then.

The parent does not say *You can't go just now because Granny and Grandpa are coming and you've got to be here to say 'Hello'*. Nonetheless the child understands perfectly that her mother is refusing permission and tries a new argument. The child might have put a different interpretation on the mother's statement, namely that she can go but must be back by half past two. With that interpretation the child might have said *OK. I'll make sure I'm back by then*. The *but* in the child's second contribution in (5) signals that the child is proposing an alternative. With the second interpretation the child is going along with what she thinks her mother is communicating but is relying on her mother accepting that she will remember to look at her watch and will be able to tear herself away from Freya at about twenty past two.

A slightly different example of unspoken but communicated information is in (6).

6   I've got a simple recipe for steak pie from that cookery programme.
   Even Angus could make it.

Even without any knowledge of the people involved, competent listeners infer that Angus is a pretty poor cook. They confidently make this inference because of their knowledge of *even*. Examples like (5) and (6) caught the attention of logicians. A central concern of logic is **entailment**, the relationship between sentences (actually, as we will see in a moment, between the propositions expressed by sentences) such as (7a) and (7b).

7   a   James has just painted the door red.
      b   The door is red.

8   James has not just painted the door red.

We assume that in both sentences, the phrase *the door* refers to the same door. When we say that (7a) entails (7b), we mean that if (7a) is true, then (7b) is also true. If we make (7a) negative, to give (8), we break the relationship; in fact, we leave the two sentences unconnected. But note that (8) does not entail *The door is not red*, because someone else could have painted it red. Importantly, we can make (7b) negative, to give (9).

9   The door is not red.

This sentence entails *James has not just painted the door red*. How could he have, if the door is not red?

What are **propositions**? A proposition is the content of an assertion about some situation. *The Queen opened the Olympic Games in London in July 2012* is an assertion conveying a proposition about a particular event, at a particular time and in a particular location. The event is one of opening; the agent is the Queen (readers with access to the correct frame of information will identify her as the Queen of Great Britain and Northern Ireland) and the object opened is the Olympic Games held in London. Propositions are built on propositional content, which is information about a type of event and types of participants; thus, OPEN (Agent, Patient) is a representation of the propositional content of the above proposition. Propositional content does not relate to specific situations involving specific participants, times and places but propositions do. One and the same proposition can be expressed by two different types of clause. For example, the proposition just discussed can be expressed by the sentence *The Olympic Games in London were opened by the Queen in July 2012*. As we will see in Section 16.4, the use of a passive clause as opposed to an active clause has a number of communicative effects, but the proposition is not affected. The Narrative section of the ACE requires the identification of propositions, and the concept of propositions is implicit in several resources that score clients on 'information'.

To make the above discussion of entailment acceptable to logicians we have to say that the proposition expressed by (7a) entails the proposition expressed by (7b). With respect to the dialogue in (5), we can say that the child infers the proposition 'Do not go to Freya's house' and responds to that proposition. With respect to (6), we can say that the listener infers from *even* the proposition 'Angus is a poor cook'. Importantly, the proposition 'Do not go to Freya's house' is not expressed overtly and is not entailed by the mother's statement. The child has to be able to infer the proposition on the basis of what her mother has said plus her knowledge of the relevant frames and scripts.

To handle such examples logicians rely on the concept of **implicature**. An implicature is a component of meaning that goes beyond whatever proposition is overtly expressed by a speaker or writer. The listener or reader (other things being equal) is led to infer a proposition that is not asserted (see examples (11)–(14) below). Since speakers and writers have to choose what to say and how to say it in order to provide hints that there are implicatures to be sought, implicature is very much a feature of language production and expression. Since listeners and readers have to interpret what is actually said and decide if there are implicatures to be worked out, implicature is also a feature of language processing and interpretation.

There are two types of implicature. One is designed to deal with examples such as (6). It is known as **conventional implicature** because what is implicated is attached by convention to words such as *even* and *but*. The second type of implicature, which the child deploys in the dialogue in (5), is known as **conversational implicature**.

Conversational implicature arises in the course of conversation (which covers all types of dialogue from domestic chit-chat to formal discussions such as current affairs programmes on radio and television). The basic idea is that the participants in conversation are aware of and generally follow **maxims of conversation**. When one participant fails to follow one or more maxims, the other participants, if they are mature speakers of whatever language is being used in whatever culture, will detect the anomaly and begin working out why the maxims have not been applied. That is, they assume that the participant who produced the anomalous utterance was being cooperative, trying to contribute sensibly to the conversation and inciting the other participants to work out the unspoken proposition.

The original maxims were devised by a philosopher called Paul Grice during the late 1960s and early 1970s. His maxims related to the work done by speakers but it became clear that separate sets of maxims were needed, one for speakers and another for listeners and readers. The maxims supported a general principle, called by Grice the **co-operative principle**. The principle reflects the fact that people normally engage in conversation in order to make sense to each other. To make sense they, to put it in everyday terms, have to keep to the point, signal when they want to change the topic of conversation and avoid talking at cross purposes. (See the discussion of coherence and cohesion in Section 14.6.) As Grice puts it: make your contribution [to the conversation] such as is required, at the stage at which it occurs, by the accepted purpose or direction of the talk exchange in which you are engaged. One of Grice's maxims is the **maxim of relevance**. It simply states 'Make your contributions relevant'. The other maxims boil down to the following:**

- not saying more than you have to on any occasion;
                      [Maxim of Quantity]
- but equally not saying less than is needed for clear communication;
                      [Maxim of Quantity]
- not lying or making statements that are not backed by facts;
                      [Maxim of Quality]

- saying things briefly, unambiguously and clearly.

  [Maxim of Manner]

Grice's conversational maxims were refined by Stephen Levinson in the late 1990s into a set of three principles, each with a maxim for speakers and writers and a maxim for listeners and readers. The **Quantity Principle**, abbreviated to **Q-Principle**, enjoins speakers not to say less than is required, and listeners and readers are to assume that whatever is not said or written is not the case. The **Informativeness Principle**, abbreviated to **I-Principle**, enjoins speakers and writers not to say more than is required. What this means is that speakers do not have to spell out all the facts of a normal situation. It is enough to say, for instance, *We went to that new restaurant yesterday* without mentioning that someone gripped the handle and pushed or pulled the door open and that once inside, the speaker and others ordered a meal and ate it. The other side of the coin is that listeners and readers can assume, unless told otherwise, that a particular situation is of the normal type and that they are entitled to infer that the participants performed the usual acts in the usual sequence. The Q and I Principles should be understood as not saying less than is required, nor more and talking to the point. As we will see in the next chapter, speakers may deliberately ignore these maxims or principles in order to communicate indirectly during conversation.

Following the I-Principle is beyond the capacity of Mark Haddon's narrator with Asperger's. On p. 59 he makes the comment in (10).

10   . . . I do not always do what I am told.

And this is because when people tell you what to do it is usually confusing and does not make sense.

For example, people often say 'Be quiet', but they don't tell you how long to be quiet for. Or you see a sign which says **KEEP OFF THE GRASS** but it should say **KEEP OFF THE GRASS AROUND THIS SIGN** or **KEEP OFF ALL THE GRASS IN THIS PARK** because there is lots of grass you are allowed to walk on.

Siobhan [one of the boy's teachers] understands. When she tells me not to do something she tells me exactly what it is that I am not allowed to do.

Or, for example, she once said, 'If you want to go on the swings and there are already people on the swings, you must never push them off. You must ask them if you can have a go. And then you must wait until they have finished'.

Following the Q-Principle, if a passer-by asks where Simon Murray lives and you say *A mile along the road, on the left*, you will not have followed the Q-Principle if you omit to say that there are five houses on the left and that his is the second one the person will come to. If you then go into speculation as to whether Simon Murray is at home or whether he might have had to take his aged car for its MOT, you are failing to follow the I-Principle and are providing too much information.

The third principle is the **Markedness Principle**, abbreviated to **M-Principle**. It enjoins speakers to keep syntax and vocabulary simple, while listeners and speakers are reminded that some message that is expressed in a complicated and/or unusual way, may have been formulated thus for a reason. (The label 'markedness' comes from the idea that simple grammar and vocabulary are normal and unmarked – for present purposes we can say that they pass 'unremarked'. Complex grammar and vocabulary are very much noticed and are marked as unusual.) If you announce to someone that it is incumbent on them to provide succour for a friend, you are using marked vocabulary, lexical items that are typical of very high-flown, and possibly archaic, written language and not of informal speech, even to adults. In writing, however, you may want to use words such as *incumbent* and *succour* if you have reason to demonstrate your command of formal written English. As an SLT talking to a colleague about a client, you will use relevant technical vocabulary. Talking to the client's relatives (assuming they are not speech and language therapists), you will use non-technical vocabulary where possible.

Let us consider some further examples of implicatures involving the above principles.

11 Parent: Have you done your maths homework and packed your bag for school?
    Child: I'm just packing my bag.

The child does not say that they have done the maths homework. Any parent will note that the child has not explicitly said that they have done the homework (What is not said is not the case!) and pursue that question. The implicature created by the parent is 'Normally he would say if they had done the homework. He hasn't mentioned it. He probably hasn't done it'.

12 A   My uncle has two cars.
    B   So has my father.

If nothing further is said, A will assume that B's father has two and only two cars. That is, A will assume that B has said as much as is required. B can cancel this implicature by adding *In fact he has three*. (Of course A and B may be exaggerating.)

13 A: I tried to skype Philippa this morning. She's usually at her computer late morning.

A may leave it at that, and the listener will pick up the implicature that A did not actually succeed in contacting Philippa. But A may be saying less than is required, and may cancel that implicature by adding, after a pause, *I had to dial a couple of times but I did get through eventually*.

14 Parent: How did you get on with John? Do you want to ask him round to play?
    Child: He's got lots of Lego Technik.

The child is not replying to the parent's question but moving away from the topic. Unless he makes positive comments about John, the parent will assume that he doesn't particularly like John himself and doesn't want to ask him round to play. This implicature is justified by the fact that the child is following neither the Q- nor the I-Principle. The principles require him to say that he did or did not get on with John and that he does or does not want to invite him round to play.

Exercise 12.4

Conventional implicatures attach to particular lexical items. What meaning is contributed to the examples below by the underlined lexical items?

1. Vera <u>even</u> handed in her essay on time.
2. <u>Even</u> Vera managed to attend all the classes.
3. Louise <u>almost</u> fell over the cliff.
4. Louise <u>almost</u> bought a ticket.
5. Louise <u>almost</u> finished writing her bestseller.
6. I <u>really</u> like your theory.
7. I don't <u>really</u> know him.
8. I <u>really</u> don't know him.
9. <u>Evidently</u> they are going to sell the estate.
10. I haven't written that reference <u>yet</u>.

12.6 Explicature

We have seen from the discussion of deixis and reference in Chapter 11 and of speech acts and implicature in this chapter that listeners and readers have to fill in a large amount of information in order to interpret utterances. This is illustrated by a very common phenomenon in conversation and narrative, **ellipsis**. This is exemplified in (15).

15   Mother: Jennifer, tidy your room.
      Jennifer: I have.

Mother understands that Jennifer's reply is to be interpreted as 'I have tidied my room', and furthermore that she has done so very recently.

The central idea is that utterances typically convey directly a small amount of information, often not corresponding to a complete proposition. Consider the examples in (16)–(18).

16   A   You've got to have your passport even if you're just flying to somewhere else in Britain.

      B   I know.

17   We were just joining the motorway when a piece of timber fell off the lorry in front. It cracked the windscreen.

18   A   Have you replied to the invitation?

      B   I am – this very minute.

In (16), A has to process and fill out B's utterance so that they arrive at the proposition that would be conveyed by the complete sentence *I know that you've got to have your passport even if you're just flying to London*. A may infer that because B knows this B will make sure they pick up their passport before setting off to catch the flight. Similarly, in (18) A has to construct an utterance for processing based on B's reply: *I am replying to the invitation*. And although *this very minute* occurs after a pause, A has to interpret that noun phrase as modifying *I am replying to the invitation*. In (17) the listener or reader has, among other things, to interpret *the windscreen* as referring to the windscreen of the vehicle in which the speaker and others were travelling. This interpretation depends on the listener having a frame to do with road vehicles which contains the information that cars, lorries, buses and so on, have windscreens. Another frame, to do with motorway travel, contains the information that British motorways are full of commercial vans and lorries and that at any point in a given journey, travellers in a car will probably find themselves behind a lorry or a van. None of this information is spelled out in the utterance but has to be filled in by the listener or reader. Other obvious tasks that the listener has to carry out are interpreting the deictic *in front* as *in front of us* or *in front of the vehicle in which we were travelling*.

Ellipted material may be incorrectly reconstituted, either by honest error because the missing material is related to what has been said in quite a complex fashion, or for the sake of humour. Consider (19).

19   A   I didn't sleep with my wife before we got married. Did you?

     B   I don't know. What was your wife's name?

What A wants to know is whether B slept with B's wife before they got married. That is, B is supposed to take A's utterance and reinterpret *I* and *my* as pointing to him, B, and *we* as pointing to B and B's wife. Instead B answers as though A were asking about a relationship between his, A's, wife and B.

Listeners and readers have to resolve ambiguities in utterances. Remember the discussion of the Garfield cartoon in Section 11.4, following example (53). Readers of the cartoon probably interpret the *book* as a well-written text, a good plot and plausible characters. The phrase *The bookmark was delicious* makes them change that interpretation to a book as a physical object that can be chewed and eaten (typically by young dogs, but also by children at the teething stage, but not typically by cats, a fact that initially guides readers towards the text interpretation).

One of the sentences in the above paragraph contains an ambiguity that you probably did not notice, in the sentence *Remember the discussion of the Garfield cartoon in Chapter 11*. Is it the cartoon that is in Chapter 11 or the discussion? Since you know that there was no cartoon reproduced in Chapter 11 but that there is a description of it and a discussion, you probably interpreted *in Chapter 11* as modifying *discussion*. Other ambiguities are more noticeable, sometimes because they are intended to be humorous, like the example in (20).

20   Mike was unable to drive straight after his treatment at the hospital.

Straight can be interpreted as a modifier of *drive* and assigned the meaning 'in a straight line'. Alternatively it can be interpreted as a modifier of *after* and assigned the meaning 'immediately'. This deliberately constructed example works better in writing, of course, since in speech the ambiguity would be removed by rhythm and intonation.

Ambiguity can also be removed by frames containing information about the normal states of affairs in the world we inhabit. Halfway up the farm track leading to the second author's house, a road (unsurfaced) cuts across. At the intersection is a sign with the legend *Heavy plant crossing*. On the assumption that *The Day of the Triffids* is not based on reality, you discard the interpretation of *plant* as referring to vegetable entities. *Plant* also denotes industrial units, but industrial units are not usually mobile or transportable in one piece. That interpretation is discarded. To get at the intended interpretation you have to know that *plant* also denotes large pieces of equipment, typically static equipment. An extension from static equipment to large self-propelled pieces of equipment gets you to the interpretation. For a number of years anyone driving along the track was liable to encounter huge dumper trucks carrying coal, bulldozers, graders and diggers. (And there is another ambiguity: were the bulldozers, graders and diggers being carried by the dumper trucks as well as coal? The reader with access to a frame with information about the size and weight of bulldozers and how they are transported from one site to another will resolve the ambiguity, but it can be removed by recasting the phrase as 'encounter bulldozers, graders, diggers and huge dumper trucks carrying coal'.)

Finally, we should remind ourselves that constructing implicatures and making inferences on the basis of implicatures is a major part of interpreting utterances, as discussed in the previous section.

All the above activities – working out the correct reference, resolving ambiguities, constructing implicatures and making correct inferences – are components of what is now called **explicature**. While implicature is a feature of language production/expression, explicature is a feature of language comprehension/reception. ('Implicature' comes from the Latin verb *plicare* 'to fold' and *in* 'in' and the metaphor is of meanings folded into an utterance and not visible or audible. 'Explicature' comes from *plicare* and *ex* 'out of' and the metaphor is of unfolding an utterance to reveal all the details hidden in it waiting to be constructed or reconstructed by the reader or listener.) Explicature is the process of interpreting an utterance by mentally building all the complete propositions so that the propositions can be processed.

Exercise 12.5

What propositions can the addressee construct from the ellipses in the following examples. Note any shifts in tense, person and so on.

1 A: Have you sent Ken an e-mail?

   B: I am.

2 A: Would you like me to deliver the computer to your house?

   B: Could you?

3 I suggested he leave it till next week but he didn't agree.

12.7   Presupposition

At the beginning of Section 12.6 we mentioned entailment as a central concern of logic and logicians. The concept of implicature is also of great interest to logicians; it explains how in everyday talk humans make all sorts of correct inferences that cannot be explained by entailment and shows that the concepts of classical logic cannot by themselves be used to account for how speakers and writers communicate information and how listeners and readers interpret utterances correctly.

Presupposition is another concept that has proved essential for the analysis of communication, though it is not accepted by all analysts working on language and logic. It is related to the everyday term 'to take something for granted' but now has two major uses in linguistic analysis. It is applied to a relation between two propositions, such that one proposition only makes sense if the other one is true. (See the discussion of (21) below.) It is also applied to propositions that language users take for granted or presuppose. (See the discussion of (22)–(26).)

In the sense of a relation between propositions, presupposition was introduced into philosophy (in the early 1950s) by a British philosopher, Peter Strawson. Suppose that Ken and Angus have just been introduced at a party. Later a conversation between Angus and his wife might go thus.

21   Angus1   Ken's wife must have money.
      Wife1   Ken doesn't have a wife
      Angus2   Are you sure? He lives in a big house but he's just a lecturer. How can he afford it?
      Wife2   He sold his parents' house when his father died.

Putting it in terms of classical logic, proposition A, 'Ken's wife has money', can only be true if proposition B is true, that is 'Ken has a wife'. Equally, if Angus had been entertaining proposition C, 'Ken's wife doesn't have money', that proposition likewise can only be true if proposition B is true. The problem is that, given proposition A and proposition C, one must be true and the other one false. They can't both be true: either Ken's wife has money or she does not. But if proposition B, 'Ken has a wife', is not true, then neither proposition A nor proposition C can be true. This is a peculiar state of affairs, quite different from entailment. The proposition 'Thumper is a spaniel' entails the proposition 'Thumper is a dog', but NOT the proposition 'Thumper is not a dog'. With respect to Ken's wife having or not having money, the proposition 'Ken has a wife' is, as Strawson put it, a **necessary precondition** of both propositions. Strawson called the relationship 'presupposition'. 'Ken has a wife' is a presupposition of both 'Ken's wife has money' and 'Ken's wife doesn't have money'. If Ken does not have a wife, it makes no sense to ask if the proposition 'Ken's wife has money' is true or false. The proposition is simply not relevant to the situation in the real world, and is neither true nor false.

A number of researchers, following Strawson, take presupposition to be a relationship between propositions. Some have tried to eliminate it and to demonstrate that only entailment is needed. The only comment we need to make here is that the concept of presupposition as a relationship is alive and well and, in Strawson's original work, is clearly different from entailment. More relevant to this chapter on language and use is an alternative understanding of presupposition that is also present in Strawson's original work. Following a comment by Strawson, we might say that in producing the utterance *Ken's wife has money* Angus commits himself to the existence of a woman who is Ken's wife. In other words, presuppositions can also be seen as actions performed by speakers and writers in taking some state of affairs for granted (presupposing some state of affairs). Angus takes it for granted, or presupposes, that Ken has a wife.

It is important to be able to recognise and, if necessary, challenge the presuppositions made by participants in a discussion. It is also important for each of us to recognise the presuppositions that we are making, sometimes unconsciously, in our dealings with others. An introductory textbook for SLT students is not the place to discuss these issues, but it is the place to point out links between presuppositions and choice of grammar and vocabulary. Consider (22a) and (22b).

22 a Did you remember to turn off the computer?
    b Did you remember turning off the computer?

The speaker uttering (22a) makes no presuppositions about whether the computer was turned off or not. The speaker uttering (22b) presupposes that the addressee did turn it off. The difference in presupposition is reflected in the use of the infinitive *to turn off the computer* in (22a) and the gerund *turning off the computer* in (22b). There is an even more obvious difference in meaning between (23a) and (23b).

23 a I didn't remember turning off the computer (and had to go back to check).
    b I didn't remember to turn off the computer. (It probably didn't use too much power while we were away.)

The signalling of different presuppositions via the use of infinitive or gerund is tied to specific lexical items in specific constructions. The verb *regret* allows a different pattern, as shown by (24a) and (24b).

24 a I regret leaving them standing at the side of the road. (But what could I do? There was absolutely no room in the car).
    b I regret to leave them standing at the side of the road – oh, what the hell, maybe we can squeeze them in.

The speaker uttering (24a) presupposes that they have no alternative, while the speaker uttering (24b) is not so convinced by their presupposition and changes their mind. (For some speakers 'regret to' is confined to phrases such as 'I regret to inform you that . . . ' and 'We regret to report that . . . '. However, the distinction in meaning shown in (24a) and (24b) is also found with 'be sorry about' and 'be sorry to'. 'I'm sorry about leaving them standing at the side of the road' can be used to talk about an event that actually happened or about an event that is about to happen and for which there is no alternative. 'I'm sorry to leave them standing at the side of the road' relates to an event that is about to happen, but the speaker can still have a change of heart.)

Note too the difference in meaning between (25a) and (25b).

25 a I imagine him making his fortune in Australia (and hope that it doesn't change him).

b I imagine him to be making his fortune in Australia (but I'm not going to take anything for granted until he tells me that he has succeeded).

The speaker uttering (25a) presupposes that the person referred to is indeed making his fortune, while the speaker uttering (25b) is making no such presupposition.

Presuppositions are reflected in the choice of lexical items, as in (26).

26 A So, you managed to submit your tax return online and before the deadline.

B There was no question of 'managing'. I've done it before and I had all the figures ready to type in.

The use of *managed* signals that A had doubts about B's ability to deal with the online system for submitting tax returns and about B's being organised enough to get all the data together in time. B rejects these presuppositions.

Chapter summary

Section 12.3 discusses frames and scripts, frames being bodies of information about specific types of situation, their settings and types of participants. Scripts contain that sort of information together with information about typical sequences of actions.

Section 12.4 deals with various types of utterance that are not to be interpreted at face value: metaphor, irony, sarcasm. The role of jokes in communication is briefly commented on.

Section 12.5 analyses implicatures, the information that is not overtly coded in an utterance but which the listener or reader reconstructs and uses to make inferences about what the speaker or writer is really saying. There are two major types of implicature: conventional implicatures attach to specific words such as *even* and *but*; conversational implicatures are reconstructed by the listener or reader on the assumption that the speaker or writer has followed the maxims of conversation.

The Quantity Principle, or Q-Principle, enjoins speakers not to say less than is required, and listeners and readers to assume that whatever is not said or written is not the case. The Informativeness Principle, or I-Principle, enjoins speakers and writers not to say more than is required. What this means is that speakers do not have to spell out all the facts of a normal situation. The Markedness Principle, or M-Principle, enjoins speakers to keep syntax and vocabulary simple, while listeners and speakers are reminded that some message that is expressed in a complicated and/or unusual way, may have been formulated thus for a reason.

Section 12.6 discusses the general phenomenon of explicature, taking an utterance and creating a set of complete propositions that can be interpreted to reach the meaning conveyed by speaker or writer, which goes well beyond what is overtly encoded in any typical utterance.

Section 12.7 deals with presupposition. There are two concepts both called 'presupposition'. One is a relationship between propositions and the other is both the act of taking something for granted and the proposition that is taken for granted. This second concept is important for the correct interpretation of conversation and narrative. It also affects choice of vocabulary.

Exercises using clinical resources

12.6. In this chapter we introduced the concepts of frames and scripts. Look at the manual and materials of the TALC. For which materials are these concepts relevant? At what level are children expected to be able to use this information?

12.7. In the CAPPA, which of Levinson's principles is examined in question 21?

12.8. In the Sheffield Screening Test for Acquired Language Disorders, which item most obviously requires the client to access a script?

12.9. Which section(s) of the MCLA ask(s) about comprehension of metaphor?

12.10. Look at the CCC-2 and identify items that focus particularly on the following:
   a. Jokes
   b. Irony
   c. Scripts
   d. The I-Principle

12.11. In the ASDS, identify items that focus particularly on
   a. Jokes and sarcasm
   b. Levinson's principles

Further reading

'Chapter 11.3: Metaphor' and 'Chapter 18: Conversational implicatures (including enrichment or explicature)' in Cruse (2004).

13 Language in Use 3: Speech Acts, Conversation

> **Clinical resources that will be referenced in this chapter:**
>
> ADI-R – Autism Diagnostic Interview – Revised
> ASDS – Asperger Syndrome Diagnostic Scale
> CAPPA – Conversation Analysis Profile for People with Aphasia
> CAPPCI – Conversation Analysis Profile for People with Cognitive Impairment
> CCC–2 – Children's Communication Checklist
> CELF-4 – Clinical Evaluation of Language Fundamentals
> Manchester Pragmatics Profile
> MCLA – Measure of Cognitive-Linguistic Abilities
> Pragmatics Profile
> SULP-R – Social Use of Language Programme (Revised)
> Understanding Ambiguity

13.0 Introduction

Speakers do not just acquire and learn the patterns of a particular linguistic code and the vocabulary that goes with it. They also learn a large number of linguistic practices governed by the conventions in force at a given time in a given community. They have to learn that they do not just break into a conversation to talk over someone else but have to take their turn. To do this successfully, they must learn to recognise when a current speaker is finishing their turn, they must practise seizing their turn when appropriate and they must learn to signal that their turn has come to an end and that they are handing the floor to the next speaker. Mature speakers of a given language do not simply ask questions using whatever yes–no or wh interrogative constructions are available and when formulating a request or suggestion or command they are just as likely to use another construction than the straightforward imperative one described in the grammars of the language.

Introductory Linguistics for Speech and Language Therapy Practice, First Edition. Jan McAllister and Jim Miller.
© 2013 John Wiley & Sons, Ltd. Published 2013 by John Wiley & Sons, Ltd.

In this chapter we will look at what are called **speech acts**, using language to make statements, ask questions and issue commands, requests and so on in an appropriate fashion. We will then discuss the business of taking part in a **conversation**: opening and establishing an interaction with one or more interlocutors, keeping the conversation going by taking one's turn and not interrupting someone else's turn and closing an interaction.

13.1   Why do SLTs need this knowledge?

SLTs need to know about speech acts and how conversation is organised because these are central to successful participation in a given community. Not all children learn to do conversation or speech acts; these are beyond the skill and comprehension of many speakers with developmental language difficulties. And adult speakers who have mastered these skills and applied them throughout their lives may lose them as the result of a stroke, an injury or a brain tumour. The loss of these skills, or the failure to master them, at the very least significantly reduces a speaker's capacity to engage in social and business relationships.

Many clinical resources focus on the skills required for smooth conversational interaction, including the CAPPA, CAPPCI, CELF-4, Manchester Pragmatics Profile and SULP-R.

13.2   Learning objectives

When you have read this chapter and completed the exercises, you should be able to:

- Understand and explain the concept of conversation management: taking turns, holding one's turn and finishing one's turn;
- Understand and explain the organisation of conversation and the concept of sequencing;
- Understand and explain the concept of speech act;
- Begin applying these concepts in your clinical work.

13.3   Frames, scripts and norms

We saw in Section 12.3 that frames and scripts are essential tools for understanding how listeners and readers correctly interpret deictics and definite noun phrases, fill out the meagre information conveyed by the utterance of a clause or even two clauses and make correct inferences. Frames and scripts are also relevant to all types of social and business interactions. The speakers of any language have to learn many routines, conventions and norms governing interactions, domestic and institutional, private and public. The term 'interaction' covers every sort of linguistic act, from asking a question or answering a question to competence in job interviews, as interviewer or interviewee.

Interactions are governed by two types of norm (which vary from culture to culture). **Sociopragmatic norms** govern who is entitled, or even required, to perform what speech act in a particular situation. The norms relate to properties of the interlocutors: their gender and relative age, their social class and occupation and their role and status in the interaction. They control such matters as who talks when in school classrooms, who says what and when in encounters with, for instance, medical personnel or passport control officers and in family gatherings or at job interviews. School students (or some of them) learn that it is unwise to hold private conversations during an exposition by the teacher. Small children learn that they cannot just interrupt a conversation when they feel like it. (This lesson may take many years to be assimilated.)

The second set of norms is **pragmalinguistic**. They govern, in a given society, which linguistic structures are appropriate in a given sociopragmatic context. Take a simple type of situation such as addressing strangers who turn up at your door. The second author and his wife live in an ex-farmhouse up half a mile of farm track. Not many strangers arrive at the farmhouse but when someone does turn up the second author or his wife go out and say *Hallo. Can I help you?* These words are uttered in a cheerful tone of voice and with a smile and possibly with an upwards nod. This formula is recognised as an indirect invitation to the strangers to explain themselves as well as an offer of help. In many cases the overt offer of help is taken up – people want to know if they can drive further along the track or where some other farm is. On the other hand, when driving through the grounds of a castle in the Scottish Borders (legitimately, since a son rents the old kitchen garden and was working there that day), the second author and his wife stopped at an intersection of two tracks where a woman was standing with her dogs. She addressed them somewhat abruptly with *Who are YOU?* She may have felt that she could dispense with the niceties, given her status not just as owner but as a member of the family that has owned the castle for several centuries and given that the various houses on the estate that are targets for burglars.

In the above type of situation either the stranger or the resident(s) can speak first. Suppose the stranger makes it as far as the door of the house and knocks or rings the bell. When the person in the house opens the door, they will probably say *Hi* or *Hallo* but it is then up to the stranger to explain themselves, using formulas such as *Sorry to bother you. I'm looking for X* or *I wonder if you could help me. I'm looking for X and I seem to have lost my way* or, more formally, *Good morning. I'm just up to have a look round the farm buildings* (not owned by the second author and his wife but by the estate on which their house is situated).

Information about sociopragmatic and pragmalinguistic norms is stored in frames and scripts. In frames, because each frame holds information about the typical participants in a particular type of situation and the relationships between the human participants. That is sociopragmatic information. In scripts, because situations evolve. Scripts contain information concerning who speaks first, who speaks next, who can take a turn at a particular point in the interaction and so on.

The four technical terms – sociopragmatic norm, pragmalinguistic norm, frame, script – are not much used in SLT materials but the concepts are well known and are central to the Pragmatics Profile in the CELF-4 Record Form mentioned in Section 13.1. The clinician has to evaluate a client's knowledge of rituals and their conversational skills. The CELF-4 is designed for assessing developmental language abilities, but other clinical resources target the conversational skills of adult speakers and the extent to which they observe the rituals. (The concept of 'rituals' is what we have been calling sociopragmatic and pragmalinguistic norms – who says and/or does what and in what order. The word 'ritual' seems rather high-flown for something as mundane as answering the door, but the point is that there are set scripts that members of a given culture usually follow. Sometimes people are described as following a script religiously.)

13.4   Speech acts

'Speech act' is no longer the buzzword it was in the 1970s and 1980s but the concept is essential in the analysis of language in use and the term is very useful, reminding us that in our daily lives we perform all sorts of acts with language. The concept of speech act was originally quite narrow. A primary interest of philosophers is with truth and falsity: in what circumstances (under what conditions) is a given proposition true or false? What is the structure of valid arguments in which a sequence of steps leads from an initial assumption to a true conclusion?

These are important questions, but in the late 1940s a British philosopher, John Austin, realised that many utterances conveyed sentences having nothing to do with truth or falsity. Many public ceremonies can only be performed if a particular sentence or formula is uttered: the religious ceremonies of christening, marrying and burying (whatever the religion and keeping in mind that there are non-religious forms of these ceremonies) are properly carried out only if the correct words are spoken; passing sentence in the law courts and launching ships likewise require particular sentences to be uttered. (In the 1970s the BBC broadcast a play, *The Bar Mitzvah Boy*. The principal character is a young Londoner, a Jewish teenager, who is about to go through the important ceremony called *Bar Mitzvah*. He is reluctant to take part, mainly because it means being the centre of attention of his immediate family, a large circle of relatives and family friends. The rabbi comes across the boy in the local park and reminds him that what is crucial is that the correct words be spoken. It doesn't matter who else is present or where the ceremony takes place. The boy relaxes and goes through the Bar Mitzvah in the park without the pressures and expectations exerted by family and family friends.)

Of course, the uttering of sentences in such public and highly formal ceremonies has to be done by people with the authority to carry out the acts. There was an instance some years ago of a person pretending to be a minister of religion who performed marriage ceremonies that were subsequently deemed to be invalid. In a university setting, a student handing in a piece of work late will be asked who said they could have an extension. It won't do to mention the Departmental Secretary, who may reign over the academic staff but does not have the power to grant extensions. If the lecturer giving the course has given permission, that may be enough, but in some departments it may be necessary for the Head of Department to have sanctioned an extra day or two. The written equivalent is a piece of paper with a declaration in the appropriate form of words and with the right signature.

Austin subsequently realised that many kinds of acts were carried out in ordinary conversation. The basic act, called a **locutionary act,** was to produce an utterance in whatever language was appropriate to the context. (*Locutionary* derives from *locution*, meaning a phrase or way of expressing some idea. It derives in turn from the Latin *locutio* 'speech, pronunciation, mode of expression', connected with *loquor* 'I speak'.) Another kind of act, called an **illocutionary act,** was to produce an utterance, not just for the sake of producing some sounds, but to make a statement, ask a question or give a command (in the most general sense). (*Illocutionary* derives from *in* + *locution*. The statement, question and so on, reside in the locution.) A third kind of act had to do with the (intended or unintended) effect of an utterance on the listener, who might interpret a statement as a threat or warning or promise. A command or request might provoke the calm response *I'll do it right now* or a bad-tempered outburst *Go and do it yourself*. This is called a **perlocutionary act.** (*Perlocutionary* comes from *per* 'through' and *locution*. It has to do with the effect produced through the locution.)

The theory of speech acts was taken up by many analysts. As it was applied, it was extended. In particular, the idea took hold that the typical direct speech act was carried out by means of clauses containing first person pronouns and verbs and the simple present tense, as in (1).

1   a   I <u>sentence</u> you to two years imprisonment.
    b   I <u>promise</u> to repay you next week.

Although these so-called performative **utterances** (or **performatives**) have the declarative clause structure that is typically used for making a statement such as describing a state of affairs, such utterances do more than just describe reality; producing them actually changes reality. So by uttering (1a), the judge who produces the utterance changes the person they are addressing from someone who was not sentenced to two years' imprisonment into someone who is so sentenced, and by the very act of uttering (2b) the person who utters it has made an undertaking to repay the addressee by next week. Austin noted the use of *hereby* in performatives, as in (2).

2   a   I <u>hereby sentence</u> you to two years imprisonment.
    b   I <u>hereby promise</u> to repay you next week.

Hereby is actually typical of legal documents but quite untypical of everyday speech. *I hereby promise to repay you next week* sounds more like a sentence from a legal document than someone borrowing money informally and making a spoken promise. *Hereby* does not occur in some of the classic performatives noted by Austin. The locution that accompanies the launching of a ship in the United Kingdom – *I name this ship 'Pugwash'. May God bless her and all who sail in her* – excludes *hereby*, as does the locution that accompanies baptisms – *Eileen Jean, I baptise you in the name of the Lord*. Neither of these performatives is part of a legal agreement, which reinforces the idea that *hereby* is typical of legal documents.

Another idea, which has proved very tenacious, is that each type of speech act is expressed by a particular verb or verbs, known as **performative verbs**. Examples are *promise*, *suggest*, *authorise* and *complain*. Even *refuse* turns out to have a performative function, as in *I refuse to have anything to do with this scheme.*

Exercise 13.1

Which of the following verbs, and the examples containing them, are performatives?

Can *hereby* be inserted into any of them?

1. I bet on the horses but only occasionally.
2. I bet you fifty quid her horse will win.
3. A   What did Brian say just now?
4. B   He bets you fifty quid that Alice's horse will win.
5. Louise says she speaks French but I bet she's never been near the country.
6. I'm asking you politely not drop your rubbish in my garden.
7. I ask you: have you ever seen such a mess?
8. I give you notice that you are no longer a member of the club.
9. I'm giving you notice that you are no longer a member of the club.
10. I apologise for any delay but air traffic control have just asked us to go into holding.
11. I'm apologising for the loss of your luggage but not for the delay in landing.

Speech acts are subject to **felicity conditions** which have to be met if a speech act is to be completely **felicitous**, to use Austin's term. These are the conditions that must be in place for the speech act to achieve its purpose. If the conditions are not in place, then, keeping Austin's terms, a speech act can **misfire**, can be **abused** or can simply not be carried out, in spite of appearances. If a speech act is not to misfire, various **preparatory conditions** must be met, that is, various conditions that prepare the scene for the performance of the speech act. Above, we referred to a person who had not been ordained as a clergyman but carried out marriage ceremonies. The preparatory conditions for pronouncing the marriage formulae had not been met. To take an everyday example, a speaker who instructs a colleague to do something must have the authority to issue instructions and must believe that the colleague is able to carry out the instruction. Of course, the speaker must also believe that whatever they want to have done has not already been done. In domestic situations a parent can ask a child to set the table or put dishes into the dishwasher. The parent, in principle, has the authority to ask the child to do household tasks and the child must be old enough to carry out the task. There is no point in asking a 2-year old to set the table. Of course, if it turns out that the table has already been set or the dishwasher loaded, the child will take great delight in telling the parent that they got it wrong. If preparatory conditions are not met, a given speech act has simply not been carried out. The act is said to have **misfired**.

Preparatory conditions differ according to context. In the United Kingdom a member of the public is entitled to ask police officers questions about the location of buildings and streets and so on. A suspect being interviewed in a police station is not entitled (or is not seen by the police as being entitled) to ask the police questions. Hence the cliché from police dramas *We're asking the questions!* (*We* refers to the police officers conducting an interview.) In a television interview the preparatory conditions (or conventions) are that the interviewer asks the questions and the interviewee gives answers. Preparatory conditions may be laid down before an event. Some presenters at seminars do not object to questions being asked during the talk and will say so. Other presenters request the audience to wait until the talk is finished before asking questions.

A speech act can be abused. A speaker who asserts *Don't worry. I promise you'll get the books back next week* but has every intention of hanging on to the books as long as possible is breaking the **sincerity condition** and abusing the locution *I promise*. A child who declares *The dog ate the biscuits* knowing that the dog had nothing to do with it is breaking a sincerity condition attached to assertions: only assert what you believe to be true. (Compare the Maxim of Quality in Section 12.5.) A speaker who says *I'm sorry* but is not in the least sorry is likewise being insincere. When a speaker carries out a speech act but breaks the relevant sincerity condition, the act is performed but an **abuse** has taken place. Addressees may only discover much later, or perhaps never, that an abuse has occurred.

Essential conditions have to do with the speaker making sure that a particular utterance counts as a question, a command, a promise, an apology and so on. The word *Sorry* muttered in a grudging tone of voice does not usually count as an apology. When a speaker asks a question they must intend the utterance to count as an attempt to elicit an answer from the addressee. That is, they make the addressee recognise the utterance as a real question. We all know that some questions do not count as such an attempt. A recognised and innocuous type has its own label, **rhetorical question**. Rhetorical questions do not expect an answer or rather the person uttering such a question does not – *Who knows when it will stop raining?* Other questions are mischievous, as when the leader of the British Labour Party, Ed Miliband, asked the members of the Cabinet who among them was not going to benefit from a reduction in the top rate of tax. He was not asking a question to which he expected an answer but taunting the Government and the question was put in such a way that the members of Cabinet present had no doubt as to what he was doing.

Exercise 13.2

What are the preparatory and sincerity conditions for the questions below?

1. Have you received the cheque I posted to you last week?
2. Who helped Fiona to organise the party last Saturday?
3. Do you think we're made of money? (Parent to child)
4. Why can't we buy a Wii? Everybody else has one.
   (Child to parent for the nth time)

5. The car won't be ready till tomorrow, will it?
6. The car will be ready tomorrow, won't it?
7. The car won't be ready till tomorrow, won't it?
8. Can you close the window?

We return to the syntax of performative utterances. The idea that performatives have special features of syntax turned out not to be very helpful. There are indeed verbs that are typically used performatively, but mainly in institutional settings, say a chief constable saying (3) to an inspector.

3   I authorise you to take whatever steps you think necessary to find the killer.

In writing, the authorisation might read as in (4).

4   Inspector X is authorised to take whatever steps he/she thinks necessary to find the killer.

Of course, the chief constable might simply say *Do whatever is needed to find the killer* and the inspector will interpret this utterance as giving the necessary authority.

That is, speech acts are not necessarily carried out by means of clauses with first person verbs in the simple present tense. In fact, some speech acts are carried out by means of utterances containing no verbs, as in *One spade*, *Three clubs*, *Check*, *No entry*. And policemen directing traffic, say at the scene of an accident, do so without words; the conventional hand signals are sufficient. The theory that speech acts involve the use of performative verbs in the first person singular is not incorrect but it does not apply to the way speech acts are often carried out in real interactions. For example, not many promises are made by means of *I promise* unless they are part of some ritual, such as the promise made by boys and girls joining the Scouts, or the promises made during baptisms in church. In informal conversation, speakers simply say things such as *I'll pay you back next week*, which is understood by the addressee to be a promise.

The way people make suggestions has provided interesting material for analysis. The original theory of speech acts correctly points out the major difference between (5a), with a first person verb in the simple present tense, and (5b), with a verb in the progressive.

5   a   I suggest you put that topic aside and focus on the policies.
     b   I'm suggesting you put that topic aside and focus on the policies.

Sentence (5a) can be uttered by someone making the suggestion. Sentence (5b) is appropriate if the speaker has already made the suggestion. The addressee has not understood what the speaker was doing and the speaker is explaining what speech act they were performing. An analysis of recordings of business meetings showed that in five or six meetings lasting 5 hours or so in total only two suggestions were made by the use of *I suggest*. Both suggestions were made by a senior person from the headquarters of a large firm talking to the less senior employees of a smaller firm owned by the larger one. The suggestions are in (6) and (7). (The transcription has no punctuation or capital letters, apart from *I*. The long dash marks a medium pause.)

6 Could I also suggest that we agree — you guys agree who's going to talk to the customer.

7 I would suggest that X's trained to speak to these customers.

Note that the senior person does not just say *I suggest* but uses an interrogative construction in (6), *could I also suggest*, and another modal verb in (7), *I would suggest*. Of course, since it is a senior management person who is talking, nobody supposes for a second that the question in (6) could be answered with *No you couldn't* or that the use of *would* is to be taken as signalling that the speaker is not actually making a suggestion. The pragmalinguistic norms of hierarchical institutions permit senior figures with power to put suggestions in this way to junior figures with less power, but not somebody addressing a person of the same rank or somebody senior. A junior figure could ask *Can I make a suggestion?* but would wait for permission to be given – *Sure, go on*. The recordings of the business meetings show that in the other 269 chunks in which some action was recommended as being desirable or bringing some benefit, the speakers used different grammar and vocabulary. Examples are in (8).

8 a I think we could stretch ourselves a lot more than we do
   b but also I think today maybe we could establish what X's job requirement's gotta be
   c and why don't you tell 'em that you'll no be accepting anything unless it's through the system?
   d and everyone's in a rush and if we can turn that around you know

In (8a,b) the speakers use *I think* (i.e. it's just my personal opinion) and *could* (I'm putting this tentatively). In (8c) the speaker uses a wh interrogative, leaving it open for the other people at the meeting to give reasons why the proposed action is not desirable. In (8d) the speaker uses a conditional clause, *if we can turn that around*, which is also a very tentative way of putting the idea, and signals the need for the addressees to confirm that they agree with the use of *you know*. *You know* is an appeal for solidarity. It is worth repeating that the speakers and addressees are of equal status in the firm. Any suggestions can be argued against and rejected.

It is not always straightforward to figure out what act a speaker is performing with an utterance. The pleasing literary example in (9) comes from Helen Dunsmore's novel, *The Betrayal*.

9 The mother pauses, holding the door handle, and looks back at Andrei. 'He's my only one,' she says, and he can't tell from her tone if it's a plea, a threat or a warning.

He's my only one is a declarative clause conveying a statement. It's what the speaker is doing with the statement that the listener, a hospital doctor, can't determine. In Terry Pratchett's novel *Snuff*, a blacksmith is co-opted into a rural police force.

The one member of that force, who has the exaggerated rank and name of *Chief Constable Upshot*, writes on the badge the legend in (10).

10   Constable Jefferson works for me. Be told! (Chief Constable Upshot)

What is the force of *Be told!*? It makes sure that people reading the badge do not dismiss it as a piece of playacting and signals that the statement has not been made idly but is a serious warning.

Speech acts are not a simple phenomenon. Nonetheless, they are an integral part of everyday communication and children very quickly learn about commands, such as *Don't touch, Stay there, Give it to Mummy/Daddy* and so on. Austin distinguished between **direct** and **indirect speech acts**. *Shut the door (please)* is a direct speech act, a command delivered by means of an imperative clause, the principal function of imperative clauses being to convey commands. In contrast, in the right circumstances the interrogative clause *Can you feel a draught in here?* can be understood as an indirect request to shut the door or window. Children too learn about indirect speech acts. Typical ones are *Hot!* or *Sharp!* Accompanied by mimes and exclamations such as *Ow!*, these function as indirect commands not to touch something. (Some children, alas, feel compelled to find out for themselves and touch something hot, usually only once.) Some indirect speech acts are highly conventional. Recently, the second author had to explain to a 10-year-old granddaughter that the question *Do you know we have a dishwasher?* was not a direct request for information but an indirect request to carry the dirty crockery and cutlery over to the dishwasher and load it.

We end this section with some remarks on speech acts and grammar. The analysis of speech acts, right from the initial work by Austin, has focused on situations in which the uttering of some formula is either one essential component of an action or by itself constitutes the action. The actions are public ceremonial rituals such as baptising and sentencing in court and the associated performative utterances are said to have various forces, including **illocutionary force**, to do with whether an utterance conveys a statement, a question or a command. We can take a slightly different view and consider making statements, asking questions and issuing commands as in themselves actions and indeed speech acts, each type with its special construction. There are three other speech acts that are intimately bound up with grammar. We touched on one of them in the previous chapter when we saw that denotation is the set of entities a given lexical item connects with in the world outside language. **Reference**, in contrast, is an act, the use of language to draw listeners' and readers' attention to some entity.

In very traditional terms, a speaker or writer refers to some entity, sets it up at the beginning of a clause, and then assigns some property to it. Thus, in *The dog barked* the property of barking at some time in the past is assigned to the dog. In *The dog is black* the property of being black is assigned. The traditional label for this action, in linguistics and logic, is **predication** – speakers predicate a property of some entity. The third action is **modification**; having set up an entity and predicated a property of it, speakers can add information about the entity or about the predicated property. In *the black dog we saw yesterday* the extra pieces of information are conveyed by *black* and *that we saw yesterday*. In *The dog barked excitedly* the extra information is conveyed by *excitedly*. Depending on what the modification applies to, the speaker chooses an adjective, relative clause, prepositional phrase (for nouns) and adverbs (for verbs). To signal an action of reference, speakers choose nouns; to signal actions of predicating, they choose verbs. The actions of referring and predicating are so central and essential to communication that all languages have ways of signalling which action has been performed, either by the choice of different lexical items traditionally called nouns and verbs and/or by special grammatical markers, such as definite articles for referring.

13.5   Conversation: scripts and routines

Our earlier discussion of scripts focused on who says what and when in formal inter-actions such as consulting a doctor, explaining to police or going through security checks at airports. Perhaps surprisingly, what we consider 'ordinary' conversation is also controlled by scripts, though not so rigidly. Scripts for conversation include information about turn-taking, about sequences of utterances such as question and answer, request and response, about initiating and finishing conversations, about catching someone's attention and so on.

13.5.1   Turn taking

Turn-taking has to do with the participants in a conversation taking turns to be speaker and listener. (Speaker and listener are roles played by the participants.) Typically a speaker finishes what they have to say and allows the listener to have a turn at speaking. The speaker is said to '**yield the floor**' to another participant. This is achieved by a long silent pause and/or by a fall in intonation to signal the end of an utterance. The handing over of the turn may be done by verbal means, asking a question such as *Do you think that's OK?* or by using a tag question, *We could go tomorrow afternoon, couldn't we?* The 'handover' effect can be increased by having a long pause between the statement *We could go tomorrow afternoon* and the tag question *couldn't we?*

Instead of waiting until the speaker finishes and yields the floor, the listener can **claim the floor**. That is, the listener can interrupt someone's turn, preferably without offending or annoying the current speaker. To do this the listener has to indicate their wish to speak by making eye contact and perhaps by a head nod or a hand movement, and by uttering *ahem* or *Excuse me* or even, in more formal situations, *Can I just say something?* The speaker may of course refuse to yield the floor, increasing their rate of speech and the amplitude and perhaps signalling by a hand movement that the other interlocutor should wait. The speaker may also say *Could I just finish this sentence?* or *Just let me finish this sentence.* The second author had a colleague who would become disfluent when their turn was threatened. This was a very effective deterrent to anyone wishing to claim the floor.

There is no point in beginning to speak unless the intended listener is listening. Would-be speakers need to know how to catch attention. Small children often do this by taking hold of a parent's clothing or by saying *Mum, Dad, Grandpa* and so on. A speaker claiming the floor after a period of silence may attract attention by saying the intended listener's name, and the person addressed may signal that they are listening, as in (11).

11   A1   Margaret.

    B1   Uh-huh.

    A2   Have you seen the blue scissors?

A longer attention-getting token is at A1 in (12).

12   A1   Hey Margaret, look at that!

    B2   What?

    A2   Look what the dog is barking at!

A person wishing to break into an ongoing conversation is expected to offer an apology and may even wait for consent to be given, as in (13).

13   A   Sorry to interrupt but something urgent has come up.

    B   No problem. On you go.

    A   Can you give advice to a customer?

    B   Sure.

13.5.2 Adjacency pairs

Turn-taking is influenced by the phenomenon of **adjacency pairs**. These are generally recognised sequences of turns in which the first turn normally obliges the listener to respond with a second turn, and to a large extent determines the nature of the second turn. Commonly occurring adjacency pairs are question and answer, invitation and acceptance (or refusal), greeting and greeting, offer and acceptance. A straightforward example of question and answer is in (14).

14   A1   Excuse me.

    B2   Yes.

    A2   Can you tell me if the Linguistics books are on this floor?

    B2   Yes. They're at the far end of the stacks.

The question–answer pair are A2 and B2. The yes–no question at A2 elicits a *yes* and further information. A doesn't explicitly ask for this information but B realises that A does not know the layout of the library. Note that A2 is prefaced by the attention-getting token *Excuse me*. This is a very simple question–answer pair, but in many situations the person requesting information may not understand the reply and has to ask for clarification or confirmation, while the person giving information may check that the information is understood. Consider the exchange in (15).

15 A1 Can you tell me how to get to the train station?

    B2 Yes. You go straight down this street and at the far end you turn right and then take the second street on the left. Just after the café with the blue door.

    A2 OK. So, turn right and then the second street on the left?

    B2 That's right.

A2 is a request for confirmation. Sometimes checking and confirming are achieved by very short utterances, as in (16).

16 A1 Do I go round the building on the left or the right?

    B1 The left.

    A2 The left.

    B2 OK?

    A3 Yeah.

OK at B2 is a check that A understands the information and *Yeah* at A3 is what is known as a **back-channel**, confirming non-verbally that the information has been received and understood. Examples such as (15) and (16) may appear trivial to competent adult speakers but they require skills that children have to learn. The Manchester Pragmatics Profile includes these skills on its list of capacities that should be assessed in by SLTs and it has been shown that cooperation in carrying out tasks is more successful if the participants in the tasks ask for confirmation and clarification and verify that information has been understood.

13.5.3 Expansions

Conversational exchanges are often intricate. To handle the intricacies, the concept of adjacency pairs has to be supplemented with the concept of **expansion**. **Pre-expansions** precede adjacency pairs in a conversation. They consist of utterances produced to ascertain whether, for instance, an invitation will be accepted, or a request granted or to explain why a particular request is about to be made. A pre-request is exemplified at A1 in (17).

17 A1 Excuse me, do you know the town?

    B1 I do. I live here.

    A2 Could you tell me how to get to Findlay Street?

    B2 Uh-huh. You see the second set of pedestrian lights? Turn left there.

An adjacency pair may be expanded by utterances following them. This is known as a **post-expansion**, exemplified at A2 in (18).

18 A1 Can you come and have a meal with us on Friday evening?

    B1 We'd love to, provided we can come after seven.

    A2 That's great. We'll expect you at eight.

A third type of expansion is found. This type, known as an **insertion** or **insert expansion,** is inserted between the first and second items in a given adjacency pair. It is exemplified at A2 in (19).

19   A1   Excuse me, can you tell me how to get to Findlay Street?

    B1   What building are you looking for?

    A2   The new Post Office.

    B2   Right. You go down here and take the second street on the left.

The adjacency pair of question and answer is in A1 and B2. The insertion consists of the question at B1 and the answer to that question at A2.

13.5.4   Preference organisation

Speakers ask questions feeling fairly certain that their questions will elicit reasonable answers. People issue invitations in the hope that the invitation will be accepted, and requests are made in the hope that they will be granted. The relationship between turns and the behaviour of speakers and writers, listeners and readers, is governed by expectations and conventions known as preference organisation. Positive responses are **preferred** and negative responses are **dispreferred**. Mature, healthy speakers have an intuitive understanding of this **preference structure**. Interlocutors who find themselves in the position of making a dispreferred response typically signal ahead that their response is negative, either by a delay in replying or by a filler such as *uhm, well, dunno* plus an excuse. Examples are in (17) and (18).

17   A1   Will you be driving to Manchester tomorrow?

    B1   [Silence]

    A2   It doesn't matter if you're not. I can easily drive over to your place
        and pick you up.

A is wondering if B will drive him to work the next day. When it becomes clear that B can't or won't drive to Manchester, A avoids a disagreement by stating that it doesn't make any big difference who does the driving. B does not offer an excuse, but does in (18).

18   A1   Any chance you can help me move to my new flat this evening?

    B1   [Silence] Thing is, I've got to take the kids to their judo practice.

    A2   No problem. I think my brother is coming over anyway.

The person making a request or issuing invitation can avoid disagreement by making a **pre-invitation** or a **pre-request**. That is, before inviting or requesting, they test the water by asking another question, as in (19).

19   A1   Are you busy this weekend?

    B1   I'm going to visit my sister. I haven't seen her new flat yet and she
        moved in six months ago.

A does not issue an invitation but ascertains whether B is going to be busy. B does not answer bluntly *yes* but provides an account of why they are going to be busy. A's question is relatively indirect but is still recognised by B as a possible precursor to some invitation or request. A could have asked *Are you free this weekend?*, which is an undisguised lead-up to an invitation or request. The essential point is that by making a pre-invitation A avoids the unpleasantness of B turning down the invitation, even if for genuine alternative commitments.

The final skill we consider here is the ability to begin, continue and finish a conversation. Young children do not have these skills but simply say what they have to say when the urge takes them. Learning not to interrupt an ongoing conversation can take some time. Finishing a conversation smoothly and without giving offence is likewise a skill that children take time to learn. Some adults do not have these skills either. The second author knows an adult male with mild Asperger's who never initiates a conversation but will reply, sometimes at length, to questions.

13.5.5   Opening a conversation

Healthy adult speakers are able to open a conversational interaction, even with strangers. One might even consider the ability to open a conversation with strangers as particularly valuable, since everyone from time to time finds themselves having to engage with strangers. Typically, the potential participants in a conversation cooperate in its opening. This is achieved by linguistic but also by paralinguistic means such as getting eye contact, making some welcoming gesture with arm or hand and smiling. The opening linguistic contribution to the conversation may refer to something worthy of talk, such as a newspaper headline, as in (20a), or something salient in the context such as a dog, as in (20b).

20 a   Do you think petrol prices are going to go up again?
    b   She's very friendly. How old is she?

It may be about supremely obvious topics such as the weather (*Nice day – makes a change.*) or the local environment (*Great view*). The opening phase of a conversation is a social negotiation. It allows friends and acquaintances to renew their relationship; it allows strangers to engage with each other and escape social loneliness. The rather exotic technical term for such exchanges is '**phatic communion**'. ('Phatic' is based on the Greek *phatos* 'said' and *phatis* 'a common saying, speech'.) The term was originally defined as a type of speech in which ties of union were created by the mere exchange of words. Later definitions talk of physical and psychological contact between people. Phatic communion also covers techniques of ending conversations, whether with strangers, acquaintances or friends. A close friend can say *Well, I'm off. I'll send you an e-mail* and depart. With strangers or acquaintances the pragmalinguistic norms in Britain are that bringing the conversation to a close requires careful handling. One speaker can say *I'm sorry. I've got to go now. I'm meeting my wife.* With this utterance the speaker offers an apology and an explanation. (It's not that I'm tired of your company. My wife is waiting for me.) And only to a close friend is one likely to say *Well, can't stand around talking all day – things to do – see you.*

An opening can of course be rejected, a signal that there could be trouble and that a conversation is best avoided. A good example of an extreme rejection is the following (real) exchange that took place at a short Saturday morning concert for subscribers to a particular orchestra. The concert hall was not full. A middle-aged woman sat down next to an elderly man sitting with his wife. The man did not respond to a smile and seemed put out that someone had occupied the seat next to him. At the end of the concert, the man and his wife stood up. The middle-aged woman put on her coat, helped by her husband, and started to collect her handbag, hat and gloves and scarf, which she had put under her seat. She smiled apologetically at the elderly man and said *Just gathering my bits and pieces*, to which he replied in an unfriendly tone *I'm in a hurry*. No point in continuing that conversation.

13.5.6   Politeness

The above routines are learned by typically developing young speakers and practised by adults with a normal competence in the language. The routines also require a competence in **politeness**, a property that some people seem to possess naturally, that other people have to work at and that some people do not bother with except when talking to people more powerful in some respect than they are. Being polite begins with children learning to say *Please* and *Thank you*, at least in English-speaking cultures but that is just the first step in acquiring a large network of routines, tactics, appropriate phrases and gestures. The general principles are not to make others lose face, to handle disagreements tactfully and to be sympathetic when necessary. The principles do not necessarily apply between seniors and juniors in institutional settings such as the army and police, or financial organs and industrial enterprises, but they do smooth interactions in many other contexts. *Excuse me, could you tell me where the Post Office is?* is more polite as an opening to a stranger than *Where's the Post Office?* and *I'm sorry, I didn't catch that* is much more polite, and in some contexts much safer, than *Don't mumble!*

13.5.7   Topic management

At this point we anticipate the discussion of **coherence** in Section 14.3. That section focuses on narrative and the fact that narratives cannot be followed and interpreted unless they present events that are related and involve the same characters and unless new characters are properly introduced into the story. Similar restrictions apply to conversation. Interlocutors cannot participate in a conversation if everyone talks about something different and if each interlocutor ignores what the others are saying. In everyday terms, interlocutors have to stick to the topic of conversation, or, if they want to bring in new topics of conversation, they can switch to a topic that is related in some way to the current topic or they can announce a completely new topic, possibly asking the other interlocutors if they have any objections.

Topics of conversation are controlled by conventions of **topic management**. They include conventions for **topic maintenance**, that is, making sure the interlocutors keep to the current topic, and conventions for **topic shift,** that is, moving from the current topic to a new one. They also include conventions for **topic introduction,** that is, proposing and establishing an initial topic in a conversation.

In many conversations topic maintenance is not difficult. There is an overarching topic, sometimes called a **supertopic,** and the interlocutors move through a series of **subtopics** related to the supertopic, slipping easily from one subtopic to the next. Consider the conversation in (21). It is an edited version of a real conversation recorded as part of a research project some years ago. The names of people mentioned have been changed and the name of the firm referred to in B8 is fictitious. The two participants have just graduated from university. Both were married students with families. The supertopic of the conversation is 'Married University Students' and the subtopics are

A1–A2   'Children'
B2–A3   'Participant's ages'
A4–B4   'Age at marriage and birth of first child'
B4–B6   'Financing one's studies'
B6–B7   'Earning money while studying'
A8–B10 'Getting a job after graduating'

21 A1   Have you got any children?

    B1   Yes. Carole is ehm three.

    A2   Three?

    B2   Yes. I was married young.

    A3   You must've been. How old are you anyway?

    B3   I'll be twenty three in July.

    A4   So you got married when you were at university?

    B4   I got married in my second year. Third year the baby arrived. I didn't get any extra grant you know.

    A5   No. That's right. You've got to be twenty six or something.

    B5   In fact I was still under parental contribution you know. Absolutely ridiculous.

    A6   Well there's another guy I know that was in exactly the same situation. In fact he was married before he went to university. He'd been married for years and he was the same thing: applied parental contribution.

    B6   My mother wouldn't have accepted that she should still fork out for me but we managed all right. My wife worked a lot and she's good with money. We managed fine really. And I had a part time job for all the time I was at university, practically.

    A7   Did you? Yes, I remember once you were talking about you and Phil Watson tiling roofs or something. Is that right?

B7   Yes. It was Phil. Actually I didn't get on that well with Phil so I didn't apply for the roofing job. I only knew him because of this other guy that I used to mess about with. He knew Phil quite well.

A8   I see. How did you get this job then? Was it advertised or was it just . . .

B8   No, it wasn't advertised. They asked me to come and do it. I had a job as a trainee sales manager with British Flours.

A9   But this is better.

B9   This is a much better job. It's more interesting.

A10   Well, it's something to do with the degree you've got.

B10   The only thing is, it's a temporary job. I'll soon have to look for something else.

The changes from one subtopic are so smooth that the interlocutors show no sign of being aware the topic shifts or of trying to prevent any of them. The topic shifts are not even easily spotted by external analysts working on the transcription. In contrast, consider the extract of conversation in (22). This is taken from a real conversation recorded as part of the same research project as (21). We looked at it in Section 11.3.8 when discussing deixis; we will see that the use of *this technician* in A4 is related to topic-maintenance.

22   A1   So how long were you off for

B1   four days

A2   four days oh dear

B2   it was great fun – I I didn't have any appetite so I existed on oranges and I lost about three pounds

A3   goodness me

C1   you'll have put it back on by now

B3   I know – start putting it back on again – eating a bit more yeah it's unfair – that technician – I think he ought to be shot

C2   yeah cause we're getting these films at

B4   very interesting films with any luck

C3   sex education

B5   they're boring at the beginning

C4   and he must have slept in or something

B6   and the roads were icy – we were late – I was late in – the car was all over the place

C5   my Mum was going awful slowly

A4   so what's this technician got to do with it?

It is difficult to see a supertopic. The interlocutors start with B's illness and absence from school. At B3, B suddenly changes to a second topic with the utterance *it's unfair* and the introduction of the technician with *that technician*. From C2 to B5 there is discussion of a third topic, the sex education films. From C4 to B6 there is a fourth topic: the technician might have been late because of the icy roads. B6 to C5 has a fifth topic, a sidestep in the conversation: B and C's parents had difficulty getting them to school in their cars. Finally, at A4, A switches the conversation back to the second topic, the technician. A does this by using *so*, which can be glossed as 'OK'. You've mentioned the technician and talked about the icy roads and the problems your parents had. Let's get back to the technician *what's this technician got to do with it?* The point made in Section 11.3.8 is that *this* presents the technician as close, in the sense that he is to be the topic of conversation. A signals that he does not want B and C to move away from that topic.

A failure to manage topic successfully can make a speaker seem disinterested, uncooperative or self-obsessed. Many SLT clients need help with learning effective topic management. Resources with items that target topic management include the CAPPA, CAPPCI, CCC-2, MCLA and Pragmatics Profile.

13.5.8 Repair

Conversations do go wrong and normal mature adult speakers have a number of **repair strategies**. Communication typically goes wrong in noisy surroundings; when engaging with non-native speakers; when talking with someone whose hearing is impaired; when talking to someone who cannot judge the emotions and intentions of others. (See the passage from Mark Haddon's novel in Section 13.6.) The need for **repair work** may be signalled by an interlocutor other than the current speaker asking for clarification, as in (23).

23 A1 What time does the Glasgow bus leave?

   B1 Nine fifteen.

   A1 Sorry. Is that nine fifteen or nine fifty?

   B2 Nine fifteen.

   A1 OK. Thanks.

The request for clarification at A1 is called an **other-initiated other repair**. 'Other-initiated' means that an interlocutor other than the current speaker sets in motion the process of repair and the repair is not carried out by that participant in the dialogue but by the other participant, who has been speaking. In (23) A initiates the repair process but the repair is to be done by B. What is to be repaired is called the **trouble source** or, less elegantly, the **repairable**.

A repair process may be initiated by the interlocutor who has miscommunicated. The repair may be a simple one, as when the speaker begins a word, stops and utters another word, as in *She said there were fif- sixty guests at the party*. More complex repairs may involve the repetition of a longer utterance and the substitution of one complete word, or even phrase, for another, as in (24). This type of repair is called a **self-initiated self repair**. The speaker him- or herself notices the error and initiates the repair process.

24   A1 Jennifer might come along to help.

    B1 I can't do it all by myself.

    A2 No, no. It's OK. Jennifer is definitely coming to help.

The miscommunication occurs at A1, where the speaker gets the message wrong. B does not explicitly ask for a repair but expresses dismay and A repairs the message at A2. Repair work may be required by difficulties in finding the appropriate lexical item, or in manipulating a tricky piece of syntax, or in turn-taking, as in (25), based on a real example.

25   A1 The university came up with...

    B1 They said Dorothy would be paid – sorry, I interrupted you there.

    A2 Yes. You did. Anyway, the university said they would pay my salary up to the end of month although I was leaving on the 8th. Turned out I hadn't taken my holiday entitlement.

B1 cuts across what Dorothy is saying but realises the mistake and does some hasty repair work with *sorry, I interrupted you there*.

Failure to repair trouble in conversation can seriously affect listeners' comprehension and can lead to social tensions between interlocutors. For this reason, repair is the focus of items in many clinical assessments, including the CAPPA, the CAPPCI and the MCLA.

Exercise 13.3

This exercise is based on the transcription of a real conversation recorded as part of a research project. A was the research assistant conducting the conversation and B and C were sixth-year school students. The original transcription has no punctuation or capital letters but they have been added to this extract to help you follow the conversation. The extract begins 10 minutes after the interlocutors began to chat. One or two utterances are in round brackets in the middle of another speaker's utterance. These are utterances produced by one speaker as another speaker was talking.

Questions

1. Is there a supertopic?
2. What subtopics are there? Where do they begin and end? (e.g. from A31 to C40)
3. Find examples of topic introduction? How are the new topics introduced?
4. How is topic-shifting accomplished?
5. Find examples of repair. Are the repairs **other-initiated other repair** or **self-initiated self repair**?

6. The production of narrative is regularly a joint effort. Find examples of joint production. What characteristics mark the joint productions?
7. Find examples of ellipsis.

Conversation

A1   What about eh what aspirations do you have you know for University? What kind of life do you think you'll have when you get there? You must have some views about it.

B1   I don't know.

A2   Don't you have a picture in your mind of

C1   Not really

A3   None?! What about you? Do you have anything . . .

B2   I think it'll be quite interesting you know. There's so much to do – not just the academic work, but there's lots of clubs and sports and things that you can get involved in.

A4   Are you interested in sport?

B3   Well certain things. Like we were at an activities – an outdoor education centre

C2   At Garelochhead for a week in september (A: uhhuh) and

A5   What did you do?

C3   Well the first day we went canoeing and

B4   and I capsized

C4   and talked to the nuclear submarine base

B5   and got some nice comments about being after sailors and things like that.

C5   and the next day we canoed round Loch Lomond which was a good day

B6   Yeah. It was great

C6   And they decided they would take us camping overnight and it was one of those huge rucksacks and tents and the food and everything and walking about just about on your knees

B7   except we had to hillwalk up a hill with the rucksacks on

C7   It was like a mountain

B8   It just about killed us

C8   And the weather was really bad

B9   Yeah. it was

C9   It was good at night. We went abseiling the next day which none of us had ever done before (A: what?) – abseiling – you've got all your ropes and you come down the cliff face at ninety degrees

A6   Yeah. I've heard that word before. How do you spell that word? I've often wondered.

B10 a-b-s-e-i-l

A7   Is it a german word?

B11 Yeah.

A8   Yeah. I've heard someone – my brother did it before.

C10 it was great

A9   Is it?

C11   Oh yeah. Great

B12   Except I'm a bit of a coward and I didn't go down a big face

C12   I did.

A10   What was that like.

C13   It was good. I was frightened until i actually got over. Getting over the top's the worst part. Once I was over it was better.
It was good.

B13   We're going on a school camp at the end of May which should be similar – the same type of thing.

A11   How many people'll be going on that?

C14   Eight sixth year are going as far as I can make out.

B14   And the rest'll be third year, so we don't mind.

A12   What is your sixth year like? You know, what kind of personalities?

C15   There's only twelve of us – the smallest sixth year ever known i think

B15   And there's one girl – she's a real extrovert you know.

C16   She's mad. There's only four boys.

B16   I think she's the one that livens up the whole place. She sort of dives on the tables and things like that.

A13   There's only four boys?

C17   Yeah, but they just do strange things – like putting vaseline and oil on door handles. You put your hand on it and (A: yugh) yes

13.6 Paralinguistic signals

So far the discussion of conversation and other types of linguistic interactions has focused on language: who says what and when in an interaction. All face-to-face interactions also make crucial use of **paralanguage**. Paralanguage consists of non-linguistic signals. They may be **vocal**, such as sighs, exclamations like *Ouch!* or the one that is usually represented as *aargh!* (a whistle, or an in-breath accompanied by very audible friction as the ingressive air stream passes over the teeth). They may be **non-vocal**, such as **head movements**, **gestures** of hand or arm, general **body posture**, **proxemics** (keeping the appropriate distance from one's interlocutor), **facial expressions**, **eye contact** and **gaze**. The use of vocal and non-vocal paralinguistic features is governed by conventions and each culture has its own conventions. It is only too easy to misinterpret paralinguistic signals produced by members of other cultures or to fail to understand them. The following comments are based on conventions followed by the second author.

Head movements, facial expressions and eye contact play an essential role in the smooth progress of conversation. Nods are used to signal agreement and encourage the speaker to continue. There are two types of nod: moving the head up and down several times in succession signals straightforward agreement; a nod consisting of two or three movements of the head forwards and downwards indicates encouragement to a speaker who is hesitating, or working out an answer to a problem. It can be glossed as 'That's right. Keep going. You're almost there'.

Shaking the head from side to side once or twice signals negation, refusing a request or giving a negative answer to a question. A slow movement of the head from side to side three or four times signals disbelief that someone could be so stupid, that somebody could have created such a silly set of rules and so on. An single upward nod accompanied by a brief smile signals collusion between two interlocutors in their attitude to a third; such signals can be glossed as 'Here we go again', 'We've heard this rubbish before', and so on.

Without eye contact a conversation will not start, or will flounder. Eye contact is typically in short bursts, but may be prolonged when the interlocutors are two people in love. Lack of eye contact indicates unwillingness to talk, lack of interest or, in the worst case, lying. Not for nothing do parents instruct children 'Look at me when I'm talking to you' or 'Look at me and tell me what happened'.

Facial expressions signal the emotions and attitude of both speaker and listener. Smiles signal friendliness, frowns indicate disapproval, the mouth going down at the corners indicates sadness, and so on. Like language, facial expressions can be made with different intentions and typically developing children learn to guess their interlocutors' intentions. An adult may frown or scowl, not to signal disapproval or annoyance, but to restore a scowling child to good humour.

Vocal but non-linguistic signals are also an integral part of conversation. A sharp in-breath can indicate pain or, if made by a listener, can signal sympathy as the speaker relates some accident or injury. It might be glossed as 'I feel your pain'. A sound that is represented in writing by 'oh' can be uttered with rising pitch and drawn out. This signals 'This is very interesting'. The sound can be pronounced with low pitch and not drawn out. This signals surprise at something unexpected and not entirely welcome. A sigh can signal exasperation at an interlocutor's obtuseness. In one task-related dialogue being analysed by the second author, one participant was giving instructions to another participant. After several exchanges, the second participant asked for more information and then said *What?* This question was puzzling until, after listening to the audio recording very carefully a number of times, the second author picked up a sigh produced by the instruction-giver. The latter was clearly annoyed at having to repeat the instructions several times.

When discussing facial expressions, we said that typically-developing children learn to guess their interlocutors' intentions. Some children do not acquire this skill. In Mark Haddon's novel (see Section 12.4), Christopher Boone, the teenager with Asperger's Syndrome, says

> *'I find people confusing.*
>
> *The first reason is that people do a lot of talking without using any words.*
>
> . . .

> *Siobhan also says that if you close your mouth and breathe out loudly through your nose it can mean that you are relaxed, or that you are bored, or that you are angry and it all depends on how much air comes out of your nose and how fast and what shape your mouth is when you do it and how you are sitting and what you said just before and hundreds of other things which are too complicated to work out in a few seconds'.*

Christopher also finds it impossible to interpret facial expressions, except the most obvious ones of happiness and sadness. This in turn means that he often does not understand what people are trying to say and he either asks them to repeat it (which normal speakers find odd) or he walks away (which normal speakers find both odd and irritating).

The subtle messages that are conveyed by paralanguage may be very difficult for some SLT clients to interpret, even though healthy adults and older, typically-developing children can do so apparently effortlessly. For this reason, they are the focus of items in many clinical resources, including the ASDS, CAPPA, CAPPCI, CCC-2, CELF-4, MCLA and Pragmatics Profile.

Chapter summary

Section 13.3 discusses the role of scripts as containing information about who can perform which speech acts in which kind of situations, and what the typical steps are in carrying out particular kinds of interaction. Section 13.4 deals with speech acts, beginning with the central acts that are built into the grammar of any language, namely making statements, asking questions and issuing commands, and setting out the distinction between the locutionary act of producing sounds or marks on a surface, the illocutionary acts of stating, questioning and commanding, and per-locutionary act of producing some effect, such as a listener interpreting a question or statement as a warning. Another central distinction is between direct and indirect speech acts. Direct speech acts are performed by means of constructions that are typical of such and such an act; commands are held to be typical of imperative clauses. Speech acts can be performed via constructions not primarily associated with them; commands can be issued by the use of a question. Section 13.5 discusses the patterns that occur in conversational interaction: turn-taking (yielding the floor, claiming the floor, keeping the floor), the sequences of turns known as adjacency pairs such as invitation–acceptance and question–answer, the conventions known as preference organisation that regulate interactions and enable interlocutors to avoid disagreements, and the important skill of phatic communion, which enables strangers to open conversations, maintain them and bring them to an amicable close.

Exercises using clinical resources

13.4. Identify items in the CCC-2 that particularly refer to
   a. Conversational openings
   b. Politeness

   c. Paralinguistic skills
   d. Topic management

13.5. Identify items in the CELF-4 Pragmatics Profile that particularly refer to
   a. Opening conversations
   b. Closing conversations
   c. Turn-taking
   d. Adjacency pairs and preference structure
   e. Paralinguistic skills
   f. Topic management

13.6. Identify items in the ASDS that particularly refer to
   a. Opening conversations
   b. Paralinguistic skills
   c. Turn-taking

13.7. Identify items in the CAPPA that particularly refer to
   a. Opening conversations
   b. Repair
   c. Turn-taking
   d. Topic management

13.8. Identify items in the MCLA that particularly refer to
   a. Opening conversations
   b. Turn-taking
   c. Paralinguistic skills
   d. Topic management

13.9. Look at the section entitled 'Inconsistent Messages of Emotion' in the manual of the Understanding Ambiguity resource. Using terminology introduced in this chapter, how would you describe the ways in which the emotional content of the utterances is conveyed?

Further reading

Cheepen (1988).

'Chapter 17: Speech acts' in Cruse (2004).

Hutchby and Wooffitt (2008).

14 Narrative 1: Introduction – Coherence and Cohesion

14.0   Introduction

The programme overview of the Narrative Intervention Programme makes a per-suasive case for the importance of narrative, pointing out its role in creating social and cultural bonds, transmitting knowledge and allowing individuals to organ-ise experience and develop insight. Children whose ability to produce or fully comprehend narrative is limited are thus at risk on many fronts – social, emo-tional, and educational. For adults who lose these abilities, the impact is similarly wide-ranging.

Speakers do not usually produce just one clause or even one sentence at a time. Most of the clauses and sentences they produce fit into a context consisting of other clauses and sentences. These may have been produced by the same speaker or writer, as in the telling of a story, but they may have been produced by other speakers, as in dialogues of all sorts such as conversations and interviews, or by other writers, as in exchanges of messages on Skype.

A word about terminology is required at this early point in the discussion. The term 'narrative' is most frequently applied to stories, whether pieces of literature

Introductory Linguistics for Speech and Language Therapy Practice, First Edition. Jan McAllister and Jim Miller.
© 2013 John Wiley & Sons, Ltd. Published 2013 by John Wiley & Sons, Ltd.

or children's relating of what they did at the zoo. The term has been extended to texts presenting theories or analyses; journalists in particular talk of the political narrative, or the narrative about examinations and so on. The more frequent term in linguistics is simply '**discourse**' and the analysis of all sorts of texts is known as **discourse analysis**. The German term is 'Textlinguistik', which appears in English as 'text linguistics'. Some scholars have proposed to apply 'discourse analysis' to the investigation of spoken texts and 'text linguistics' to the analysis of written texts. The proposal has not caught in, at least in the United Kingdom, where 'discourse analysis' remains the general term for the analysis of any text, spoken, written or signed.

Adults produce and interpret many different types of narrative text and dialogue in their daily lives: spoken and written. Children too have to deal with many different types of text and have to learn how to take part in conversation, how to follow a narrative and how to organise their own narratives, beginning at the beginning and setting events out in order. This skill is necessary for such everyday narratives as how a toy got broken, how a hand got hurt and what happened in the school playground, and is one of the prerequisites for following and understanding a narrative related by another speaker. In this chapter and the following two we will be looking at the structure of narratives.

14.1   Why do SLTs need this knowledge?

Many SLT resources address narrative skills, including the ACE, CELF-4, ERRNI, MCLA, Narrative Intervention Programme, Peter and the Cat, Pragmatics Profile, Sheffield Screening Test for Acquired Language Disorders, Squirrel Story and Renfrew Bus Story. In this chapter and the next two we introduce concepts that will allow you to analyse narrative and use these resources.

Narrative is a key focus in the UK National Curriculum for studying English. The strategy for English repeatedly emphasises the need for students to demonstrate clear organisation in their written and spoken communication. The topics that we cover in this chapter are fundamental to achieving this organisation.

14.2   Learning objectives

After reading this chapter and doing the exercises, you should:

- Have a general understanding of how narratives are organised;
- Understand and be able to explain the role of conceptual coherence in creating a narrative;
- Understand and be able to explain the role of various types of markers signalling that two or more clauses are interconnected and form (part of) a narrative;
- Be able to apply the concepts of coherence and cohesion to real narratives.

14.3   Tasks for speakers and writers

Speakers carry out various tasks when they organise clauses and sentences into a text:

- They signal what a text is about.
- They signal what a clause or sentence is about.
- They introduce new entities such as people, things and events that have not been mentioned before and new topics of conversation.
- They talk about entities that have already been mentioned and are familiar to the listeners.
- They talk about entities that are salient or prominent in the context.
- They highlight information that they consider important.

The different clause constructions that we discussed in Chapters 7, 8, 9 and 10 enable speakers to carry out the above tasks successfully. A number of clause constructions that we have not yet examined enable speakers to highlight information as required in different contexts. We will look at these constructions in Chapter 15. We will see that the many different clause constructions are essential tools for the understanding and production of narrative.

14.4   Concepts for analysing narrative

We require the following concepts in order to analyse the organisation of narrative:

- theme
- focus
- end focus
- end weight
- given and new
- coherence
- topic
- cohesion
- reference
- predication
- modification

We will address each of these concepts in this chapter and the next two, but we give a brief outline of each of them here.

Theme

We begin with the basic fact that phrases at the beginning and end of a clause are more prominent than phrases in the middle. The initial phrase in a clause is called the **theme**, and the choice of theme is not random. The position occupied by the theme is the **theme position**.

End focus

The final phrase in a clause (strictly, the final lexical item) is the **end focus phrase**, which is in **end focus position**. Other things being equal, the major stress in a clause falls on the stressed syllable of the final major lexical item. In (1a) this is *Ca* in *Canada* and in (1b) it is *mor* in *tomorrow*.

1   a   I've just posted that parcel to Canada.
    b   Sue is going to phone tomorrow.

End focus is the major stress in a clause, but it does not involve special highlighting for contrast or emphasis. This comes under the heading of **focus**, which is signalled by stronger stress and higher pitch or by the use of special constructions, as in *It's tomorrow that Sue is going to phone* and *What I've just posted to Canada is that parcel*.

End weight

End weight is the phenomenon of long and/or complex phrases being placed at the end of clauses. Consider the sentence in (2).

2   <u>That the team were not going to progress beyond the group stages</u> quickly became obvious.

As a subject it has a long complement clause (underlined). This causes two difficulties for listeners (and to a lesser extent for readers): they have to wait until the speaker reaches the end of the clause before finding out that the structure of the main clause is 'X quickly became obvious'; they also have to process the long complement clause before processing the rest of the main clause: *quickly became obvious*. The second version, in (3), is more conveniently organised for listeners.

3   It quickly became obvious <u>that the team were not going to progress beyond the group stages.</u>

Sentence (3) allows the listener (or, more likely, the reader) to grasp that the clause is about something becoming obvious and then to process the underlined chunk knowing that it denotes whatever became obvious and without having to wait for an important phrase somewhere beyond the chunk.

Given and new

The concept of **given** has to do with what the speaker thinks the hearer can easily pick up from the context (in the broadest sense) and **new** has to do with what the speaker thinks the hearer cannot pick up. The decision as to whether some piece of information is to be treated as given or new affects how the speaker (and writer) refers to an entity: compare (4a) and (4b).

4   a   The <u>guy in the green pullover and blue trousers</u> is the owner.
    b   He's the owner.

The underlined phrase provides much more information, and help, to the hearer than *he*.

Coherence and cohesion

Coherence has to do with the content of a text. In a conversation you are supposed to stick to the topic or signal if you want to change the topic. A good narrative presents a story that typically progresses from a beginning to a conclusion and is about at least a constant central cast of characters. A **coherent** story moves in an orderly fashion from one event to another and avoids contradictions. **Cohesion** is the gluing together of the text in which a narrative is presented. It reflects the coherence of a given content, even by the use of very basic organising devices such as *First of all . . . , next . . . , then . . . , finally . . .*

Topic

The word 'topic' was used in the previous paragraph. This term occurs frequently in discussions of sentences in narrative. 'Topic' is a necessary term but we will confine it to the content of a text, what a text is about. In the case of clauses it so happens that the phrase conveying what the clause is about may come first in the clause. When it does, the topic phrase is also the theme phrase (see above), but when it does not come first the theme and topic phrases are different.

Reference, predication, modification

Reference, as discussed in Sections 11.3 and 11.4, is a central part of creating a text. It is an act carried out by speakers and writers who wish to direct their audience's attention to entities and who have to decide how best to do it in a given context. Predication and modification are also acts performed by speakers and writers. The speaker refers to some entity, brings it to the listener's attention and says something about it. In traditional analyses the speaker is said to predicate a property of some entity, to assign a property to it. Thus, in *That snake is very aggressive* the speaker brings the snake to the listener's attention and predicates a property of it: *is very aggressive*. Modification is another act. To modify something is to change it. In language use this is the addition of more information, say by adding an adjective – not just *snake* but <u>black</u> *snake* or <u>black</u> *snake* <u>sunning itself in the middle of the path</u>. The addition of an adverb is also modification – not just *spoke* but *spoke* <u>loudly</u> and <u>angrily</u>.

14.5 Spoken text

Consider the dialogue in (5). Parent and child keep each utterance short, but the six contributions to the dialogue make up a **text** in which the six contributions are interconnected. (The text in (5) is written, a transcription of speech. The term 'text' was originally applied to writing but in contemporary linguistics it is applied to writing, speech and signing.)

5 Parent1: Freya, are you ready?
   Freya1: Just coming.
   Parent2: Where's your shoes?
   Freya2: I left them at the front door.
   Parent3: Well, they're not there now. Where's your schoolbag?
   Freya3: I've got it.

The text has a general topic. It could be labelled 'Going out' or 'Going out to school'. There are three sub-topics: the stage reached in Freya's preparations, the whereabouts of Freya' shoes and the whereabouts of Freya's schoolbag. The utterances connected with each sub-topic are linked. Parent1 contains the proper noun *Freya*; parents need to know that their children know that they are being addressed and that they are paying attention. (That is, the parent uses an attention-getting token as mentioned in Section 13.5.) Freya1 has no subject noun phrase. Freya could have said 'I'm just coming' but in context she doesn't need to mention herself as it is obvious who she is talking about. She simply mentions the information that is new and important, 'Just coming'.

Parent2 contains the noun phrase *your shoes*, but in her reply Freya just uses the pronoun *them*. The shoes have been introduced into the exchange in Parent2 and can be referred to as economically as possible. In Parent3 the shoes are again referred to by the pronoun *they*, but another item is brought into the conversation, the schoolbag. A full noun phrase is needed, *your schoolbag*, since this is the first mention of the bag but in her response Freya just uses the pronoun *it*, since she and her parent know what this part of the conversation is about.

Parent and Freya keep to each sub-topic. If Freya2 had been *Can I listen to my music for two minutes?* that would have been a deviation from the topic. The continuation of the topic is signalled in the language by the missing subject in Freya1, the connection between *your shoes* in Parent2, *them* in Freya2 and *they're* in Parent3, and between *your schoolbag* in Parent3 and *it* in Freya3.

Sentence (5) is a text, but a particular kind of text, unplanned domestic dialogue. Such dialogue has typical features that are not (often) found in other types of text. The lack of a subject noun phrase in Freya1 is very typical, as is the use of *Where's* with the plural noun *shoes*. (And the use of *there's* with plural nouns is equally common, as in *There's two policemen waiting outside*.)

Another feature of this type of text is the simple construction of the clauses and phrases: very simple noun phrases consisting of one word – *Freya*, *I* and *you* – or two words, as in *your shoes*, and no subordinate clauses. A narrative relating the events could be slightly more complex or a lot more complex depending on the storyteller. A possible version is in (6).

6   Freya's Mum shouted to her to ask if she was ready to leave. Freya answered that she was just coming downstairs. Her Mum asked where her shoes were. Freya replied that she had left them at the front door but her Mum said they weren't there now. At least Freya was able to tell her Mum that she had her schoolbag.

The noun phrases are still not too complex – the most complex are just two words long, as in *Freya's Mum, Her Mum, her shoes, the front door, her schoolbag*. The sentences contain complement clauses – *if she was ready to leave, that she was just coming downstairs, where her shoes were, that she had left them at the front door, they weren't there now, that she had her schoolbag*. There is a non-finite clause – *to ask if she was ready to leave*. And narrators can add phrases indicating their attitude to the narrated events, such as *At least* in the final sentence.

14.6   Coherence and cohesion

14.6.1   Coherence

Coherence is a major and essential property of well-constructed narratives and dialogues. Without it, a text can either not be interpreted at all or only with difficulty. To achieve a coherent text narrators have to keep to the topic, keep to a central set of participants and relate events in order. Participants in dialogues likewise have to keep to the topic, announce any changes in topic, relate their contributions to what other participants have said, respond to questions and so on.

In more general terms, coherence derives from a good relationship between text and context. All language activity takes place in a context, or perhaps we should say 'contexts'. There is the immediate context in which a particular instance of language activity occurs: the setting (domestic, institutional, workplace), the participants (child and parents, work colleagues, teacher and students, narrator and audience), the purpose of the activity (telling a bedtime story, describing symptoms to a doctor or nurse, explaining how to play a game). There is also a wider context: the background culture of the participants and their knowledge of it, their general knowledge of the world, their shared knowledge of previous events. All these factors play a part in determining whether a text is coherent.

An important ingredient of coherence is topic, which is what a piece of text is about. Consider the following two texts:

7   There are splendid examples of eighteenth- and nineteenth century architecture in Britain. Edinburgh has wonderful buildings from the late eighteenth- and early nineteenth centuries.

8   Perhaps the best-known city in Scotland is Edinburgh. Edinburgh has wonderful buildings from the late eighteenth- and early nineteenth centuries.

Both texts contain the same second sentence *Edinburgh has wonderful buildings from the late eighteenth- and early nineteenth centuries*. The topic of the text in (7) is 'splendid examples of eighteenth and nineteenth century architecture in Britain'. In the second sentence the phrase that picks up this topic is *wonderful buildings from the late eighteenth- and early nineteenth centuries*. But this phrase is at the end of the sentence, which begins with *Edinburgh*. The two sentences in (7) do not make up a text with coherence because it is not clear what the topic of the text might be. In contrast, the topic of the text in (8) is 'Edinburgh' and in the second sentence the first phrase is indeed *Edinburgh*.

The second sentence in (7) can be rephrased as (9) to reflect more clearly that the topic of the text is not Edinburgh but buildings of a particular period.

9   There are wonderful eighteenth-century buildings in Edinburgh.

Sentence (9) is an example of the existential construction. It is sometimes called the **existential-presentative** because speakers and writers use it to assert that some thing exists and to present the thing to the listener or reader. The construction is introduced by *there* + *be* followed by a noun phrase, here *wonderful eighteenth-century buildings*. In formal written English *be* and the noun in the noun phrase agree in number: *there is a building*, *there are buildings*. In spoken English *there's* is what typically turns up, and the clients of SLTs will typically use that form: *There's a building*, *there's buildings*. The construction will turn up again in the discussion of given and new.

Discourse topics help listeners and readers to interpret texts. Sentence (10) is an adaptation of a well-known, but contrived, example.

10   He lay on the mat, planning his escape. He hated being held, especially since the charge against him had been weak. He considered the lock. It was strong, but he thought he could break it.

The passage is understood quite differently depending on whether you know that the discourse topic is 'The law and prison' or 'Wrestling heroes'. In real language use, listeners and readers depend on knowing the topic of a given text when interpreting lexical items. *Landing* is understood differently according to whether a text is about a journey by plane or a voyage by ship. *Treatment* is given one interpretation in (11a) and another in (11b). The former has to do with medical procedures, the latter with the general care and attention (or lack of it), such as feeding and exercising the animals.

11   a   The practice nurse will see you in the treatment room.
     b   The treatment of the dogs was shocking.

Basin in *There was a basin in the far corner of the room* is interpreted differently from *basin* in (12), from Charles Darwin's *Journal during the Voyage of HMS Beagle round the World*.

12   After crossing many low hills, we descended into the small land-locked plain of Guitron. In the <u>basins</u>, such as this one, which are elevated from one thousand to two thousand feet above the sea, are two species of acacia.

We can sum up the discussion of coherence thus. Sentences that form a text 'hang together' because they have various properties.

  i They share a topic and a purpose.
 ii They do not contradict the listeners' or readers' knowledge of the world or what they take for granted in their culture.
iii They display logical and consistent development and structure.

The last property takes us on to cohesion, which has to do with how the development and structure are signalled.

14.6.2   Cohesion

Cohesion is perhaps more associated with the properties of different glues (or bonding substances) but that gives us a good metaphor for understanding the role of cohesion in texts. The clauses and sentences in texts have to be glued or bonded into a structure that can be understood. The glue is provided by the choice of lexical items, grammatical constructions and discourse particles.

Logical progression through a text is signalled by means of adverbs such as those in (13):

13 First   then   immediately   now   next   then

The following instructions from a cookery book illustrate their use. The adverbs are in bold.

14 **First** prepare the chicken by chopping it into small pieces. **Then** mix with the sauce ingredients. **Next** heat the oil until smoking and then add the chicken. **Now** stir until cooked. Serve **immediately**.

The adverbs take the reader through the sequence of events, and in cooking instructions events have to be presented in strict order. You do not heat the oil until it is smoking and then start mixing the sauce ingredients unless you are being shown how to deal with disasters in the kitchen. In children's stories the same device is used, as in (15).

15 **First** the puppy chewed a shoe. **Then** she knocked over a lamp. **Finally** she carried a packet of bacon into the garden and ate the whole lot.

Sentence (16) shows how another set of words, the determiners *most* and *some* and the adverb *only*, can be used lead listeners or readers from the more general – *most politicians* – to the more specific – *some local councillors* – to the very specific – *only one*.

16 **Most** politicians draw the line at such tactics. **Some** local councillors openly condemn what has happened. **Only** one councillor has failed to speak out.

Cohesion may supplied by adverbs conveying contrast and similarity, such as *on the other hand* and *so*, or *too* or *so too*, as in (17).

17 a They won the battle. **On the other hand**, they lost the war.
    b The students were feeling the pressure. **So (too)** were the staff/The staff were **too**.

In texts setting out an argument or presenting an analysis, sentences may be chained by adverbs that overtly signal the connections between them, as in (18) and (19).

18 **Initially** it was thought that the penguins were being attacked by a virus. **Subsequently** scientists discovered that the fish on which they fed were diminishing. **In addition** the number of leopard seals was increasing. **Finally** they published a very pessimistic report.

19 Evolution is often thought of as a ladder. **Yet** this can be misleading. **Indeed** ladders allow only for single-file ascent. **Therefore**, the ladder image can lead to the wrong assumptions about humans evolving from apes.

The connections in (18) are straightforwardly temporal: a first hypothesis (*initially*), a later development (*subsequently*), an extra fact (*in addition*) and the last action (*finally*). The connections in (19) are more subtle. *Yet* signals that while many people use the metaphor of a ladder when discussing evolution, the fact that many people use it does not make the metaphor appropriate. *Indeed* highlights the property of ladders that destroys the usefulness of the metaphor. *Therefore* signals that this property – ladders only allowing people to climb them one at a time – can cause people to form mistaken ideas about the evolution of humans from apes.

A narrative may be presented as a stack of units, with the layers in the stacks being indicated and identified by phrases such as *in the paragraph below* and *in the above example*.

Finally, adverbs that give cohesion to a text may simply express the speaker's or writer's attitude to a particular fact or to a previous speaker's or writer's assertion. In (20) *surprisingly* conveys the speaker's attitude to the fact that his father-in-law had a sharp mind: often the consumption of much alcohol and the smoking of cigarettes cause cerebral damage.

20   My father-in-law was ninety seven when he died. He had smoked between the ages of sixteen and eighty one and enjoyed red wine and whisky until the last week of his life. **Surprisingly**, his mind remained razor-sharp.

In (21) *well* signals that the speaker does not accept either that Katarina's mathematical ability is unexpected or that all the members of her family are innumerate.

21   a   Katarina is really good at maths. Yet she comes from a family of innumerates.
       b   **Well**, her grandmother had a degree in maths.

Pronouns play an important part in holding sentences together in a text and signalling the interconnections. The typical pattern is that some entity is first mentioned by means of a full noun phrase while the two or three subsequent mentions are done through pronouns, as in (22).

22   **A young man** holding a book answered the door. **He** wasn't pleased at being disturbed. **He** wouldn't even tell us how to get back to the main road.

He in (22) is said to have anaphoric reference. ('Anaphoric' comes from a Greek word meaning 'carrying up'. The metaphor is of a reader holding a scroll vertically and being taken back up the scroll to some full noun phrase.) Some pronouns are said to have cataphoric reference, 'cataphoric' coming from a Greek word meaning 'carrying down'. In modern terms, they point forward to some upcoming noun phrase, as in (23)–(25).

23   Trudy abandoned her original courses and enrolled in **the following**: Physics, Computer Science and Maths.

24   I heard a story today. Let me tell you, **this** will scare you witless.

25   OK, let's give up the previous idea. What about the **following** idea? We'll sell all the shares and invest the money in property.

In (24) *this* points forward to a story that is about to be told. In order to point back to stories that have just been told or news items that have just been reported, *that* is used, as in (26) and (27). The connection with spatial deixis is that a story that is about to be told is conceived as nearer than a story or news report that has been told and is receding into the past. Note the formulas such as *This is the BBC News at Ten* (at the beginning of the programme) and *That was the News at Ten* (at the end of the programme).

26   **That** was a great tale they told. I'd like to hear more.

27   **That** was Gavin Hewitt reporting from Athens.

Pronouns such as *this* and *that* and spatial deictics such as *here* are mainly used anaphorically, as in (28).

28   a   Consider the account of the Russian Revolution. Here we find many errors of fact.
     b   We received his plan that evening. We quickly saw that this was not going to work.
     c   The king imposed a new tax. It was very unpopular.

Others, such as *this*, are used mainly cataphorically. There are pronominal phrases such as *the foregoing* that are only anaphoric, and pronominal phrases such as *the following* that are only cataphoric.

Finally, we should note that ellipsis creates cohesion. Ellipsis is the deletion of material that is repeated, as in (29) and (30).

29   Bill always tidies his room but John doesn't.

30   a   Have you written your essay?
     b   I have.

In (29) *John doesn't* is the ellipted form of *John doesn't tidy his room*, where the repeated and ellipted material is *tidy his room*. The repeated material does not have to be an exact copy of the chunk that stays behind: *(Bill always)* **tidies** *his room* versus *(John doesn't)* **tidy** *his room*. In (30) the ellipted material is *written my essay*, which is not an exact copy of *written your essay*. In an example such as *John is working in the garden. Bill is too*, what has been ellipted is *working in the garden*, and exactly the same phrase occurs in the first clause.

Ellipsis and the use of pronouns allow speakers and writers to produce economical texts which allow listeners and readers to construct interpretations while processing a small amount of text. Ellipsis and pronouns are not always interpreted in accordance with the speaker's intentions. Sentence (31), repeated here from Section 12.7, is an example of ellipsis being deliberately misinterpreted in the interests of humour.

31   A   I didn't sleep with my wife before we got married. Did you?
     B   I don't know. What was her name?

A expects B to restore the ellipsis as in (32), but B restores it as in (33).

32   Did you sleep with your wife? (i.e. Did B sleep with B's wife?)

33   Did you sleep with my wife? (i.e. Did B sleep with A's wife?)

Pronouns likewise can be misinterpreted, but not necessarily in the interests of humour. Particularly in dialogue, topics of conversation or discussion change. At the beginning of a dialogue, speakers and listeners centre or focus their attention on some entity or set of entities but as the topic changes they have to recentre or refocus their attention. Speakers can signal that they are recentreing their attention on another topic and that their listeners should follow suit. The cohesive devices in (18) were discussed with respect to cohesion but one way in which they contribute to cohesion is by signalling recentreing from virus to fish to leopard seals.

One of the tasks of speakers (and also writers) is to try to ensure that listeners and readers understand their intentions and also are paying attention to the same topic and entities. Especially in dialogue, speaker and listener can end up at cross-purposes because their attention is centred on different things. Consider the narrative in (34) from a primary school teacher.

34 I took my class to the park to look for birds. One of the boys shouted:
    'Hey Miss, here's a bird. It's eating a biscuit!'
    I rushed over, bird book in hand.
    'What kind is it?'
    'Don't know, Miss. I think it's a digestive!'

There are some small boys whose attention would be first and foremost on the bird but, particularly after a walk in the open air, most small boys are more interested in biscuits than in birds. The teacher's attention, however, was on the bird. Hence two different interpretations of *it* in *What kind is it?*

Exercise 14.1 Cohesion

Fill in the gaps in the following narrative with these words:

after, already, how, however, the, so, such as, these, to, where, which, why.
Each gap requires one word and each word fits just one gap.
Note that the list of words contains conjunctions connecting a given sentence with the preceding text, items signalling the speaker is treating information as given and items that point to other items in the text (deictics).

I decided to try and write a popular book about space and time _____ I gave the Loeb lecture at Harvard in 1982. There were _____ a considerable number of books about the early universe and black holes, ranging from the very good, _____ Steven Weinberg's book, *The First Three Minutes*, _____ the very bad, _____ I will not identify. _____ I felt none of them really addressed _____ questions that had led me to do research in cosmology and quantum theory: _____ did the universe come from? _____ and _____ did it begin? Will it come to an end and if _____, how? _____ are the questions that are of interest to us all.

Chapter summary

Section 14.3 lists the tasks speakers and writers face in the production of organised narrative: signalling what a whole text is about; signalling what a clause or sentence is about; introducing new entities such as people, things and events and new topics of conversation; talking about given entities; highlighting information that they consider important.

Section 14.4 lists the concepts required in the analysis of narrative: theme; focus; end focus; end weight; given and new; coherence; topic; cohesion; reference; predication; modification.

Section 14.6.1 gives an account of coherence: keeping to the topic, the set of participants and presenting events so that the temporal and causal relationships between them are clear.

Section 14.6.2 discusses the various devices that give cohesion to a text, signalling the relationships between the clauses and sentences.

Exercises using clinical resources

14.2. In which section of the MCLA is coherence recorded?

14.3. Look at the story scripts in the following narrative assessments and identify the linguistic devices that are used to create cohesion.
  a. Renfrew Bus Story
  b. Peter and the Cat

Further reading

'Chapter 9: What is text? Cohesion' in Collins and Hollo (2000).

15 Narrative 2: Given and New, Theme, Focus

> **Clinical resources that will be referenced in this chapter:**
>
> ERRNI – Expression, Reception and Recall of Narrative Instrument
> FAST – Frenchay Aphasia Screening Test
> Renfrew Bus Story
> VAST – Verb and Sentence Test

15.0 Introduction

This chapter deals with three aspects of narrative and dialogue that are interconnected. Theme phrases often convey given information and what is focused or highlighted is often new information. The distinction between given and new information affects the choice of referring expression, as discussed in Sections 11.3 and 11.4 and below in Section 15.3. New information is typically conveyed by full noun phrases, while given information is conveyed by deictics, particularly pronouns. Theme phrases often contribute to the cohesion of a narrative, as discussed in Chapter 14. And the account of focus will show that, like other languages, English possesses a number of syntactic constructions enabling speakers and writers to make phrases salient, which in turn gives salience to the information they carry.

15.1 Why do SLTs need this knowledge?

Like the concepts introduced in Chapter 14, the concepts introduced in this chapter are central to the study of how children who are acquiring their first language learn how to take part in conversations, to listen to rhymes and stories and tell stories themselves. The handling of given and new information is an essential narrative skill. New information needs to be presented clearly, while given information can be expressed very succinctly or even not at all. The choice of theme, the first phrase

Introductory Linguistics for Speech and Language Therapy Practice, First Edition. Jan McAllister and Jim Miller.
© 2013 John Wiley & Sons, Ltd. Published 2013 by John Wiley & Sons, Ltd.

in a clause, makes a vital contribution to the cohesion of a narrative, or any other kind of text. Children also have to learn how to highlight words and phrases in a narrative. This is the function of the focusing words and constructions in English (and of prosodic factors like loudness and pitch).

15.2   Learning objectives

After reading this chapter and doing the exercises you should:

- Have extended your understanding of how narratives are organised;
- Understand and be able to explain how speakers and writers handle given and new information in narrative;
- Understand and be able to explain the choice of theme phrases;
- Understand and be able to explain how speakers and writers highlight/focus on pieces of information and their choice of focus construction;
- Be able to apply the concepts of given and new, theme and focus in the analysis of real narratives;
- Understand and be able to apply the clinical assessments of skill in understanding spoken paragraphs and understanding and producing narratives.

15.3   Given and new information

Information that the speaker/writer presents as recoverable is called **given information**. By 'recoverable' we mean that the speaker/writer assumes that the listener/reader knows who or what is referred to. The who or what might have been already mentioned in the dialogue or narrative, or might be considered available in the immediate context or from world-knowledge. (Speakers/writers can make incorrect assumptions.)

Given entities are referred to by means of a **definite noun phrase** such as *the match*, *this player* or *that programme*, a personal pronoun such as *he, I, they*, demonstratives such as *this* and *that*, or a proper name. These phrases signal that the speaker/listener is presenting information as given. Examples are in (1). The noun phrases conveying given information are underlined.

1   a   <u>The book you asked about</u> is being published in <u>January</u>
     b   [Speaker skyping from Norwich]
          Hi. What's <u>the weather</u> like in <u>Edinburgh</u>?
     c   Are <u>her parents</u> still alive?

In (1a) the speaker uses the definite noun phrase *The book you asked about*, which makes it clear that the book has already been mentioned, and by the current listener. In (1b) the speaker is entitled to treat the weather as given because every place on our planet has weather. And the speaker in (1c), knowing that everyone has parents, can treat the third person's parents as given. *January* and *Edinburgh* are proper names. The first is assumed to be identifiable on the assumption that all adult users of English know the names and sequence of the months. *Edinburgh* is known, since that is where the recipient of the e-mail was.

Sentence (2) is an example from a children's book. It demonstrates that mentioning something for the first time is not the same as treating something as new.

2 When Mr Bump was a postman he got his hand stuck in the pillarbox, and they had to fetch the fire brigade to come and set him free.

Roger Hargreaves *Mr Bump* 1971 London: Fabbri.

Mr Bump has already been introduced. Pillarboxes and fire brigades have not been mentioned but the author uses definite noun phrases, *the pillarbox* and *the fire brigade*. The reason lies in the frames that the author assumes are possessed by readers. In Britain, pillarboxes are a prominent part of what architects call street furniture and pushing letters into pillarboxes and watching postmen taking mail out of them are activities that small children enjoy. Fire brigades are prominent through the use of fire engines, whose noise and colour impinge on small children very early in their lives. British children listening to *Mr Bump* identify the pillarbox as the one Mr Bump, in his capacity as postman, was taking mail out of, and the fire brigade as the brigade belonging to the town where Mr Bump was working. A listener from a different country and culture might have difficulty in making the identification.

All this can be summed up by saying that, as discussed in Section 12.3, the native speakers of a given language typically share lots of frames and scripts from the culture that 'goes with' the language. There are, however, native speakers of English who do not share the frames and scripts absorbed by, say, a child in Norwich. There are children whose first language is English but are brought up in Brussels because that is where their parents work. There are children whose first language is English but are brought up in an English-speaking country but not in Britain. The cultural frames and scripts available to English-speaking children in New Zealand differ considerably from those learned by English-speaking children in Britain. And of course a child with a first language other than English but being brought up in Britain may acquire a large number of the relevant frames and scripts.

In contrast with given information, **new information** is presented by the speaker/writer as not recoverable by the listener. The speaker uttering (3a) mentions the student for the first time in the conversation and uses the indefinite noun phrase *a student*. To make it quite clear that a new entity is being mentioned the speaker can use the existential-presentative construction as in (3b).

3 a A student was looking for you this morning
   b There's a student looking for you

An entity that is new for the listener may or may not be new for the speaker. The speaker uttering (4a) does not make it clear whether they are looking for any notebook at all. If they are, the continuation in (4ai) is appropriate. But they might be looking for a specific notebook, in which case continuation in (4aii) is appropriate.

4 a I'm looking for a notebook.
   ai Where can I buy one?
   aii I'm sure I left it on my desk

Exercise 15.1 Given and new

The following narrative is from a catalogue (probably not of any great interest to the typical SLT student). The narrative is placed to the left of a colour photograph of a model wearing the items described.

Q: In the narrative, what things are treated as given and what are treated as new? Why do you think the writer feels able to present some things as given but others as new?

Silk–Cotton Blouse
Always lovely, this rather light silk–cotton mix gives you all the style and breathability you demand. Exquisitely finished with notch neck, neat Mandarin collar, gentle pleating from the shoulder and self-covered buttons.

Stylish Silk Trousers
Pure Fuji silk trousers with a matt sandwashed finish. With discreet back elastication for total comfort, smart flat front and two side pockets, this classic straight leg trouser is your perfect summer outfitter.

Exercise 15.2 Given and new

The following piece of narrative is from Terry Pratchett's (1998) *The Last Continent*, p.12. It contains ten instances of third person pronouns, *he*, *him* and *his*.

 i. How many people are referred to by the pronouns?
 ii. How do we know who is referred to any given instance?

The Bursar has been shouting at a university porter making a loud noise outside the window of the Librarian's sickroom.

'That man really makes me want to swear,' said the Bursar. He [1] fumbled in his [2] pocket and produced his [3] little green box of frog pills, spilling a few as he [4] fumbled with the lid.' 'I've sent him [5] no end of memos. He [6] says it's traditional but, I don't know, he's [7] so … boisterous about it … ' He [8] blew his [9] nose. 'How's he [10] doing?'

'Not good,' said the Dean.

The Librarian was very, very ill.

15.4   Theme

The **theme** of a clause is whatever phrase is in first position. First position in a clause is important because it is the starting point of a message or some portion of a message and is relatively prominent. The other relatively prominent position is the final one in a clause, but the middle of a clause is not prominent and is usually occupied by material that is relatively unimportant.

In neutral clauses, in which no item is specially emphasised, first position is occupied by the subject noun phrase. We saw in Chapter 8 that English has various constructions that speakers can use when talking about situations involving a state or event and two (or more) participants. The active construction is used to present both participants, typically as agent and patient respectively. The agent noun is the subject and linked closely to the verb by person and number agreement. The passive constructions are all used to make the patient noun the subject. The patient noun being subject and the starting point of the message, a particular event is presented from the perspective of the patient and not of the agent. The agent can be omitted, as in (5a,b).

5   a   The car was wrecked.
    b   The car got wrecked.

Alternatively, the agent can be included but presented as a secondary participant by means of a path phrase with *by*, as in (6).

6   The car was wrecked <u>by a reckless roadhog</u>.

The middle construction presents one participant as neither agent nor patient but as controlling a given event, as in (7).

7   a   The cutlery polished up very nicely.
    b   The cutlery is polishing up very nicely.

The noun denoting the controller is in first position and is the subject, though, because of number agreement between the noun and the verb, the noun's status as subject is more obvious in (7b). To sum up, these three central constructions, active, passive and middle, present events from different perspectives. This is made possible by the fact that they allow either the agent or patient or controller noun phrase to be in first position, to be the grammatical subject, to be the starting point of the message and to be clause theme.

There are examples in English of two active constructions that describe the same situation but allow a different noun to become theme and grammatical subject, thereby providing a different perspective. Examples are in (8) and (9).

8   a   A head of the hydra is missing.
    b   The hydra has a head missing.

9   a   The sun melted the ice-cream.
    b   The ice-cream melted in the sun.

The examples in (5)–(9), whether active, passive or middle, are all neutral. No word or phrase is given special emphasis by the syntax and all the constructions are said to be unmarked. Other constructions allow non-agent phrases to be made clause theme. They are not neutral and are said to be marked. The first example is in (10).

10   Sprouts I can't stand.

The theme of the clause is *sprouts*, which is not the grammatical subject of *stand* but the direct object. In neutral declarative active clauses, the direct object follows the verb; in (10) it is a long way from its usual position, the construction is unusual, and is marked. Why have a direct object noun phrase as theme? If we think of a context in which (10) might plausibly be used, the following comes to mind.

11   A: What do you eat for Christmas dinner in your house?

    B: Oh, the usual – carrots, onions, beans. I like all these. <u>But sprouts I can't stand</u>. Horrible taste and usually hard as bricks.

In (11) *sprouts* is in theme position for two reasons. One is to give it prominence because it is being contrasted with *carrots, onions, beans*. The other is because it is acting as a bridge between its clause and previous clauses. *Sprouts I can't stand* is a negative clause, but such theme noun phrases occur in positive clauses too, as shown by (12). The direct object noun phrase *The cake* is theme and the clause is positive: compare *I can eat cake all day*.

12   A: Don't you want a piece of cake?

    B: Yes, but without icing and marzipan. They're too sweet. <u>Cake I can eat all day</u>.

The marked clauses in (11) and (12) can be avoided by using a construction known as a WH cleft. We will discuss WH and other clefts in Section 15.5 below. For the moment we look at one example, in (13), but without explanations and only in order to say what a WH cleft is.

13   What everybody wants is warm sunshine.

The 'WH' in the name of the construction comes from the chunk with a wh word, here *What everybody wants*. As explained in Section 9.4.1 on relative clauses, this chunk is a free or headless relative clause. The content expressed by (10) and (12) could be expressed by (14) and (15).

14   What I can't stand are sprouts.

15   What I can eat all day is cake.

If we put these in context we get (16) and (17).

16   Oh, the usual – carrots, onions, beans. I like all these. <u>But what I can't stand are sprouts.</u>

17   A: Don't you want a piece of cake?

    B: Yes, but without icing and marzipan. They're too sweet. What I can eat all day is the actual cake.

Another construction is obtained by taking a WH cleft and swapping the wh phrase and the final noun phrase. Thus, (18) can be converted into (19).

18   <u>What I can't stand</u> are **sprouts**.

19   **Sprouts** are <u>what I can't stand</u>.

Sentence (19) is an example of what is called the reverse WH cleft. It allows the speaker to put into theme position a noun phrase that would otherwise be the direct object of the verb, as in *I can't stand sprouts* and *I can eat cake all day*. (20) provides a plausible context for the former example.

20   Susan told everyone that I don't eat cauliflower. That's rubbish.

      Sprouts are what I can't stand.

Sprouts, in theme position at the front of the clause, acts as a bridge back to *cauliflower*, with which it is in contrast. It is prominent by virtue of being the first phrase in the clause, and for additional highlighting can be assigned emphatic stress. But the construction as a whole is unmarked because this is the normal order for the reverse WH cleft.

Items in theme position often play a role in making a set of sentences cohesive. A good example is (14) from Section 14.3.2 on cohesion, repeated here as (21).

21   First prepare the chicken by chopping it into small pieces. Then mix with the sauce ingredients. Next heat the oil until smoking and then add the chicken. Now stir until cooked. Serve **immediately**.

The underlined words take the reader through the sequence of actions and act as bridges to the preceding clauses: *then* signals that this clause follows on from *First prepare the chicken by chopping it into small pieces*. *Next* signals that its clause follows on from *Then mix with the sauce ingredients*, and so on.

The examples so far in this section have been carefully chosen to avoid complications, but one complication must be discussed because it arises from examples that are perfectly normal, occur regularly and are typical of everyday spoken and written English. Consider (22a–d).

22   a   Hopefully, they will change their minds about wave power.
      b   Surprisingly, nobody objected to the huge building.
      c   Understandably, she finds curling quite exciting.
      d   Regrettably, the team keeps losing.

The initial words in (22a–d) are known as **sentence adverbs**. That is, they are adverbs that modify an entire sentence (in traditional language) or an entire clause. They express the speaker's or writer's attitude to some situation. In writing they are often separated from the following chunk by a comma, and the following chunk is a complete clause. In the above examples, the adverbs *Hopefully*, *Surprisingly*, *Understandably* and *Regrettably* look like the themes of the clauses, but what are we to do with examples such as (23a–c)?

23   a   They changed their position on nuclear power. **Surprisingly**, about wave power they didn't change their minds.
      b   She doesn't watch football. **Understandably**, curling she finds quite exciting.
      c   **Regrettably**, at the meeting he refused to negotiate.

The examples in (23a–c) all begin with a sentence adverb, in bold. Each sentence adverb applies to the whole following clause. But the following clauses also have marked themes, indicated by underlining. In (23a), the prepositional phrase *About wave power* is at the front because it acts as a bridge back to *nuclear power* and continues the topic of generating electricity. The phrase also contrasts with *on nuclear power*. In (23c), the prepositional phrase *at the meeting* would function as a bridge to a previous piece of text, as in (24).

24   When we had our preliminary discussions in London the Foreign Secretary seemed well-disposed towards the proposal. **Regrettably**, <u>at the meeting</u> he refused to negotiate.

From the fuller narrative in (24) we can see that *at the meeting* is a bridge back to the phrase *in London*, with which it contrasts. In (23b), the direct object *curling* is a very marked theme, right out of the normal direct object position. The discourse reason for this is clear: *curling* looks back to *football* in the previous clause and the topic of watching sport. It also contrasts with *football*.

The point of the examples in (22) and (23) is that we need to recognise two types of theme. In each example the sentence adverb is a theme, being in first position in the whole clause. But the rest of each example, beyond the sentence adverb, is a complete clause and the initial phrase in each remainder is a theme with the normal functions of themes – continuing topics and therefore carrying, in part, given information, and possibly conveying a contrast. Useful labels are 'outer theme' for the sentence adverbs and 'inner theme' for the theme in the remainder of the clause. Note that the sentence adverbs are not always (outer) themes. The label 'outer theme' applies only to sentence adverbs in first position. Consider (25a,b).

25   a   He decided, regrettably, not to negotiate.
      b   About wave power they didn't change their minds, surprisingly.

In (25a) the adverb *regrettably* modifies the whole clause or sentence *He decided not to negotiate*. It is clearly a sentence adverb but is not in first position and is therefore not a theme. Likewise in (25b), *surprisingly* modifies the whole clause that precedes it but it is in final position and is not the clause theme. It is, however, a sentence adverb.

We finish this discussion of theme by looking again at the interplay between theme and cohesion. We saw in (21) that the theme of a clause can be an adverb such as *first*, *next*, *then* and *now*. When they appear in successive clauses, they mark out the order of events and make an important contribution to cohesion. Theme phrases typically carry given information and consist of pronouns. Pronouns hook up with phrases occurring earlier in a given text, and thereby help to hold the various clauses and sentences together. However, the term pronoun is not sufficient, because we are dealing not just with items such as *this*, *they* or *she*, which hook up with noun phrases but with items such as *so* and *do* which hook up with other types of phrase. This is shown by the examples in (26).

26   a   He wasn't polite to his neighbours. **So** they didn't help him.
      b   Susan is going to be a doctor. **So** is Helen.
      c   Ken is obnoxious. **So** is his friend.

In (26a), *so* links with the previous clause *He wasn't polite to his neighbours*, referring to the situation described by that clause. In (26b), *so* links up with *going to be a doctor*, which is a verb phrase inside the bigger verb phrase *is going to be a doctor*. *Is* is repeated. In (26c), *so* links up with the adjective *obnoxious*.

A final twist to the tale of the theme comes from the way in which given information is often treated, especially in spoken dialogue: it is simply ellipted. That is, it is cut out. This is shown by the examples in (27)–(31). The material that we can think of as having been ellipted is in italics. (The classic instruction in school exercises to reply in complete sentences goes right against a major set of habits in speech and in much writing.)

27 A: Who was driving the red Audi?

    B: Ken (*was driving the red Audi*).

28 A: What was Ken doing?

    B: (*Ken was*) driving the red Audi.

29 A: What was Ken driving?

    B: (*Ken was driving*) the red Audi.

30 A: Where was Ken going?

    B: (*Ken was going to*) Sheffield.

31 A: When is Ken going to Sheffield?

    B: (*Ken is going to Sheffield*) tomorrow.

In (27) *was driving the red Audi* is given, since that chunk of syntax is part of the wh question. It is quite permissible for the person replying to utter a whole clause *Ken was driving the red Audi*, or *Ken was driving it*, but mostly speakers cut out the given information, or at least the chunk of syntax that would otherwise carry it. Similarly, in (28), the fact that Ken was doing something is given; it is what the person asking the question takes for granted or presupposes (see Section 12.7) and the answer excludes *Ken was* but provides the chunk carrying the new information *the red Audi*. In the same vein, *Sheffield* in (30) and *tomorrow* in (31) convey the new information and all the given information is omitted. One way of thinking about these examples is to say that the person replying has omitted what would have been the theme if they had uttered a complete clause. The bits that are left carry new information, which is untypical of themes but very typical of **rhemes**; a rheme being the chunk of clause that is not part of the theme. Thus, in (27)–(31), we can regard B's clauses as not having a theme.

Some questions permit very short answers, as in (32).

32 A: Is Ken driving the red Audi to Sheffield tomorrow?

    B: Yes.

Some questions call for longer answers, as in (33).

33 A: What's happening?

    B: Ken is driving the red Audi to Sheffield tomorrow.

The answer in (33) consists of a complete clause in which all the phrases carry new information. Obviously the clause has a phrase in first position, *Ken*, but many analysts regard such clauses as not having a theme or a rheme but as a special construction, known as a **thetic sentence** or **thetic clause**. (The term 'thetic' comes from the Greek verb 'to put/place' and the underlying metaphor is that the speaker puts down for consideration a chunk of syntax carrying only new information. If a discussion ensues, some or all of the new information will end up as given information.)

Exercise 15.3 Theme

In the following narrative, purporting to be from a guidebook, pick out the theme of each clause. For each clause, explain the choice of theme phrase. Are there any outer themes?

The Entrance Hall

Entering the room the visitor immediately notices the sturdy columns and rounded arches that divide the room into three. The single column on the right carries two arches, and has an octagonal capital, in contrast to the two plainer columns on the left, which support three arches. Above the fireplace a decorative map shows the town as it was in the seventeenth century. Unfortunately the map suffered water damage in the flood of 1981.

Going through the door to the right of the fireplace the visitor enters the kitchen. It has a surprisingly wide stone fireplace. Inside the fireplace is a nineteenth-century kitchen range. Beside the range is an early eighteenth-century settle in elm. The wall clock is by a local clock maker. Another item of note is a Flemish iron-bound oak coffer with a domed lid.

15.5   Focus

Focus has to do with speaker or writer highlighting particular bits of information and the words, phrases or clauses carrying that information. In speech, a highlighted item stands out because it carries an emphatic accent. In both speech and writing special syntactic constructions can be used, or discourse particles such as *only* or *just*. In fact, such devices have to be used in written text, although writers can also signal highlighting by means of underlining, capitals, bold or italics.

15.5.1   Focus: tonic accent

In speech, focus or highlighting is frequently signalled by what is called the **tonic accent** or simply the **tonic**. (Another label is '**focal accent**'.) In examples such as (33), there may be a number of tonics, since all the information carried by the clause is new. Thus, in *Ken is driving the red Audi to Sheffield tomorrow* there can be tonics on *Ken*, *driving*, *red*, *Audi*, *Sheffield* and *tomorrow*. A particular speaker may produce fewer tonics and different speakers may utter the clause with different rhythms and different patterns of pauses. Speakers typically produce simple clauses, such as *Ken's driving to Sheffield*. In such clauses, the most frequent pattern is for the tonic to be on the stressed syllable of the last major lexical item, here *Sheff* in *Sheffield*. In *Ken's driving the red Audi* the tonic would typically be on *Au* in *Audi*.

A more settled pattern is also typical of examples such as (30) and (31). Suppose that in (30), the question *Where was Ken going?* is not answered by the one word *Sheffield* but by the whole clause *He was going to Sheffield*. In this clause, the words and phrases carrying given information do not normally carry the tonic; it falls on the head of the phrase carrying the new information, namely *Sheffield*. Similarly, if the question *When is Ken going to Sheffield?* elicits the answer *He's going to Sheffield tomorrow*, the chunk *He's going to Sheffield* conveys given information and does not carry the tonic; the tonic is placed on *tomorrow*, which does carry new information.

The tonic can be placed on lexical items elsewhere in a clause, but such a pattern is not neutral, being used for extra emphasis or for contrast. For the same purposes the tonic can be placed on non-lexical items such as auxiliary verbs and determiners. Thus the question *Where was Ken going?* can be answered by *He was going to Sheffield*, but the tonic stress on *was* signals that the speaker, without saying anything explicitly, is inviting the listener to infer that the plan has changed, or that the speaker is about to state some contrast explicitly: *But he's now going to Manchester instead* or *But Sue is going instead* or *But he's in bed with flu*. Note how the tonic/focal accent occurs on different words in (34) depending on which items are in contrast. Each example consists of a question and reply and the word carrying the tonic is underlined.

34   A: What's on the agenda for today?

  B: My sister is looking at <u>houses</u>.

B's reply is a thetic clause; all the information is new and the tonic falls on the last major lexical item.

35   A: Is your sister going to buy a house?

  B: She's more interested in <u>flats</u>.

Flats carries the tonic on three counts: it is the last major lexical item, it conveys new information and it contrasts with *house*.

36   A: Is your sister going to buy an old house?

  B: No, she's looking at <u>new</u> houses.

New contrast with *old* and carries the tonic.

37   A: Is your sister going to buy a house?

  B: No, she's going to <u>rent</u> a house.

Rent contrasts with *buy* and carries the tonic.

38   A: Is your brother looking at houses today?

  B: My *sister* is looking at houses.

Sister contrasts with *brother* and carries the tonic. In a real dialogue, the speaker would probably use a construction called the IT cleft (discussed in Section 15.5.2) and say *It's my <u>sister</u> that's looking at houses.*

The final point in this discussion of the placing of the tonic/focal accent is that it can be carried by non-lexical items, as in (39)–(42). The underlined words carry the tonic and they are all auxiliary verbs.

39   A: Why haven't you fed the cat?

    B: I <u>have</u> fed the cat.

40   I thought you fed the cat. You <u>haven't</u> fed her at all!

41   Ah ha! So you <u>did</u> buy me a birthday present. (I thought you might but wasn't quite sure.)

42   You've misunderstood. I <u>will</u> be helping at the party.

15.5.2   Focus: IT clefts

Words and phrases can be focused by means of syntax. We have already seen examples, connected with the choice of theme, in (10), (12) and (23b), repeated here as (43a–c).

43   a   <u>Sprouts</u> I can't stand.
    b   <u>Cake</u> I can eat all day (but icing and marzipan are too sweet).
    c   (She doesn't watch football. Understandably,) <u>curling</u> she finds quite exciting.

Sprouts in (43a) is the direct object of *stand*, *cake* in (43b) is the direct object of *eat* and *curling* in (43c) is the direct object of *finds*. These direct objects are out of their normal position, which gives them prominence. They become even more prominent by being at the very beginning of the clause. In speech, *sprouts*, *cake* and *curling* would carry a focal accent/tonic. (43a-b) are active declarative clauses that are marked because they have an unusual order of words. English has special focusing constructions, known as clefts, that allow words and phrases to be highlighted without an unusual order of words. (44) is an example of an IT cleft.

44   Everybody ran to the window. It was <u>Freya</u> who ran outside to help.

Why is the construction called an IT cleft? The idea behind the name is that you take a basic declarative clause – *Freya ran outside to help*. You decide what word or phrase you want to make prominent, here *Freya*. You cleave the clause into two bits, one bit being *Freya*, the other bit being *ran outside to help*. You construct part of a copula clause, that is, a clause constructed round the verb *be*: It *was* (or *It is* or *It will be* as required), you put the first bit of the cleft clause next to *was* to give *It was Freya*, and you turn the second bit of the cleft clause into a relative clause: thus, *ran outside to help* becomes *who + ran outside to help* (or *that ran outside to help*). Whatever word or phrase follows the copula is said to be focused or in focal position; in (44) it is *Freya*, which in speech would carry the focal accent. The words in focal position in IT clefts are often, but not necessarily, contrasted with something else; *Freya* as opposed to the other people looking out of the window.

The same process can be applied to direct objects or oblique objects. Consider (45) and (46).

45   We saw Freya opening the car door.

46   We are meeting Freya in Beirut.

47   We are going to New Zealand in February.

To focus on *Freya* in (45) we cleave the clause in two to give *Freya* and *We saw [] opening the car door*. We construct part of a copula clause, *It was*. We position *Freya* next to *was*: *It was Freya*. We turn the second bit of the cleft clause into a relative clause: *who + we saw opening the car door*. All these steps give us the IT cleft in (48).

48   It was Freya who we saw opening the car door.

Remember the discussion of relative clauses in Section 9.4.1. The relative clause could be introduced by *that*, as in (49), or by zero, as in (50).

49   It was Freya that we saw opening the car door.

50   It was Freya [] we saw opening the car door.

We can follow the same procedure with (46) and (47). From (46) we obtain the three chunks *It is + in Beirut + that we are meeting Freya*. These combine to give the IT cleft in (50).

50   It is in Beirut that we are meeting Freya.

From (47) we obtain the three chunks *It is + in February + that we are going to New Zealand*. These combine to give the IT cleft in (51).

51   It is in February that we are going to New Zealand.

In (50) *in Beirut* is focused; in (51) *in February* is focused. These examples can be contrastive: *in Beirut, not in Ankara* and *in February, not in July*. Many examples of IT clefts with place or time adverbs in focus are not contrastive but merely emphatic, as in (52). Writers often use such IT clefts simply to begin a narrative and to give a place or time a little prominence. Such opening sentences occur regularly in newspaper reports and articles, possibly to catch the reader's attention.

52   It was in 1984 that the approaching comet was noticed by astronomers.
     There was great excitement as it was going to pass very close to Earth . . .

It should be mentioned that, while (50) and (51) are the structures described in grammars of English, by far the most common structure in speech, and now frequent in writing, is the one in (53) with *where* and *when* instead of *that*.

53   a   It was in Edinburgh <u>where</u> they met (not Glasgow).
     b   It's in February <u>when</u> they go to New Zealand (not July).

These are the types of cleft that SLTs are most likely to hear in their clinics (and elsewhere).

Exercise 15.4 IT clefts

Consider this sentence:

Jane Austen wrote *Pride and Prejudice* in the sitting-room of the parsonage at Chawton round about 1805.

Convert it to an IT cleft focusing on:

  i. Jane Austen;
 ii. *Pride and Prejudice*;
iii. in the sitting-room;
 iv. round about 1805.

In each of your four IT clefts, what information is treated as given and what information is treated as new?

Is it possible to convert the sentence into an IT cleft focusing on the prepositional phrase *at Chawton*?

15.5.3   Focus: WH clefts

Another cleft construction is the WH cleft, exemplified in (54).

54   a   What I dislike is his arrogance.
    b   What they're doing is driving to Nice.

We begin our discussion by introducing a construction called a **free relative clause**. The exact structure of free relative clauses is controversial. They are considered to be relative clauses that are free because they are not tied to a noun. They do not modify a noun, but function as subjects or objects. For present purposes we concern ourselves only with free relative clauses introduced by *what*, as in (55) and (56). (The free relative clauses are underlined.)

55   <u>What was bothering Sabrina</u> was the heat.

56   Sabrina explained <u>what was bothering her</u>.

In (55) the free relative clause is the subject of *was* and in (56) it is the direct object of *explained*. (You will come across the label 'headless relative clause'. This just reflects the idea that these clauses do not modify a head noun in a noun phrase. Other descriptions use the label 'fused relative clause'. This reflects the idea that *what* represents a fusion of *that* + *which*.)

As with IT clefts, the idea behind the label is that a basic clause, such as *I dislike his arrogance*, is cleft in two. *I dislike* is made part of a free relative clause – *what I dislike*. This clause is connected to the original direct object of *dislike* by *is* (or *was* or *will be*) – *is* + *his arrogance*. The meaning of the example can be glossed as 'I dislike something and that something is his arrogance'. (54b) is slightly different. The basic clause is *They're driving to Nice*. It is cleft in two, to give *they're* +

driving to Nice. They're is made part of a free relative, with the dummy verb *do* and *what* as the direct object of *do*: *What + they're + doing*. This free relative clause is then connected by *is* with the other chunk of the cleft clause, *driving to Nice*: *What they're doing + is + driving to Nice*.

It is the final phrase in the WH clefts that is focused: *his arrogance* in (54a), *driving to Nice* in (54b) and *the heat* in (55). WH clefts have three main uses. They introduce and highlight a new entity (*his arrogance*) or a new event (*driving to Nice*). There may be a contrast: if we hear *What they're actually doing is driving to Nice* we can be sure that the speaker is contradicting a previous assertion, but even without *actually* a contrast is possible. In dialogues they are used to draw a line under a discussion and move on to a new piece of dialogue. This is illustrated in (57).

57 A1: How are we going to get to the airport?

  B2: We could drive down early in the morning.

  A3: But we can't take our car. Jennifer needs it.

  B4: Oh. That's a pain. Our car needs a big repair.

  A5: What we'll do is ask James to drive us down.

  B5: That's a good idea. He's a good driver and that way we can relax.

The WH cleft in A5 (the free relative clause is underlined) draws a line under the discussion about how to get to the airport and moves the conversation on to other topics.

WH clefts are regularly used to begin lectures and talks, as in (58).

58 What we're going to do this afternoon is consider the treatment of aphasia. You've all heard of aphasia but you may not have come across anyone with the condition . . .

In all three uses the final phrase in the WH cleft is the one that is in focus.

15.5.4 Focus: TH clefts

The final type of cleft construction that we will look at here is the TH cleft, as in (59).

59 a That's what you need to do.
  b That's why we don't take the car abroad.
  c That's where you should go on holiday.

TH clefts begin with a deictic th word, typically *that*, but *this* does occur. *That or this* is followed by some form of *be*, most frequently *is* or *was*. Following *be* is a free relative, *what you need to do*, *why we don't take the car abroad*, *where you should go on holiday*. TH clefts are used to point back at some entity that has been mentioned in a text (written or spoken) and to highlight it as something to be done or the reason for (not) doing something and so on.

Exercise 15.5 Focus constructions: use and misuse

Assume that the narrative below is the opening paragraph in a novel. It contains a number of constructions whose function is to focus on words and phrases: clefts, marked word order, passives. Are they used appropriately? If not, why not? And can you rewrite the paragraph so that it reads more acceptably?

What Fiona Dalhousie wanted to enter was the diplomatic service and at university she studied languages. It was her father who died before she completed her degree. Also dead was her mother so her own efforts had to be relied on and earn her living was what she had to do. Foreign travel she was always keen on and heaven and earth were moved by her to get a job as a courier with a large travel firm. It was her knowledge of several foreign languages that was in her favour, plus her experience of several Alpine ski resorts. To India she had also travelled. There was a vacancy that arose, the post was applied for by her, and to the post she was appointed.

15.6   Conclusion

Spoken English has a wide range of devices enabling speakers to given prominence to an assertion or question, or to some characteristic. Instead of baldly stating *The plan won't work without Fiona* or baldly asking *How are you going to persuade them?*, speakers can utter the examples in (60).

60   a   <u>The problem is</u>, the plan won't work without Fiona.
     b   <u>The problem is</u>, how are you going to persuade them?

Alternatively they use the *thing* is construction, as in (61).

61   a   Thing is, nobody knows where he put the documents
     b   The annoying thing about Ken is that he's never around.

Such highlighting devices are very typical of informal speech but occur in informal written texts such as personal letters, and even in formal written texts such as textbooks or newspaper editorials. (It all depends on the attitude of the writer to such devices.)

We finish this look at focus by drawing attention to a word that will certainly be used by (older) children and adults in speech therapy clinics and that is *like,* as in *She like didn't blink an eyelid* or *He bought like a really expensive watch.* This word is generally scorned by grammarians and arbiters of language style. It has been written off as a passing quirk of teenagers' language and as a mere pause filler. Another view is that *like* is also a focusing device. This is not the place for a detailed assessment of the data and the analyses but it is worth pointing out that *like* is used by adults, is seldom accompanied by a pause and in many recorded examples does highlight a following word or phrase.

Exercise 15.6 Focus in a written narrative

In the following excerpt from a catalogue, how are the words and phrases focused (highlighted) that are to be emphasised for the reader?

Look at choice of clause construction (e.g. do they all have verbs?), the choice of clause theme, the choice of active versus middle, the choice of subject.

A warm welcome to our summer silk collection!

Nothing beats the luxurious feel of natural fibres against your skin and summer is the perfect time to try our range of exquisite fabrics. From cosy cotton nightwear to comfortable stylish daywear we have something for everyone.

Travelling is made easy, silk tees pack away to nothing and keep you cool and fresh always. In fact, our silks are so light, easy to wash and slow to crease that you can travel light and still have plenty of room for souvenirs.

Crisp cottons and silk dresses see you through a casual day out or a special event. Or treat yourself to our very popular nightwear and silk knitted underwear range.

We're proud to offer genuinely personal service backed by our 100% satisfaction guarantee.

Chapter summary

Section 15.3 discusses given and new information. Speakers and writers present all sorts of entities as given (people, things, places, events) if they think listeners or readers can work out what they are. This might be because the entities are prominent in the context without being mentioned or because they have already been mentioned in the narrative or dialogue.

Section 15.4 deals with the concept of theme, the initial phrase in a clause. Such phrases are not chosen at random but typically contain given information, provide a connection with a preceding chunk of narrative or dialogue or make a phrase prominent.

Section 15.5 presents the concept of focus. Bits of text can be highlighted for emphasis or contrast by means of special constructions such as clefts or by means of particles, and keeping to the topic, as discussed in Sections 14.6.1 and 14.6.2, involves speakers and writers keeping the same entities in focus in their capacity as topic.

Exercises using clinical resources

15.7. In this chapter we have introduced several kinds of cleft structure. What sort of cleft is included in the Grammaticality Judgement section of the VAST?

15.8. The FAST includes a River Scene picture that is used to test comprehension and Expression. Here is a description of the scene that illustrates some of the concepts that were discussed in this chapter. (This is clearly not the sort of description that would be produced by a client.) Identify instances of the following:

Given
New
FM = first mention
D = deixis
FR = information from frame
P = perspective

For example, the first referring expression *The picture* could be classified as [given FM].

The picture shows a landscape. In the foreground is a river and there are hills in the background. Right in the front of the picture there is a man. He is walking his dog. The dog is standing still looking at something out of the picture. The man is waving to another man on a barge. This man is standing at the stern holding the tiller. Close to the bank is a kayak paddled by a boy. Just beyond the barge there is a rowing boat. The oars are very long compared with the paddle being used by the person in the kayak. This rowing boat is going upstream and is about to go under a bridge. The bridge is built of stones and has the shape of an arch. On this side of the bridge there are steps going up to a road or path and there are two tall trees. Between the rowing boat and the barge there is a duck swimming and close to the spot where the man is walking there are two more ducks. On the opposite bank from the man is a warehouse, and beyond the bridge, partly hidden by a tree, is a house. No smoke is coming out of the chimneys and the trees have all their leaves. The man walking his dog is in his shirtsleeves, so it is probably a summer day.

Further reading

'Chapter 8: Information structure in the clause', 'Chapter 10: Text and context' and 'Chapter 11: Text analysis' in Collins and Hollo (2000).

'Chapter 13: Clauses, sentences and text' in Miller (2008).

16 Narrative 3: Syntax and the Organisation of Text

> **Clinical resources that will be referenced in this chapter:**
>
> Boston Diagnostic Aphasia Examination
> CELF-4 – Clinical Evaluation of Language Fundamentals
> ERRNI – Expression, Reception and Recall of Narrative Instrument
> The Squirrel Story
> The Renfrew Bus Story

16.0 Introduction

We have already looked at syntax and the construction of narrative and conversation. In Sections 15.5.2, 15.5.3 and 15.5.4 we discussed the role of IT, WH and TH clefts in text and took time to analyse the syntactic structure of the various clefts. In Section 15.4 we considered the choice of clause theme, the position of the theme phrase at the beginning of clauses and how to analyse clauses with initial sentence adverb followed by a marked order of words, with the direct object noun preceding the subject and the verb: *Regrettably, sprouts I can't stand*. In this chapter we begin, in Section 16.3, by looking at tense and aspect in narrative. In Section 16.4 we analyse four narratives analogous to narratives used in clinical assessment materials. They contain the same syntactic constructions but the characters, the vocabulary and some of the events are different. Finally, in Section 16.5, we give an account of some concepts and phenomena that are important in the general theory of discourse organisation but are not commonly targeted in clinical resources. But anybody wishing to claim an understanding of discourse analysis and the organisation of narrative text should be aware of them.

16.1 Why do SLTs need this knowledge?

The same general reasons apply as are set out in Sections 14.1 and 15.1. Among the skills tested by clinical assessment materials are whether a given client can

Introductory Linguistics for Speech and Language Therapy Practice, First Edition. Jan McAllister and Jim Miller.
© 2013 John Wiley & Sons, Ltd. Published 2013 by John Wiley & Sons, Ltd.

listen to a story and reproduce the key points and whether they can construct a narrative based on a series of pictures. Tense and aspect are crucial in presenting events as completed or ongoing, in presenting one event as taking place and being completed while another event is taking place, and in correctly presenting one event as happening before or after another one. The analysis of test narratives in Section 16.4 goes to the heart of any clinical work. The narratives parallel four narratives used in real clinical assessment. Section 16.4 takes you through the process of analysis that you will have to carry out, and carry out competently, as a qualified SLT.

16.2   Learning objectives

After reading this chapter and doing the exercises, you should:

- Understand the basic function of tense in narrative;
- Understand the basic function of aspect in narrative;
- Understand, and be ready to apply, assessments of narrative skills;
- Be ready to begin analysing the narratives produced during clinical assessment.

16.3   Tense and aspect in narrative

16.3.1   Tense and aspect: reminder of the main points

In Chapter 5 we outlined the system of tense and aspect in English. Tense has to do with the location of an event in past, present or future time. Aspect has to do with an event being presented as in progress or as completed. The central tense–aspect contrasts in English are exemplified by the verb forms *bakes* versus *baked* (Present Tense vs. Past Tense), *baked* versus *was baking* (Simple Past vs. Progressive) and *bakes* versus *is baking* (Simple Present vs. Progressive). The Simple Past is typically used to present a single event as completed (*Sabrina baked a cake yesterday*), while the Progressive is used to present a single event as ongoing or in progress (*Sabrina was baking a cake when we arrived, Sabrina is baking a cake just now and can't come to the phone*). The Simple Present can be used to present a single event as completed, but only in sports commentaries or stage directions (*Messi beats the centre back, hits the ball with his left foot and scores*). Its typical use is to present an event as habitual or repeated (*Sabrina bakes cakes for birthday parties*).

Speakers use the future tense to present events as taking place in future time. The Future Tense is constructed with the modal auxiliary *will* (much more rarely with *shall*) and the bare verb (*Sabrina will bake a cake on Saturday*).

The Present Perfect Tense is constructed from the present tense of *have* plus a past participle. The participle denotes the result of an event — *written, baked* and *has* and *have* denote possession: *Sabrina has baked a cake* presents Sabrina as possessing the result of a baking. *Sabrina baked a cake* is interpreted as saying that at some time in the past Sabrina baked a cake but the cake may have vanished.

Sabrina has baked a cake is interpreted as saying not only that Sabrina baked a cake at some time in the past but also that she has the cake ready to be displayed and eaten.

16.3.2 Simple Past versus Progressive in narrative

In a narrative two strands can be recognised that affect the choice of the Simple Past or the Progressive. There is typically a strand of major **foregrounded events** that take place one after the other and move the narrative forward. The example in (1) is from *The Runaway Tractor* story in Section 16.4.1. Irrelevant bits of text are omitted and the Simple Past forms are underlined.

  1   The tractor <u>raced</u> down the steep field. . . . he <u>tried</u> to stop . . . he <u>fell</u> in the pond with a splash and <u>got</u> stuck in the mud.

The second strand in narratives consists of **backgrounded** events that do not move the narrative forward but set up the background for major events. *The Runaway Tractor* story also has an example of this, shown in (2).

  2   While his driver <u>was shutting</u> a gate into a field, the tractor decided to go off on his own.

The major event in the narrative is the tractor deciding to go off: *the tractor decided to go off on his own*. The background event is the driver shutting the gate: *while his driver was shutting a gate into a field*. The background event is presented as in progress and the time occupied by the major event is contained in the time occupied by the background event. The adverbial clause of time *While his driver was shutting a gate into a field* could be introduced by *as* or *when*: *As/when the driver was shutting . . .*

Sequences of major events presented by means of simple verb forms are also to be found in the two stories *A Visit to the Safari Park* and *School Sports Day*. These forms are part of future tense verbs: *will see, will meet, will have, will play, will get*. The sequence of events moving the narrative forward is nicely highlighted by the use of adverbs such as *first, next* and *then*.

16.3.3 Perfect

The aforementioned three stories together with the story *The Hungry Squirrel* offer only one example of a Perfect, and not a Present Perfect as discussed in Chapter 6 but a Past Perfect, shown in (3).

  3   Yesterday lightning had struck the wood.

Why the Past Perfect? The Past Perfect is used to present an event as taking place in past time, but further back in past time than some other event. Three events are mentioned: the squirrel ate her last meal of seeds, the squirrel jumped from branch to branch, the squirrel fell asleep in a hole in a tree. The event of the lightning striking the wood preceded all these events.

16.3.4   Tense and aspect: problems of usage

The example with the Past Perfect leads us into a brief account of variation in use that SLTs need to be aware of, in order not to misdiagnose clients. The problem is that the clinical assessments are based on the patterns of tense and aspect described in grammars of English. Grammars of English deal not just with the standard variety but with the standard written variety. Many clients do not speak the standard variety of English; if they are young children they will certainly not have much knowledge of written English, and even many older children and adults do not do much reading or writing.

Why is this important? Picking up example (3) with a Past Perfect, the Past Perfect is typical of written English and is not very frequent in informal spoken English. Many speakers just use the Simple Past. Clients may have no difficulty understanding a narrative such as *The Hungry Squirrel* but may well not use the Past Perfect if asked to repeat the story.

Grammars of English devote a lot of space to the differences between the Present Perfect and the Simple Past. The difference is relevant to written English, especially formal written English. In spoken English, whether non-standard or standard, the Simple Past is used where grammars say the Present Perfect is used. In speech, Simple Past is used for all the interpretations of the Perfect except the extended now. Examples are in (4a–c).

4   a   I never visited New York in my life. (Experiential Perfect)
     b   Your mother just arrived five minutes ago. (Hot-News Perfect)
     c   Lucie cooked the meal. Come and eat. (Result Perfect)

But note (5).

5   We've been waiting since two o'clock.

It is generally claimed that the above uses of the Simple Past are typical of American English. They are also frequent in all varieties of British English and SLTs will come across them in the production of narratives.

The use of the Progressive is changing. The accepted account, repeated in grammars of English, is that speakers use the Progressive to present a single event as ongoing and do not use it with verbs denoting states such as *understand*, *see* (= 'consider') and *believe*. Sentence (6) is an example of a verb in the Progressive denoting a habitual or repeated event and (7) shows verbs in the Progressive denoting states. Importantly, three of these examples are from written texts.

6   a   ... it may be that internal linguistic factors... are governing the Choice. (Sali Tagliamonte 2004. *Have to, gotta, must*. Grammaticalization, variation and specialization in English deontic modality. In: Hans Lindquist and Christian Mair (eds), *Corpus Approaches to Grammaticalization in English*, pp. 33–55. Amsterdam: John Benjamin)
     b   The code is often changed and students are forgetting the new number. (Minutes of final year Staff-Student Liaison Committee Meeting, University of Edinburgh)

7 a   Department Y <u>is still not really understanding</u> what it is that X needs to
       do. (University of Auckland, e-mail from a committee chairperson)
   b   She lives in a house which <u>is dating back 200 years</u>.
       (BBC photography programme, 17th June 2007, 9–9.30 pm)

Clients in SLT clinics are likely to produce examples with the Progressive that would
not be approved by grammars of English or by teachers and university academics.
That does not mean that the clients have failed to master aspect in English, merely
that they use a different system of aspect.

The final problem in analysing the use of aspect in clients' production relates to a
combination of aspect and clauses introduced by *when*. Consider (8).

8 a   When we <u>were watching</u> television, our neighbours called in.
   b   When we <u>left</u> the office, we locked the door.

In (8a), the *when* clause contains a Progressive and presents a backgrounded event.
The time occupied by this event includes the time occupied by the event of our
neighbours calling in. The latter event is foregrounded and moves the narrative
on. In (8b), the *when* clause contains a Simple Past. It does not background the
event: the *when* clause and the main clause present one event as being followed by
another. SLTs will come across combinations of *when* clause and main clause like
the example in (9).

9   We came round the corner when we suddenly saw a ghost.

The order of clauses is changed. The main clause comes first, and both it and the
when clause contain Simple Past verbs. As in (8b), the two clauses present one
event as being followed by another, only it is the main clause that presents the first
event, *We came round the corner*. In such examples the *when* clause is more like a
main clause and *when* functions like *and*. This construction is very common, may
well be used by clients telling or retelling a narrative, and is not an error. It is not
non-standard but is not recognised in grammars of English.

16.4   Analysing clinical test narratives

In this section we will see how the concepts discussed in this chapter and in Chapters
14 and 15 apply to the sorts of narratives that occur in the tests of narrative competence used in speech and language therapy clinics. We emphasise the phrase 'sorts
of'. Thanks to a very rigorous application of copyright we are not allowed to quote
the actual texts in published clinical assessments, even for teaching purposes. The
narratives discussed in this section, however, use the same syntactic constructions
and discourse devices as the real assessment narratives. We begin with a narrative
that bears a passing resemblance to Catherine Renfrew's Bus Story.

16.4.1   The runaway tractor story

THE RUNAWAY TRACTOR

1. On a farm there was a very big tractor. He didn't always do what his driver
   said. While his driver was shutting a gate into a field, the tractor decided to go
   off on his own.

2. He ran along the main road beside a huge lorry. They made funny faces at each other and raced each other. But the tractor had to go on alone, because the lorry went into a supermarket. He hurried into the next town, where he met a policeman who waved his arms and shouted, "Stop, stop".
3. But the runaway tractor paid no attention and ran on, back into the country. He said, "I'm fed up of running on hard roads". So he drove through an open gate into a steep field. He passed a cow, who said, "Moo, I don't believe it".
4. The tractor raced down the steep field. As soon as he saw there was water at the bottom, he tried to stop. But he didn't know how to put on his brakes. So he fell in the pond with a splash and got stuck in the mud. When the driver found where the tractor was, he phoned for another tractor to pull him out and put him back on the grass.

The first clause in paragraph 1 has an outer theme, *On a farm*. The rest of the clause is thetic; all the information is new, and the construction is the existential, that is, it is the classic construction for presenting new information.

The second sentence consists of an adverbial clause of time, *While the driver was shutting a gate*. This clause describes an ongoing event in the middle of which the tractor decides to run away. Verbs in the progressive, such as *was shutting*, generally provide background information but do not move the narrative on. Simple past tense forms, such as *decided*, or *ran*, *drove* and *passed* in paragraph 3, are what move narratives on.

The tractor is referred to by the indefinite noun phrase *a very big tractor* in the first clause, which introduces and establishes the tractor, but thereafter the tractor is referred to by a definite noun phrase *the tractor* or by the pronoun *he/him*. The first reference to the driver is by means of the definite noun phrase *his driver*. It is assumed that listeners will apply their knowledge of the world, i.e. the relevant frame, which includes the fact that all vehicles are controlled by drivers.

In paragraph 2 the tractor is referred to by *he*, having been mentioned three times. A second participant is introduced, the lorry, by means of an indefinite noun phrase, *a lorry*. In the third sentence the narrator uses a full definite noun phrase, *the tractor*. *He* will not do because there are now two participants in the situation and *he* could refer to either the tractor or the lorry. The theme of the third sentence is *the tractor* and this is continued in the fourth sentence by *he*. The lorry is actually mentioned in the third sentence, but in a subordinate clause, *because the lorry went into a supermarket*. Subordinate clauses do not interrupt the continuation of the clause theme from one main clause to the next.

The fourth sentence in paragraph 2 has quite complex syntax. *Town* is modified by the relative clause *where he met a policeman who waved his arms and shouted, "Stop, stop"*. The relative clause introduced by *where* contains another relative clause: *who waved his arms and shouted, "Stop, stop"*. This relative clause in turn consists of two conjoined clauses, *who waved his arms* and *(who) shouted, "Stop, stop"*.

Paragraph 3 begins with a mention of the tractor. A definite noun phrase is used, *the runaway tractor*, because the previous paragraph ended with a sentence describing the actions of the policeman. An occurrence of *he* would be taken as referring to the policeman. In any case, even where the same theme continues across a paragraph boundary, writers often re-establish the entity with a full noun phrase in theme position in the first clause of the new paragraph. Paragraph boundaries seem to disrupt the narrative flow for both author and reader. Once re-established in the narrative, the tractor is referred to by zero in *Ø ran on, back into the country* and by *he* in the remaining sentences. Note the cohesion provided by *but* at the beginning of this paragraph. *But* is to be interpreted as 'in spite of the event just described' and thus links the new paragraph to the previous one. In the third sentence *so* provides cohesion with the second sentence, since it points back to the tractor's thought 'I'm fed up of running on hard roads'.

In paragraph 4, the tractor is initially referred to by means of a definite noun phrase, since the last participant referred to is the cow. But in the following three sentences and five clauses the reference is by *he*, since the theme of the first clause continues from one sentence to the next: the tractor raced down the field → the tractor saw water → the tractor tried to stop → the tractor didn't know how → the tractor fell in the pond → the tractor got stuck. In the fifth sentence the driver is reintroduced by means of *the driver* and the tractor is referred to by *the tractor*, since the reference of *he* would be unclear. The reference of *him* in *phoned for another tractor to pull him out* is decided on the basis of context: it's the tractor that has gone into the pond, the driver can't drive the tractor out of the pond and, when not stuck, tractors can be used to pull heavy vehicles.

At this point we can usefully note two general points concerning vocabulary. The first is that it is essential to choose appropriate vocabulary. The second is that clinical assessments that remain in use for many years must be updated. The above narrative says that the driver *phoned for another tractor*. The original Bus Story narrative uses the verb *telephoned*. The Bus Story was published in 1969, some 40 years ago. The verb *telephone* is not used in speech nowadays and indeed, was not used in speech even in the 1950s or 1960s. Even in writing it is becoming very rare and marks very formal usage, as recognised by the *Cambridge Advanced Learner's Dictionary*. The word that young children are familiar with is *phone*.

Similarly, the above narrative has the phrase *fed up of running on hard roads* in paragraph 3. An earlier idiom is *fed up with running on hard roads*. Older users of British English may consider *with* the correct preposition but would not allow the phrase in writing. Nowadays, not only is the phrase used in writing but *with* has been replaced by *of*.

The syntax of the sentences in paragraph 4 is more complex than the syntax of the preceding ones. The second sentence is complex, containing an adverbial clause of time *As soon as he saw there was water at the bottom*. This clause in turn contains a complement clause *there was water at the bottom*. The complement clause modifies *saw*. The next sentence is also complex, containing the complement clause *how to put on his brakes*. This complement clause modifies *know*. The fourth sentence is compound, consisting of the conjoined main clauses *he fell in the pond with a splash* and *Ø stuck in the mud*. *So* refers back to *he didn't know how to put on his brakes*, thus providing cohesion with the preceding sentence. From a textual viewpoint it is an outer theme. It could apply to both conjoined clauses or just to the first one.

16.4.2 The safari park story

A VISIT TO THE SAFARI PARK

1. Today is a very exciting day for Mrs Macgregor's class.
2. They are going on a visit to the safari park.
3. Hui Ging Chen's mum is going along to help Mrs Macgregor look after the class.
4. At 9:00, Mrs Macgregor, Mrs Chen, and all the children will go to the safari park in a school bus.
5. At the safari park, they will see the lions and tigers.
6. Next, they will see the bears, monkeys and zebras.
7. Best of all, they will meet one of the keepers and watch a video about the animals.
8. Afterwards, they will have a picnic lunch at the playpark near the safari park.

This narrative was composed for children aged 5–6. The links between the sentences are well signposted by cohesion marking of various kinds. The last phrase in sentence 1 is *Mrs Macgregor's class*. This is the antecedent for the first word in sentence 2, *they*. In sentence 3, the phrase *Hui Ging Chen's mum* will be interpreted via a frame relating to school practice – parents of children in any given class help with school outings – and via an inference that Hui Ging Chen is a child in the class. The remainder of the narrative is tightly ordered. The sentences begin with *At 9:00, At the safari park, Next, Best of all* and *Afterwards*. These are all outer themes, separated by a comma from the rest of each clause. In their capacity as (outer) themes, they signal progression from one event to the other and provide a bridge to the preceding text. The text consists of main clauses only. There are no complex sentences and only one, relatively straightforward, compound sentence: *they will meet one of the keepers and (they will) watch a video about the animals.* All the clauses are active.

16.4.3 The sports day story

SCHOOL SPORTS DAY

1. Kelston Primary School's Sports Day will be held at the school sports field this Friday.
2. First there will be a tug-of-war.
3. Then there will be relay races.
4. After lunch, both boys and girls will play football.
5. Each class will have a red team and a blue team.
6. Pupils must remember to wear their team's colour on Friday.
7. After the last game, each player will get a prize and have ice cream.

This narrative is for children aged 7–8. As in the previous one, there is clear cohesive marking. Sentence 1 is a thetic sentence, introducing the primary school, the school sports and the day on which they are to be held. The cohesive connections between sentences 2, 3 and 4 follow the order of events: *First*, then, *After lunch*. Sentences 5 and 6 are connected by links between lexical items together with a frame relating to the structure of schools. The school is mentioned in sentence 1. Schools consist of classes, so in sentence 5 the phrase *each class* provides a bridge to the preceding text. Classes consist of pupils, so *Pupils* in sentence 6 provides a bridge to sentence 5. Sentence 7 begins with an outer theme that signals the end of the chain of events in the sports day. The clause syntax is simple, although the main clause in sentence 1 is passive, but a short passive. That is, there is no *by* phrase to complicate the process of interpretation. Sentences 2 and 3 in the above list (just a single text sentence in the narrative) contain examples of the existential construction.

16.4.4   The squirrel story

THE HUNGRY SQUIRREL

1. The little red squirrel hopped through the grass, sniffing the air.
2. The squirrel's tummy made noises as she remembered eating her last meal of seeds.
3. That had been before she jumped from branch to branch to escape the fire and fell asleep in a hole in a tree, exhausted.
4. Yesterday lightning had hit the wood and all the animals had to escape from the blaze.
5. The squirrel was very hungry.
6. Suddenly she caught the faint scent of something familiar.
7. Could it be nuts?
8. The scent took the squirrel to a hole under some leaves.

Sentence 1 is a thetic sentence; all the information is new. The free participial clause *sniffing the air* presents this action as secondary to hopping through the grass but taking place simultaneously with the hopping. In sentence 2 the squirrel is again referred to by a full noun phrase, *the squirrel's*, but this contains less information than the first mention of the squirrel, *the little red squirrel*. In the adverbial clause *as she remembered eating her last meal of seeds*, the squirrel is simply referred to by 'she'. In sentence 3, the squirrel is referred to by *she*, as the squirrel is well established as a participant and can be treated as given. In sentence 4 other animate participants are introduced, and in sentence 5 a full noun phrase is again used, *the squirrel*. This re-establishes the squirrel as the major participant and the next reference, in sentence 6, is by means of the pronoun *she*. Sentence 7 introduces nuts, and in sentence 8 the squirrel has to be re-established by means of the full noun phrase *the squirrel*.

This narrative presents complexities that the other narratives do not. In addition to the free participle non-finite clause in sentence 1, **sniffing the air**, there is the subject complement *exhausted* in sentence 3. (Some analysts would call this a small clause.)

Sentence 2 contains an adverbial clause of time, *as she remembered . . .* , and this clause contains a gerund non-finite clause, *eating her last meal of seeds*. Sentences 4 and 6 have outer themes, *Yesterday* and *suddenly*. Sentence 7 demonstrates the use of a direct question to represent a creature's thoughts.

Note that it is not explicitly stated that the lightning caused the blaze. The reader needs to have a frame of information about thunder and lightning and the capacity of lightning to set materials ablaze with a direct hit.

16.5   Some loose ends

16.5.1   End weight

The principle of **end weight** is straightforward: long and complex chunks of syntax are placed at the end of a clause or sentence. Sentence (10) has simple syntax.

10   Sabrina explained the plan to Jennifer.

The plan is a short and simple noun phrase and is next to the verb. *Sabrina explained to Jennifer the plan* sounds peculiar. Sentence (11) has the same order of words and phrases as (10) but is awkward and unacceptable.

11   Sabrina explained <u>the complex theory of evolution by small increments</u> to Jennifer.

The problem is that the direct object of *explained* is both long and complex: *the complex theory of evolution by small increments*. It is difficult for the listener (or even the reader) to work out where the phrase ends and to fit *to Jennifer* into the syntax of the clause. But, as shown by (12), putting the heavy noun phrase at the end alleviates the process of interpreting the clause (and also the process of producing the clause).

12   Sabrina explained to Jennifer <u>the complex theory of evolution by small increments</u>.

When listeners hear *Jennifer*, they know that they have processed a chunk of syntax consisting of a subject, *Sabrina*, a verb, *explained*, and the prepositional phrase complementing the verb, *to Jennifer*. They can concentrate on the following heavy piece of syntax, which they know is the direct object of *explained*.

16.5.2   End weight: extraposition

The solution to the awkwardness of (11) is simply to move the direct object phrase to the end of the clause, thereby leaving the prepositional phrase next to the verb. English also has a special construction, called **Extraposition**, that allows heavy noun phrases to be at the end of a sentence. The starting point is (13).

13   All the newspapers reported <u>that the bank had collapsed</u>.

The complement clause *that the bank had collapsed* is the direct object of *reported*. This direct object clause can be the subject of a passive, as in (14).

14   <u>That the bank had collapsed</u> was reported by all the newspapers.

This sentence is not too difficult to process, since the complement clause, *that the bank had collapsed*, is not overlong or complex. Nonetheless, the construction in (14), a passive clause with a complement clause as its subject, is not frequent either in writing or in speech. Instead, the Extraposition construction is used. The main clause is still passive, but the subject is *it*, as in (15).

15   *It* was reported by all the newspapers.

This clause is easier to process, and the speaker can either stop the clause at *newspapers* if the listeners know what *it* refers to or add content to *it* by tacking on a complement clause, as in (16).

16   *It* was reported by all the newspapers <u>that the bank had collapsed</u>.

The idea behind the label 'Extraposition' is that the complement clause is extra-position, 'extra' being Latin for 'outside of'. The complement clause was regarded as being out of its normal position because it was considered to be the 'real' subject of the main clause, as it is in (14). The fact is that examples such as (14) are very rare in informal speech and not particularly frequent even in writing. When the preferences of speakers and writers are taken into account, it makes more sense to regard (16) as an independent construction. That is, *it* is the real subject and the complement clause is not out of position but is exactly where it should be. *It* can be analysed as referring to the complement clause; that is, in (16) *it* refers to *the bank had collapsed*.

Sometimes it is strikingly obvious that the extraposition construction has to be used and that making the complement clause the subject would create an ugly monster of a sentence. Sentence (17) is a real example from a written text, and (18) is what results when the complement clause is put into subject position. The complement clause is underlined.

17   It is a disgrace <u>that at a time when so much new information is available nobody has undertaken a new assessment to determine how accurate Pytheas' account really was</u>.

The complement clause is particularly complex because it contains a relative clause modifying *time*: *when so much new information is available*. Nonetheless, the clause, which was written, not spoken, is not difficult to interpret, unlike (18). Readers of (18) would have to wait some time before they reached the end of the complement clause and realised that the clause was complete and that it described what constituted the disgrace.

18   <u>That at a time when so much new information is available nobody has undertaken a new assessment to determine how accurate Pytheas' account really was</u> is a disgrace.

Exercise 16.1 End weight

Which of the following examples can the principle of end weight make easier to interpret? How would you restructure the relevant examples?

1. Barnabas showed the new puppy to his friends.
2. Barnabas showed the new puppy they had just collected from the kennels to his friends.
3. That the Government made a mistake in downgrading the level of threat to the embassy is now beyond doubt.
4. That this is a serious error has been agreed.
5. That the directors persuaded the CEO to make illegal payments has been discovered by the inquiry.
6. Whether the attacks will succeed in dislodging the guerrillas or merely turn out to be a huge waste of resources is difficult to predict.

16.5.3   Passives in narrative text

The passive was analysed in Section 8.4 as a construction that allows speakers to focus on the patient in a given situation and to put the agent into the background, either by omitting the **agent phrase** or by expressing the agent by means of a prepositional phrase. Thus, the speaker who uses the active clause in (19) puts the agents, *the settlers*, in the prominent initial position.

19   The settlers felled many trees.

The speaker who uses the passive clause in (20) puts the patient into the prominent initial position.

20   Many trees were felled by the settlers.

The speaker who uses the passive clause in (21) makes the patient even more prominent by having no agent phrase at all.

21   Many trees were felled.

Consider now the (invented) examples in (22) and (23).

22   My sister has been writing short stories for years and she decided to enter a national competition.

23   The committee that was judging the competition had a hard job deciding which stories were best.

The examples have different topics. Sentence (22) is about the speaker's sister; (23) is about the judging committee. *My sister* is clause theme in (22) and *The committee* is clause theme in (23). There is a strong tendency in narrative for a theme to be continued from one clause to the next until there is a change in topic. A natural continuation for (22) is (24) and a natural continuation for (23) is (25).

24   She was awarded the prize, to her great astonishment.

25   They eventually awarded the prize to my sister.

In each little piece of narrative the continuation is a clause describing the award of the prize. To keep *My sister* as theme in the continuation of (22), a passive is required. That is, the cohesion of the narrative controls the choice of syntactic construction. There is no need to mention the judging committee; listeners and readers will use their knowledge of the relevant frame to infer that there must have been a person or committee judging the entries. To keep *The committee* as clause theme in the continuation of (23), an active clause is required. Since the committee has already been mentioned and is therefore given, the pronoun *they* can be used. The noun phrase referring to the recipient of the prize conveys new information and is brought in at the end of the clause, in the prominent end-focus position.

Sentence (26) is a real example of how textual pressures lead to new syntactic patterns. The relevant piece of narrative is underlined.

26   Next month the trio return to their roots, Aberdeen University – the place they first met and got together as students – where they will be conferred with honorary degrees.

The usual construction with *confer* is *confer a degree on someone* but not *confer someone with a degree* (at least, that is the construction listed in dictionaries) and the expected passive clause is *Honorary degrees will be conferred upon them*. But the clause *they will be conferred with honorary degrees* implies an active clause *X will confer them with honorary degrees*. Whatever the source of this passive clause in (26), it is clear that it is required in order to continue the clause theme: *the trio* in the first clause, *they* in the second (*they first met*) and *they* as understood subject in the third clause (*got together as students*). To keep *the trio* or *they* as subject of the fourth clause, the passive *be conferred with* is required. This pattern already exists for verbs such as *present*, as shown in (27) and (28), (29) and (30), and has been extended to *confer*.

27   They presented medals to the soldiers.
     (Parallel to: They + conferred + honorary degrees + on the trio.)

28   Medals were presented to the soldiers.
     (Parallel to: Honorary degrees + were conferred + on the trio.)

29   They presented the soldiers with medals.
     (Parallel to: They + conferred + the trio + with honorary degrees.)

30   The soldiers were presented with medals.
     (Parallel to: The trio + were conferred + with honorary degrees.)

The use of the passive construction underlined in (26), we surmise, is driven by the organisation of the narrative text. Sentence (26) is only one out of many narrative texts and the constructions *Someone is conferred with a degree* and *They conferred someone with a degree* occur regularly. Another factor entrenching the new construction in usage is the strong tendency for humans to place human participants at the centre of situations. *The university conferred a degree on Smithers* puts the university and the degree at the centre of the clause and thereby presents them as central in the situation. *The university conferred Smithers with a degree* puts the university and Smithers at the centre of the clause and presents them as central to the situation.

Another example of real narrative is (31).

31   Not long ago, workmen took down two plane trees. It had been thought that the trees might be sold as timber, but they were found to be useless for this. <u>They were still embedded with war-time shrapnel and bomb fragments.</u>

The verb *embed* describes the insertion of one thing into another: you can *embed tiles in cement* and *embed a nail in a wall*; more nastily, a bomb blast can embed shrapnel or pieces of glass in people and things. The passive construction allows the examples in (32).

32   a   The tiles were embedded in the cement (after they had been decorated).
      b   Two pieces of glass had been embedded in his leg by the force of the impact.

These are the patterns listed in grammars and dictionaries of English. The patterns in (33) are not listed.

33   a   The specialist embedded the cement with tiles.
      b   The force of the impact embedded his leg with two pieces of glass.

Yet it is this pattern that is implied by the underlined part of (31) – repeated below with the clauses split up and numbered for ease of analysis.

34   i Not long ago, workmen took down two plane trees.
       ii It had been thought
      iii that the trees might be sold as timber,
       iv but they were found to be useless for this.
        v <u>They were still embedded with war-time shrapnel and bomb fragments.</u>

As in (26), the textual pressure is clear. The topic of the text is 'taking down two plane trees'. Clause (i) introduces the whole situation and all the participants are new. This is a thetic clause or thetic sentence. (See the last paragraph in Chapter 11.2.) Clause (iii) has *the trees* as its theme. In fact the topic of Clauses (iii)–(v) is 'the trees'. The theme is continued in clause (iv) with *they*, and is picked up in clause (v), again with *they*. But this continuation of the theme calls for a passive, hence *They were still embedded with war-time shrapnel and bomb fragments*. Again the organisation of narrative text overrides restrictions on syntax.

16.5.4 Non-finite clauses

Non-finite clauses also have a role to play in the organisation of narrative. Infinitives and gerunds as in (35) are typical of spoken and written English alike. (See Chapter 10.)

35 a   Catriona wants <u>to swim the Channel</u>.
    b   Catriona loves <u>swimming</u>.

Other non-finite clauses are rare in informal spoken English but occur regularly in written English, where they are used to compress text, to convey as much information as possible in as little narrative text as possible. Non-finite clauses are regularly used by writers of guidebooks who need to pack facts and figures, instructions and route directions into books that can be easily carried by tourists. The example in (36) is a different type of text: the label on a bottle of wine, a text-site that is extremely limited. The non-finite clauses are in bold and inside square brackets. The sentences are split off from each other and numbered.

36   i   Smith and Hooper wines are sourced from two adjacent vineyard blocks **[previously owned by the Smith and Hooper families]**.
     ii   **[Once covered by the sea]**, Wrattonbully – on the limestone coast of South Australia – is today, a premium wine growing region **[blessed with a maritime climate [providing ideal ripening conditions]]**.
    iii   Rich terra rossa soil over limestone forces the vines to struggle for survival, **[ultimately producing wines of intense flavour]**.

The comma after *today* in sentence (ii) is in the original.

In sentence (i), *Previously owned by the Smith and Hooper families* is a reduced relative clause. It saves a couple of words – *that were* – but is not particularly interesting.

Rather more interesting is *Once covered by the sea* in sentence (ii). It looks like a reduced relative clause, since we could rewrite the text as *Wrattonbully, which was once covered by the sea, . . .* But relative clauses (in English) do not precede the nouns they modify. We will just accept that this non-finite clause precedes the noun it modifies.

This makes it useful in this text, because the writer can get that chunk of syntax and information out of the body of the clause, freeing up space for a prepositional phrase, *on the limestone coast of South Australia*, that is inserted into the text sentence (see Section 9.7) without becoming an integral part of the syntax. The dashes before and after this prepositional phrase signal its unattached nature and the fact that it conveys information treated as secondary and incidental.

Blessed with a maritime climate [providing ideal ripening conditions] is a second reduced relative clause, containing in turn a third reduced relative clause.

Finally, *ultimately producing wines of intense flavour* could be a reduced adverbial clause (equivalent to *so that they produce wines of intense flavour*) or a relative clause (modifying either *terra rossa* or *vines* and equivalent to *which ultimately produces/produce wines of intense flavour*.

Packing a lot of information into a small chunk of narrative is useful for documents that have to be easy to carry, such as papers for a meeting. But compressed text requires a lot of processing effort from readers (and would require too much processing effort from listeners). The non-finite clauses in (36) are not easy to process but the narrative could be much simplified, as in (37).

37   Smith and Hooper wines are sourced from two adjacent vineyard blocks that previously belonged to the Smith and Hooper families. Wrattonbully is on the limestone coast of South Australia and was once covered by the sea. Today it is a premium wine growing region with a maritime climate providing ideal ripening conditions. The vines struggle to survive on the rich terra rossa soil over limestone and therefore produce wines of intense flavour.

Sentence (37) contains 72 words as against 67 in (36). It has only one non-finite clause, *providing ideal ripening conditions*. There is one finite relative clause: *that previously belonged to the Smith and Hooper families*. The rest of the clauses are main clauses. There are no phrases in apposition. The small increase in the number of words is more than offset by the simpler syntax and the easier processing.

Chapter summary

Section 16.3 offers an account of tense and aspect in narrative, with a sub-section on uses that SLTs are likely to come across in their clinical work.

Section 16.4 contains an analysis of four narratives analogous to narratives contained in clinical assessment materials.

Section 16.5 ties some loose ends relating to the interconnections between syntactic constructions and the organisation of narrative. In particular it deals with end weight, the positioning of long and complex phrases or clauses at the end of sentences; with the role of the passive in preserving cohesion; and with the role of non-finite clauses in allowing a large quantity of information to be packed into a small amount of text.

Exercises using clinical resources

As we have seen in the last few chapters, narrative requires deployment of a wide range of linguistic devices. These exercises draw together some of these in the analysis of narratives based on pictures used in clinical resources.

16.2. Below is a description of the Cookie Theft Picture in the Boston Diagnostic Aphasia Examination (not the sort of description that would be produced by a typical SLT client, but useful for present purposes). Analyse it to identify the structures that have been discussed in Chapters 11–16; in particular, identify the following:
Progressive
Simple Present
Perf = Perfect
'be going to' Future
first mention

deixis
information from frame
perspective
generic reference
clause theme (follows the theme phrase)

Almost in the middle of the picture you can see a woman in a kitchen. Behind her are two children, a girl and a boy. The woman is standing at the kitchen sink. She's drying a plate and seems to be thinking about something else because she has not noticed that the water is pouring over the edge of the sink and on to the floor. But she will probably notice quite soon because a puddle of water has appeared round her feet and is getting bigger. On the countertop beside the sink are two small bowls and a plate. It looks as though the family have just had lunch. Along the end wall of the kitchen is a row of cupboards and in one of them, on the top shelf, is a jar of biscuits. The boy has climbed up on a three-legged stool so that he can reach the jar. He has taken one biscuit from the jar and has been handing it to the girl. Unfortunately three-legged stools are not very stable and the stool has begun to topple over. The girl is reaching out her hand to take the biscuit the boy is holding out to her but there is going to be a nasty accident. The boy is going to fall to the floor and unless he lets go, he'll pull the jar of biscuits down with him.

16.3. The following is a description based on the pictures in the ERRNI Fish Story. Identify the narrative features listed below.
Progressive
Simple Present
Perfect
Theme

The story begins in the living room of a house. A boy is standing beside a fish tank containing one fish. His mother comes into the room and he asks if he can have money to buy another fish to keep the first one company. He sets off for the shops. In the third picture he is walking along a path with grass on either side and is carrying an orange bag. In the fourth picture he has reached the town centre and is walking along a street. A motorbike passes him. In the following two pictures the boy has arrived at the pet shop and is pointing to the tanks containing fish. The shop assistant has taken a bowl of water, put a fish into it and is putting the bowl into the bag. The boy is walking home when he meets two girls he knows, an older girl and a younger girl. One of the girls is carrying a yellow bag. The boy and the older girl go to a kiosk to buy ice creams. They leave the younger girl sitting on a bench. She takes a doll out of the yellow bag and the bowl out of the orange bag but puts the doll back in the orange bag and the bowl in the yellow bag. When they have finished eating their ice creams and chatting they set off for

296 Introductory Linguistics for Speech and Language Therapy Practice

home but are going in opposite directions. The big girl is carrying the yellow bag, which now contains the fish bowl, and the boy is carrying the orange bag, which now contains the doll. In the next set of pictures the boy has arrived at his house and is taking the doll out of the bag. He realises what has happened and tells his mother. She phones the big girl's mother. In the penultimate picture the boy's mother is talking to the two girls, who have come to the boy's house to give him his fish bowl and collect their doll. The final picture shows the new fish swimming in the tank with the first fish. The boy is pointing to the tank and saying something to the girls, hopefully 'Thank you very much'.

17 Conclusion

Assuming that an introductory linguistics text is not likely to be so exciting that you had to jump to the last chapter to see how it turns out, you may well be reading this after having worked through the book chapter by chapter and having completed all of the exercises. If so, well done! We hope you feel that you have learned some useful things.

We began this book by dismantling language, in a sense. We identified different aspects of the language system: meaning, form and function, and on a more detailed level, the lexicon, morphology, syntax, semantics and so on. We took language apart in the way that one might disassemble a car engine. We were able to examine its working parts one by one. We saw how the mental lexicon contains a vast number of stored items, and we identified various features of words. We saw that many words could be broken down into smaller units via morphological analysis. We investigated the syntactic component of the language system and saw how words could be linked together to form phrases, and how phrases could combine to form clauses; we learned to recognise the different kinds of construction that were possible in English, and identified these structures in clinical resources.

If we want to understand any complex machine, from a car engine to the language system, it is useful to identify its parts in this way. But to see the system in action, we need to learn the complex ways in which these lower-level units fit back together, and how they operate in unison. We saw how speakers and writers use words, phrases and clauses in subtle ways to convey meanings above and beyond the semantic representations inherent in these components, and how listeners and readers are able to extract these subtle meanings with assistance from contextual information. We saw, finally, the complex way that the lexicon, morphology and syntax contribute to the production and comprehension of a narrative.

The clinical resources that we have been examining in this text are rather like a toolkit for working on the language system when some part of it is damaged. Some of the resources can be used to diagnose the problem, and others may help the clinician to fix it. Some of the tools are very general purpose, and others have much

Introductory Linguistics for Speech and Language Therapy Practice, First Edition. Jan McAllister and Jim Miller.
© 2013 John Wiley & Sons, Ltd. Published 2013 by John Wiley & Sons, Ltd.

more specific uses. One thing is for sure though – to get the best from your toolkit, you really need an in-depth understanding of the system that you are trying to fix. We hope that this book has gone some way towards giving you that understanding. But it is only a start. To become expert users of the toolkit you need to do a more in-depth study of the areas that we have identified. You also need to make sure that you become thoroughly familiar with the operating instructions (manuals) of the tools. And you need lots of experience of using these tools for their intended purpose, that of assessing and remedying disordered language.

Appendix A: Islands of Reliability for Determining Parts of Speech

This is a list of relatively common words whose part-of-speech label is most often the one shown here. You can never be 100% sure that this will be the word's part-of-speech in a given sentence, but it is pretty likely that it will be. You can then use the information to provide an island of (relative) reliability for working out the parts of speech of adjacent words that are more ambiguous.

a, an	Det	body	Noun
able	Adj	brought	Verb
action	Noun	business	Noun
actually	Adv	but	Conj
age	Noun	by	Prep
almost	Adv	came	Verb
already	Adv	can	Verb
although	Conj	car	Noun
always	Adv	central	Adj
am	Verb	centre	Noun
among	Prep	century	Noun
and	Conj	certain	Adj
are	Verb	child	Noun
area	Noun	children	Noun
ask	Verb	church	Noun
at	Prep	city	Noun
available	Adj	come	Verb
be	Verb	committee	Noun
became	Verb	community	Noun
because	Conj	company	Noun
become	Verb	could	Verb
been	Verb	council	Noun
began	Verb	country	Noun
behind	Prep	day	Noun
believe	Verb	death	Noun
big	Adj	development	Noun

Introductory Linguistics for Speech and Language Therapy Practice, First Edition. Jan McAllister and Jim Miller.
© 2013 John Wiley & Sons, Ltd. Published 2013 by John Wiley & Sons, Ltd.

did	Verb	important	Adj
different	Adj	in	Prep
difficult	Adj	industry	Noun
do	Verb	information	Noun
doing	Verb	international	Adj
done	Verb	is	Verb
door	Noun	it	Pron
during	Prep	itself	Pron
economic	Adj	job	Noun
education	Noun	keep	Verb
evidence	Noun	knew	Verb
eyes	Noun	known	Verb
fact	Noun	large	Adj
family	Noun	law	Noun
father	Noun	let	Verb
feel	Verb	likely	Adj
felt	Verb	little	Adj
find	Verb	local	Adj
food	Noun	lot	Noun
found	Verb	management	Noun
from	Prep	me	Pron
full	Adj	men	Noun
gave	Verb	moment	Noun
general	Adj	money	Noun
get	Verb	months	Noun
getting	Verb	morning	Noun
give	Verb	mother	Noun
given	Verb	national	Adj
gone	Verb	night	Noun
got	Verb	now	Adv
great	Adj	of	Prep
had	Verb	often	Adv
has	Verb	or	Conj
have	Verb	particular	Adj
having	Verb	particularly	Adv
he	Pron	party	Noun
health	Noun	people	Noun
heard	Verb	period	Noun
held	Verb	person	Noun
here	Adv	police	Noun
high	Adj	policy	Noun
himself	Pron	political	Adj
history	Noun	position	Noun
I	Pron	possible	Adj
idea	Noun	power	Noun
if	Conj	probably	Adv

problem	Noun	they	Pron
problems	Noun	thing	Noun
provide	Verb	things	Noun
put	Verb	think	Verb
quite	Adv	thought	Verb
read	Verb	times	Noun
remember	Verb	today	Adv
road	Noun	told	Verb
said	Verb	took	Verb
saw	Verb	towards	Prep
say	Verb	turned	Verb
says	Verb	up	Prep
school	Noun	upon	Prep
see	Verb	usually	Adv
seem	Verb	very	Adv
seemed	Verb	wanted	Verb
seems	Verb	war	Noun
seen	Verb	was	Verb
shall	Verb	water	Noun
she	Pron	we	Pron
small	Adj	week	Noun
society	Noun	went	Verb
sometimes	Adv	were	Verb
special	Adj	white	Adj
street	Noun	will	Verb
sure	Adj	with	Prep
system	Noun	within	Prep
taken	Verb	without	Prep
taking	Verb	woman	Noun
tell	Verb	women	Noun
the	Det	words	Noun
them	Pron	would	Verb
themselves	Pron	yesterday	Adv
then	Adv	you	Pron

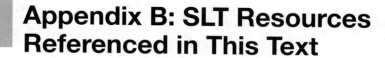

Appendix B: SLT Resources Referenced in This Text

Short title	Details
ACE	Adams, C., Cooke, R., Crutchley, A., Hesketh, A. & Reeves, D. (2001) Assessment of Comprehension and Expression 6-11. London: NFER Nelson Publishing Co Ltd.
ADI-R	Rutter, M., Le Couteur, A. & Lord, C. (2003) Autism Diagnostic Interview Revised. Los Angeles: Western Psychological.
ASDS	Myles, B., Bock, S. & Simpson, R. (2001) Asperger Syndrome Diagnostic Scale. Austin: Pro Ed.
A-STOP-R	van de Lely, H. Advanced Syntactic Test of Pronominal Reference – Revised.
BDAE	Goodglass, H. (2001) The Boston Diagnostic Aphasia Examination & Boston Naming Test. Third Edition. Austin: Pro Ed.
BOEHM 3	Boehm, A. (2001) Boehm 3 Preschool. London: Psychological Corporation.
Boston Naming Test	Goodglass, H. et al. (2001) The Boston Diagnostic Aphasia Examination & Boston Naming Test. Austin, TX: Pro-Ed.
BPVS	Dunn, L.M. et al. (1997) British Picture Vocabulary Scale.
Bracken	Bracken, B.A. (2006) Bracken Basic Concept Scales (Expressive; Receptive). San Antonio, TX: Harcourt Assessment.
Bracken Concept Development Program	Bracken, B. (1986) Bracken Concept Development Program. London: Pearson Assessment.

Introductory Linguistics for Speech and Language Therapy Practice, First Edition. Jan McAllister and Jim Miller.
© 2013 John Wiley & Sons, Ltd. Published 2013 by John Wiley & Sons, Ltd.

Short title	Details
CAPPA	Whitworth, A., Perkins, L. & Lesser, R. (1997) Conversation Analysis Profile for People with Aphasia (CAPPA). London: Whurr Publishers Ltd.
CAPPCI	Perkins, L., Whitworth, A., & Lesser, R. (1997) Conversation Analysis Profile for People with Cognitive Impairment (CAPPCI). London: Whurr Publishers Ltd.
CAT	Swinburn, K., Porter, G. & Howard, D. Comprehensive Aphasia Test. Hove, UK: Psychology Press.
CCC-2	Bishop, D. (2003) Children's Communication Checklist. London: Psychological Corporation.
CELF-4	Wiig, E., Secord, W. & Semel, E. (2006) Clinical Assessment of Language Fundamentals, 4 (UK). London: Harcourt Assessment.
CLIP	Semel, E. & Wiig, E. (1990) Clinical Language Intervention Program. London: Pearson Assessment.
CELF-Preschool	Wiig, E., Secord, W. & Semel, E. (2006) Clinical Assessment of Language Fundamentals, Preschool 2 (UK). London: Harcourt Assessment.
DASS	Howell, B. (2003) Dorset Assessment of Syntactic Structures. Ponteland: STASS Publications.
Derbyshire Language Scheme	Knowles, W. & Masidlover, M. (1999) Derbyshire Language Scheme. Derbyshire County Council, UK.
Don't Take it So Literally!	Legler, D. (1991) Don't Take it So Literally!: Reproducible Activities for Teaching Idioms. ECL Publications.
ERB	Seeff-Gabriel, B. Chiat, S. & Roy, P. (2008) The Early Repetition Battery. London: Pearson Assessment.
ERRNI	Bishop, D. (2004) Expression Reception and Recall of Narrative Instrument. London: Harcourt Assessment.
FAST	Enderby, P., Wood, V. & Wade, D. (2006) Frenchay Aphasia Screening Test. Second Edition. Chichester: John Wiley & Sons Ltd.
LIST	Lloyd, P., Peers, I. & Foster, C. (2001) The Listening Skills Test. London: Pearson Assessment.
Living Language	Locke, A. (1985) Living Language. London: nferNelson Publishing Co Ltd.
MCLA	Ellmo, W., Graser, J., Krchnavek, E., Calabrese, D. & Huack, K. (1995) Measure of Cognitive-Linguistic Abilities. Vero Beach: The Speech Bin Inc.
Narrative Intervention Programme	Joffee, V. (2011) Narrative Intervention Programme. Bicester: Speechmark Publishing Ltd.

Short title	Details
LARSP	Language Assessment, Remediation & Screening Procedure. See Crystal, D., Fletcher, P. & Garman, M. (1989) *Grammatical Analysis of Language Disability* (2nd edn). London: Cole & Whurr.
PALPA	Kay, J., Lesser, R. & Coltheart, M. (1992) Psycholinguistic Assessment of Language Processing in Aphasia. Hove, UK: Psychology Press.
Peter and the Cat	Leitao, S. & Allan, L. (2003) Peter and the Cat. Keighley, UK: Black Sheep Press.
PLS-3	Zimmerman, L., Steiner, V., Pond, R., Boucher, J. & Lewis, V. (1997) Pre-School Language Scale 3. London: Psychological Corporation.
PPVT	Dunn, D. & Dunn, L. (2007) Peabody Picture Vocabulary Test. Third Edition. San Antonio: Pearson.
Pragmatics Profile (children)	Dewart, H. & Summers, S. (1996) The Pragmatics Profile of Everyday Communication in Children. Windsor, UK: Nfer Nelson.
PTT-20	Conti-Ramsden G., Durkin K., Simkin Z., Lum JA, & Marchman V. (2011) The PTT-20: UK normative data for 5- to 11-year-olds on a 20-item past-tense task. International Journal of Language and Communication Disorders, 46, 243–248.
Pragmatics Profile (adults)	Dewart, H. & Summers, S. (1996) The Pragmatics Profile of Everyday Communication in Adults. Windsor, UK: Nfer Nelson.
Pyramids and Palm Trees	Howard, D. & Patterson, K. (1992) Pyramids and Palm Trees Test. London: Harcourt.
RDLS-III	Edwards, S., Hughes, A., Fletcher, P., Letts, C., Garman, M. & Sinka, I. (1997) Reynell Developmental Language Scales Iii. London: Nfer Nelson.
Renfrew Action Picture Test/RAPT	Renfrew, C. (1997) Renfrew Language Scales – Action Picture Test. Bicester, UK: Speechmark.
Renfrew Bus Story	Renfrew, C. (1997) Renfrew Language Scales - Bus Story. Bicester, UK: Speechmark.
Renfrew Word Finding Test	Renfrew, C. (1995) Renfrew Language Scales – Word Finding Vocabulary Test. Bicester, UK: Speechmark.
Semantic Links	Bigland, S. & Speake, J. (1992) Semantic Links. Ponteland, UK: Stass Publications.

Short title	Details
Sentence Processing Resource Pack	Marshall, J., Black, M., Byng, S., Chiat, S. & Pring, T. (1999) The Sentence Processing Resource Pack. Bicester: Speechmark Publishing Ltd.
Sheffield Screening Test for Acquired Language Disorders	Snyder, D. (1993) Sheffield Screening Test for Acquired Language Disorders. London: NFER Nelson.
Squirrel Story	Carey, J., Leitao, S. & Allan, L. (2006) The Squirrel Story. Keighley, UK: Black Sheep Press.
STASS	Armstrong, S. & Ainley, M. South Tyneside Assessment of Syntactic Structures. Ponteland, UK: STASS Publications.
SULP-R	Rinaldi, W. (2001) Social Use of Language Programme (Revised).
TALC	Elks, L. & McLachlin, H. (2007) Test of Abstract Language Comprehension. St Mabyn, UK: Elklan.
TAPS-R	van de Lely, H. Test of Active and Passive Sentences (Revised).
TOAL-4	Hammill, D., Brown, V., Larsen, S. & Wiederholt, J. (2007) Test of Adolescent & Adult Language. Austin: Pro Ed.
TOPL	Phelps-Terasaki, D. & Phelps-Gunn, T. (1992) Test of Pragmatic Language. Austin, TX: Pro-Ed.
TROG-2	Bishop, D. (2003) Test for Reception of Grammar 2. London: Psychological Corporation.
TOWK	Wiig, E. & Secord, W. (1990) Test of Word Knowledge. London: The Psychological Corporation.
Understanding Ambiguity	Rinaldi, W. (1996) Understanding Ambiguity. London: Nfer Nelson.
VAN	Webster, J. & Bird, H. Verb and Noun Test. St Mabyn, UK: STASS Publications.
VAST	Roelien Bastiaanse, R., Edwards, S. & Rispens, J. (2002) Verb and Sentence Test. London: Thames Valley Test Company.
VATT	van de Lely, H. Verb Agreement and Tense Test.
Vocabulary Enrichment Programme	Joffee, V. (2011) Vocabulary Enrichment Programme. Bicester: Speechmark Publishing Ltd.
Western Aphasia Battery	Kertesz, A. (2007) Western Aphasia Battery. San Antonio: Harcourt Assessment.

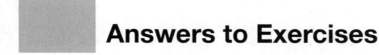

Answers to Exercises

Chapter 1

General exercises

1.1. *Is the Pope a Catholic?* Function. It looks as though this is a request for information, though in fact it is a means of answering the original question, by suggesting that the answer is obvious.
Rumours on the internets – Form.
Elbows for shoulders – a speech error involving exchange of words similar in meaning.

1.2. Car ad: semantics; alternative meanings of *drive*.
Misundersestimated: morphology; mis- is often part of word structure (e.g. mislead, misquote), but it is not appropriate here.
Is our children learning and *Literacy level are appalling*: syntax; mismatch between *is* and *children* in the first example and *level* and *are* in the second.
Were you born in a barn? Pragmatics – non-literal interpretation required.

Exercises using clinical resources

1.3. CCC-2: 12, semantics and lexicon; 15, pragmatics; 19, semantics, pragmatics; 36, morphology; 43, syntax; 54, pragmatics; 55, syntax.

1.4. Your answer will no doubt depend on the resources that you have access to. Some resources, such as the Clinical Evaluation of Language Fundamentals (CELF-4) are very comprehensive, and cover aspects of all of the areas. We will reference many other resources during the course of this book. Look at the start of each chapter to identify resources relevant to the topics covered there.

Chapter 2

General exercises

2.1. Usage of both terms increased in the early 1990s, but *mobile phone* quickly outstripped *cell phone*, and in 2008 *mobile phone* was a much more widespread term.

Introductory Linguistics for Speech and Language Therapy Practice, First Edition. Jan McAllister and Jim Miller.
© 2013 John Wiley & Sons, Ltd. Published 2013 by John Wiley & Sons, Ltd.

2.2. For example, just taking five words at random from the list:

Word	Frequency in MRC Psycholinguistic Database (out of 1 million)	Frequency in British National Corpus (out of 100 million)
apple	9	2610
beast	7	874
Flask	5	270
hoist	1	116
Mule	4	182

Obviously the scores from the British National Corpus are much larger, because the sample is 100 times bigger than that in the MRC Psycholinguistic Database; but it is interesting that the rank order is the same in both (i.e. *apple* is the most frequent and *hoist* is the least frequent).

2.3. The number of orthographic neighbours for each word according to the Washington database is as follows:

apple	3
beast	10
flask	5
hoist	4
mule	7

The average is therefore 5.8.

2.4. To access the words you need to select 'Toddler Says'; this part of the database foes up to 30 months of age. Examples are *dog, bottle, balloon, shoe, eye*.

2.5. For example, according to the Washington database *zux* has no neighbours and *gan* has 20 neighbours.

Exercises using clinical resources

2.6. Set 1: mean letters = 5.1, mean syllables = 1.5; all in the MRC Psycholinguistic database; Set 2: mean letters = 9.0, mean syllables = 3.5; only 1 in the MRC Psycholinguistic database.

2.7. Item 3.

2.8. Length.

2.9. They were matched for frequency and for length in both syllables and phonemes. It was not possible to match them for imageability.

2.10. Number 1.

2.11. Length in syllables (1, 2 or 3).

2.12. Items 1–8, 9406 per 100 million words; items 53–60, 132 (answers rounded to nearest whole number).

2.13. Length in syllables, frequency, imageability, regularity.

Chapter 3

General exercises

3.1. The matrix would need to look something like this (notice that the feature Human is no longer redundant):

	Woman	Girl	Man	Boy	Mare	Stallion	Colt	Filly
Human	+	+	+	+	−	−	−	−
Female	+	+	−	−	+	−	−	+
Adult	+	−	+	−	+	+	−	−

3.2. The underlined words belong to more than one of the semantic fields. boot, slipper, sandal, trainer (footwear); bonnet, wheel, door, windscreen (parts of a car); helmet, beret, cap, trilby (types of hat); window, ceiling, wall, floor (parts of a room).

3.3. Some of the items are grouped according to non-semantic categories, but semantic categories include the following: people, games and routines, animals, vehicles, toys, food and drink, clothing, body parts, furniture.

3.4. Examples include mother–mum, spectacles–glasses, get–obtain, choice–selection, rich–wealthy.

3.5. above/below directional opposites
odd/even complementary opposites
teach/learn directional opposites
employer/employee relational opposites
hero/villain antonyms
marry/wed synonyms
bus/vehicle hyponym/hypernym
same/different antonyms or complementary opposites, depending on viewpoint; see 'Big Bang Theory' example.

3.6. Examples as follows (with possibly more meanings than are listed here). Homonymy: *peer* (look closely/Lord), *bark* (dog noise/tree covering), *match* (sporting fixture/ignition device). Polysemy: *wood* (substance that a tree is made of/group of trees), *foot* (part of the body/lowest part of hill, mountain, etc.), *hound* (hunting dog/harass or pursue).

Exercises using clinical resources

3.7. Semantic associates; sense; semantic features.

3.8. Examples are: low imageability – condition–state, advantage–benefit; high imageability – baby–infant, meadow–pasture.

3.9. Examples are
REGULAR
maid – a female servant
bean – a sort of vegetable
hare – animal that looks like a rabbit

EXCEPTIONS
war – armed conflict
knead – get bread ready for baking

3.10. For example: Lowest age-band, sad–happy (both words are known by 80% or more of 30-month-olds in the MacArthur Bates Communicative Development Inventories, described in Chapter 2); highest age-band, commence–cease.

3.11. For example, boat – oar – tennis racquet; chef's hat – whisk – screwdriver

3.12. For example, central picture = cup, target = jug, semantic distractor = bottle, phonological distractor = cap, unrelated distractor = peg.

Chapter 4

General exercises

4.1. **a.** Agatha Christie wrote 'Death on the Nile'.
  b. Simon Doyle shoots Lynette Ridgeway.
  c. The murderer had drugged Poirot.
  d. Poirot will solve the mystery.

4.2. (Incidentally, the Agent and Patient are as shown below in the active versions of the sentences as well.)
  a. Agent = Agatha Christie; Patient = 'Death on the Nile'.
  b. Agent = Simon Doyle; Patient = Lynette Ridgeway.
  c. Agent = The murderer; Patient = Poirot.
  d. Agent = Poirot; Patient = the mystery.

4.3. Reversible passives: b and c (in these, either participant could carry out the action; it does not matter who did). Non-reversible passives: a and d ('Death on the Nile' cannot write Agatha Christie; the mystery cannot solve Poirot).

4.4. **a.** Non-reversible passive; Agent = MPs; Patient = a new law.
  b. Reversible active; Agent = Chris; Patient = Jamie.
  c. Reversible passive: Agent = the leader of the opposition; Patient = the prime minister.
  d. Reversible active: Agent = the actress; Patient = the critic.
  e. Non-reversible active; Agent = the composer; Patient = a new piece.

Exercises using clinical resources

4.5. All of the 'bad' passive sentences have an action that requires an animate agent, but they have been given an inanimate agent. In fact, if we reverse the current agent and patient in each of these items, we will get 'good' sentences.

4.6. Reversible passives are as follows:
  a. TROG-2 – block K
  b. PALPA – subtest 55, items with code RDP (16, 21, 37, 47) or RNP (10, 28, 33, 41); subtest 56, items with code RDP (25, 30, 40, 60) or RNP (6, 18, 36, 44).
  c. TAPS-R – 2, 3, 7, 19, 22, 24, 26, 27, 33, 37.

4.7. For example: puppy behind kitten; car below truck; cup on plate; star over triangle.

4.8. In the possessive structure that is used here, the entity that is mentioned before the -'s is the possessor, and the entity after it is the entity that is possessed (as it were!). But the entities that have been selected in these examples are both capable of taking either role (being either possessor or possessed). If we label the two entities X and Y, both *The X's Y* and *The Y's X* result in interpretable phrases. But in an example where X = *girl* and Y = *accident*, only *The X's Y* (*The girl's accident*) would be interpretable, while *The Y's X* (*The accident's girl*) would not.

Chapter 5

General exercises

5.1. Determiners underlined and prepositions in bold:
  <u>This</u> paragraph concerns <u>the</u> novel 'David Copperfield', which was written **by** Charles Dickens. It was published **in** <u>the</u> form **of** <u>a</u> novel **in** 1850, <u>a</u> year **after** <u>its</u> serialisation **in** <u>a</u> magazine. It is **about** <u>the</u> life **of** David Copperfield. He was orphaned **at** <u>a</u> young age and **for** <u>a</u> time worked **in** <u>a</u> factory **under** cruel conditions. **During** <u>this</u> time he lodged **with** <u>a</u> family called Micawber who were sent **to** prison **because of** <u>their</u> debts. Facing <u>a</u> life **without** financial or emotional support, <u>our</u> hero eventually escaped **from** <u>those</u> miserable conditions and was raised **by** <u>his</u> aunt, Betsey Trotwood. **Through** <u>her</u> kindness he completed <u>his</u> education and later began <u>a</u> legal career. Mr Micawber came **into** <u>the</u> story again when he provided evidence **against** <u>an</u> evil character, Uriah Heep. **Over** <u>the</u> years, David developed <u>a</u> talent **for** storytelling and observation, and later became <u>an</u> acclaimed writer.

  See notes in the chapter about *its, his* etc which are often called 'possessive pronouns' in traditional grammar; we pointed out that these forms have a 'determiner use' which is what is underlined here.

5.2. Nouns underlined:
  a. <u>Procrastination</u> is the <u>thief</u> of <u>time</u>.
  b. The <u>Queen</u> is a <u>believer</u> in the <u>sanctity</u> of <u>marriage</u>.
  c. This <u>wine</u> tastes of <u>blackcurrants</u>.
  d. Your <u>attitude</u> causes <u>problems</u>.
  e. The <u>magician</u> astonished us with his <u>performance</u>.
  f. The <u>activist's</u> <u>heroism</u> led to a <u>change</u> in the <u>law</u>.
  g. A <u>horse</u>, a <u>horse</u>, my <u>kingdom</u> for a <u>horse</u>!

h. The <u>company's employees</u> voted for a <u>strike</u>.

i. <u>Levels</u> of <u>employment</u> must rise.

5.3. Labelling personal pronouns:

Pronoun	Person	Number	Form
me	First person	singular	objective form
they	Third person	plural	subjective form
he, she, it	Third person	singular	subjective form
we	First person	plural	objective form
them	Third person	plural	objective form
him, her, it	Third person	singular	objective form
I	First person	singular	subjective form
us	First person	plural	objective form

5.4. Pronouns underlined:

Snow White's stepmother, the Evil Queen, had a Magic Mirror <u>which</u> [relative pronoun] could speak. Every day <u>she</u> [personal pronoun, third person singular, subjective form] looked at <u>herself</u> [reflexive pronoun, third person singular] in <u>it</u> [personal pronoun, third person singular] and asked, "<u>Who</u> [interrogative pronoun] is the fairest in the land?". The Mirror usually replied, "<u>You</u> [personal pronoun, second person] are, my Queen". But one day the Mirror replied, "Snow White is the fairest". The Queen was furious. <u>She</u> [personal pronoun, third person singular, subjective form] would do anything to be rid of Snow White. <u>She</u> [personal pronoun, third person singular, subjective form] called for the woodcutter and ordered <u>him</u> [personal pronoun, third person singular, objective form] to take Snow White into the forest and kill <u>her</u> [personal pronoun, third person singular, objective form]. The woodcutter was deeply shocked by <u>this</u> [demonstrative pronoun]. <u>He</u> [personal pronoun, third person singular, subjective form] did take Snow White into the forest, but <u>he</u> [personal pronoun, third person singular, subjective form] let <u>her</u> [personal pronoun, third person singular, objective form] escape.

Snow White met seven dwarves, <u>who</u> [relative pronoun] allowed <u>her</u> [personal pronoun, third person singular, objective form] to live with <u>them</u> [personal pronoun, third person plural, objective form]. "Will you [personal pronoun, second person] look after this house for <u>us</u> [personal pronoun, first person plural, objective form] while <u>we</u> [personal pronoun, first person plural, subjective form] are at work?" <u>they</u> [personal pronoun, third person plural, subjective form] asked. <u>They</u> [personal pronoun, third person plural, subjective form] went off every day to work in a gold mine. One day while <u>they</u> [personal pronoun, third person plural, subjective form] were out the Queen came along in disguise. <u>She</u> [personal pronoun, third person singular, subjective form] tricked Snow White into eating a poisoned apple.

At first Snow White was reluctant, saying, "The dwarves told <u>me</u> [personal pronoun, first person singular, objective form] not to take anything from strangers. <u>I</u> [personal pronoun, first person singular, subjective form] am not sure whether <u>I</u> [personal pronoun, first person singular, subjective form] should eat <u>that</u> [demonstrative pronoun]". But the Queen said, "See, <u>I</u> [personal pronoun, first person singular, subjective form] have cut the apple in half and <u>we</u> [personal pronoun, first person plural, subjective form] will each take half. <u>You</u> [personal pronoun, second person] eat <u>yours</u> [possessive pronoun, second person], and <u>I</u> [personal pronoun, first person singular, subjective form] will eat mine [possessive pronoun, first person]". But the half <u>that</u> [relative pronoun] <u>she</u> [personal pronoun, third person singular, subjective form] gave Snow White contained poison. As soon as Snow White bit the apple <u>she</u> [personal pronoun, third person singular, subjective form] fell into a deep sleep.

When <u>they</u> [personal pronoun, third person plural, subjective form] saw <u>her</u> [personal pronoun, third person singular, objective form], the dwarves persuaded <u>themselves</u> [reflexive pronoun, third person plural] that <u>she</u> [personal pronoun, third person singular, subjective form] was dead, and placed <u>her</u> [personal pronoun, third person singular, objective form] in a glass coffin. But a year later a Handsome Prince saw the sleeping Snow White and fell in love with <u>her</u> [personal pronoun, third person singular, objective form]. <u>He</u> [personal pronoun, third person singular, subjective form] awakened <u>her</u> [personal pronoun, third person singular, objective form] with a kiss, and said at once, "Will <u>you</u> [personal pronoun, second person] marry <u>me</u> [personal pronoun, first person singular, objective form]?" Snow White agreed, and <u>they</u> [personal pronoun, third person plural, subjective form] were married, and lived happily ever after.

5.5. Adjectives underlined:
La Pedrera is the name of a building designed in the <u>twentieth</u> century by the <u>Catalan</u> architect Antoni Gaudi. Its <u>basic</u> design was <u>controversial</u> because of the <u>curvaceous</u> forms of the façade. Architecturally it is considered <u>innovative</u> because of <u>original</u> methods used in its construction. <u>Other</u> innovations were the construction of <u>separate</u> lifts and stairs for the owners and their servants. It was built for a <u>wealthy</u> couple, Roser Segimon and Pere Milà, whose lifestyle was extremely <u>lavish</u> and <u>flamboyant</u>. Gaudi held <u>strong religious</u> beliefs and tried to incorporate <u>Christian</u> symbols in the design of the building, but the <u>local</u> government objected to this. Today La Pedrera is a venue for <u>various</u> activities and exhibitions.

5.6. Verbs underlined:
   a. This exercise <u>seems</u> easy.
   b. Towards the finish, the runners <u>quicken</u> their pace.
   c. We <u>celebrate</u> Christmas in December.
   d. The party <u>was</u> a great success.
   e. Henry <u>has</u> measles.
   f. Voters often <u>criticise</u> the government.

    g. Those flowers <u>are</u> gorgeous.

    h. *The Iron Lady* <u>concerns</u> the life and career of Margaret Thatcher.

    i. He <u>explained</u> his concerns about the plan.

    j. She <u>became</u> an MP in 1966.

    k. Leaves <u>change</u> their colour in autumn.

5.7. Auxiliary verbs underlined:

    a. I am a fan of *The Big Bang Theory*. [*am* is not an auxiliary here]

    b. *The Big Bang Theory* is about Leonard, Sheldon, Howard, Raj and Penny. [*is* is not an auxiliary here]

    c. Leonard has glasses. [*has* is not an auxiliary here]

    d. Penny <u>is</u> [primary] working as a waitress.

    e. Penny and Leonard <u>have</u> [primary] <u>been</u> [primary] dating.

    f. Sheldon and Leonard share an apartment. [no auxiliary]

    g. Why <u>do</u> [primary, dummy] Sheldon and Leonard share an apartment?

    h. Howard is an engineer. [*is* is not an auxiliary here]

    i. Sheldon <u>should</u> [modal] <u>have</u> [primary] <u>been</u> [primary] awarded the Nobel prize by now.

    j. Raj is usually shy with women. [*is* is not an auxiliary here]

5.8. Adverbs underlined:

<u>Never</u> boil an egg that you have taken <u>straight</u> from the fridge because it will <u>immediately</u> crack in the boiling water. <u>Always</u> use a small saucepan. Fill the pan with water, and when it is <u>just</u> simmering, <u>quickly</u> but <u>gently</u> place the egg in the water using a spoon. After one minute remove the pan from the heat. Use a timer to measure the next stage <u>exactly</u>. After 6 minutes the yoke should be <u>fairly</u> liquid and the white will be <u>quite</u> wobbly; after 7 minutes the white will be <u>completely</u> set and the yolk should be <u>lightly</u> cooked but <u>still</u> soft.

5.9. Conjunctions underlined:

John Fitzgerald Kennedy ("JFK") was the 35th President of the United States. He served from 1961 <u>until</u> [subordinating] he was assassinated in 1963. <u>After</u> [subordinating] he completed military service, he represented Massachusetts in the US House of Representatives. In the presidential elections he defeated Richard Nixon <u>even though</u> [subordinating] he had far less experience than his opponent. His success was partly due to his skilful use of television. <u>While</u> [subordinating] JFK looked young and handsome in televised debates, Nixon looked tense and uncomfortable and perspired freely. Radio listeners to the same debates thought that Nixon had <u>either</u> [correlative] won <u>or</u> [correlative] performed equally well.

JFK was assassinated on 22nd November, 1963, in Dallas, Texas. Lee Harvey Oswald was charged with the crime, <u>but</u> [coordinating] he was shot <u>and</u> [coordinating] killed two days later by Jack Ruby <u>before</u> [subordinating] he could be tried. JFK's assassination has been the subject of many conspiracy theories, <u>not just</u> [correlative] in the United States <u>but</u> [correlative] elsewhere in the world.

5.10.

The	children	crossed	the	very	busy	road
Det	N	Full Verb	Det	Adverb (Intensifier)	Adj	N

She	was	becoming	rather	cross
Pers pron	Primary Aux	Full Verb	Adverb (Qualifier)	Adj

The	teacher	put	a	cross	beside	the	answer
Det	N	Full Verb	Det	N	Prep	Det	N

Raise	your	hand	if	you	can	answer
Full Verb	Det	N	Subord Conj	Pers Pron	Modal Aux	Full Verb

The	cook	added	the	juice	of	an	orange	to	the	mixture
Det	N	Full Verb	Det	N	Prep	Det	N	Prep	Det	N

He	was	wearing	an	orange	suit	which	he	bought	at	Primark
Pers Pron	Primary Aux	Full Verb	Det	Adj	N	Relative Pron	Pers Pron	Full Verb	Prep	N

Long	hair	suits	you
Adj	N	Full Verb	Pers Pron

What	were	they	doing?
Int Pron	Primary Aux	Pers Pron	Full Verb

You	should	cook	the	eggs	until	they	are	very	firm
Pers Pron	Modal Aux	Full Verb	Det	N	Subord Conj	Pers Pron	Full Verb	Adverb (Intensifier)	

The	firm's	accountant	demanded	immediate	payment	from	us
Det	N	N	Full Verb	Adj	N	Prep	N

I	received	a	final	demand	in	the	post
Pers Pron	Full Verb	Det	Adj	N	Prep	Det	N

I	must	post	this	letter
Pers Pron	Modal Aux	Full Verb	Det	N

Would	you	prefer	fish	or	meat?
Modal Aux	Pers Pron	Full Verb	N	Coord Conj	N

We	could	fish	in	the	sea
Pers Pron	Modal Aux	Full Verb	Pre	Det	N

The	road	that	leads	to	my	home	is	completely	straight
Det	N	Rel Pron	Full Verb	Prep	Det	N	Full Verb	Adv	Adj

These	are	mine	and	those	are	yours
Dem Pron	Full Verb	Poss Pron	Coord Conj	Dem Pron	Full Verb	Poss Pron

That	might	have	been	the	best	solution	for	this	problem
Dem Pron	Modal Aux	Primary Aux	Primary Aux	Det	Adj	N	Prep	Det	N

Who	's	there?
Int Pron	Full Verb (uncontractible copula)	Adv

It	's	me
Pers Pron	Full Verb (uncontractible copula)	Pers Pron

Exercises using clinical resources

5.11. CAT, Section 9 'Comprehension of Spoken Sentences': items 1 & 2: Det, N, Primary Aux, Full Verb; item 3: Personal Pronoun, Primary Aux, Full Verb; items 4 & 5: Det, N, Primary Aux, Full Verb, Det, N; item 6: Det, N, Primary Aux, Full Verb, Prep, Det, N; item 7: Det, N, Full Verb (copula), Prep, Det, N; items 8 & 9: Det, N, Full Verb, Det, N; items 10 & 11: Det, N, Primary Aux, Full Verb, Prep, Det, N; item 12: Det, N, Full Verb, Det, N; item 13: Det, N, Prep, Det, N, Full Verb (copula), Adj; item 14: Det, N, Det, N, Full Verb (copula), Prep, Full Verb (copula), Adj; item 15: Det, Adj, N, Full Verb (copula), Prep, Det, N; item 16: Det, N, Prep, Det, N, Full Verb (copula), Adj.

5.12. In the TOAL-4, subtest 4 (Word Similarities), which of the 40 target items could be
  a. Nouns: 3–5, 8–10, 18, 20, 24, 27–29, 36, 38, 39
  b. Verbs: 1, 3, 6–11, 13-15, 19-23, 25, 26, 31–33, 39
  c. Adjectives: 2, 3, 12, 16, 17, 30, 34, 35, 37
  d. Adverbs: 3
  Note that 7 could be a noun (in the sense of 'taking a turn') but it is more commonly a verb.

5.13. Types of pronouns in the following:
  a. CELF-4 – possessive, personal (subjective and objective), reflexive.
  b. CELF-Preschool – possessive, personal (subjective and objective), reflexive.
  c. TROG-2 – personal (subjective and objective). Sections G and Salso contains relative pronouns
  d. ERB: personal (mainly subjective); demonstrative
  e. New RDLS – personal (objective), reflexive.

5.14. Items in the CELF-4 sub-test Formulated Sentences that can be used as:
  a. Verb: 4, 5, 8 (full verbs)
  b. Adverb: 1, 6, 7, 9, 10, 11, 12, 13, 16, 21, 24

5.15. Kinds of pronouns tested in the A-STOP-R: third person reflexive and personal (objective).

5.16. Modal auxiliaries listed under AUX on the STASS/DASS Rapid Assessment Score Sheet: will, might, could

Chapter 6

General exercises

6.1. dirt + y; first + born; ketchup; odd + ity; offer + ing; off + load + ing; paper + back; re + pay + ment; sing + er; stubborn; unit; uncle; un + clean; un + common + ly; up + market; wait + er; water.

6.2. We can find other words with the same hypothesised root preceded by pre-fixes that are found in other words, for example *consume – resume; pervert – convert – divert – revert; receive – conceive – deceive – perceive; detract – contract – retract.* There are meaning similarities among the roots in each set, although, as noted in the chapter, these meanings are very abstract and difficult to articulate precisely.

6.3. Though there are exceptions, the suffix *-ible* typically attaches to bound roots (e.g. *audible, edible, horrible, terrible, visible*), while *-able* most often attaches to free roots (e.g. *comfortable, dependable, predictable, reasonable, understandable*).

6.4. We can find the suffixes -ic, -ify, -ity and -ian in many other words, so it makes sense to analyse the words as follows: electr + ic, electr + ify, electr+ ic + ity, electr + ic + ian.

6.5. The root becomes the bound form *-cept* (deception, inception, reception, conception, conceptual, perceptual, etc).

6.6. Allomorphy:
    a. confession; distinct allomorph, change to pronunciation.
    b. secrecy; distinct allomorph, change to pronunciation and spelling.
    c. depth; distinct allomorph, change to pronunciation and spelling.
    d. decision; distinct allomorph, change to pronunciation and spelling.
    e. signifies; distinct allomorph, change to pronunciation.
    f. definition; distinct allomorph, change to pronunciation and spelling.
    g. swimming; distinct allomorph, change to change to spelling.
    h. ability; distinct allomorph, change to pronunciation and spelling.
    i. qualified; distinct allomorph, change to spelling.
    j. composition; distinct allomorph, change to pronunciation and spelling.

6.7. Compounds: for example –
A causes B: *dog-bite*
B causes A: *starvation diet*
B prevents A: *flu vaccine*
B resembles A: *Catwoman*
B is appropriate at time A: *Easter egg*
B is made of A: *hairball*
B is part of A: *shirt button*

6.8. (((wrist watch) strap) shop).

6.9. Focusing on spelling for the moment, the choice of allophone depends on the initial letter of the root, so *im-* is added to roots beginning with m, b or p (*immaterial, imbalance, impossible*); *il-* is added to those beginning with l (*illogical, illegal*); *ir-* is added to those beginning with r (*irreconcilable, irrational*); and *in-* is added everywhere else (*inescapable, indecisive*, etc.). Although *in-* is added in the written for words like *constant* or *capable*, notice that when the word is spoken the consonant at the end of the prefix is the one at the end of *sing*, not the one at the end of *sin*.

6.10. Examples: was/been; saw/seen; ate/eaten; drank/drunk; gave/given.

6.11. Lexemes versus grammatical word forms; note differences between spoken and written language:

BLACK – black (base form), blacker (comparative), blackest (superlative) – three forms.

DECORATE – decorate (base form), decorates (third person singular, present tense), decorated (past tense, past participle), decorating (progressive) – four forms.

HARD (adverb) – hard (base form), harder (comparative), hardest (superlative) – three forms.

FROG – frog (base form, singular), frogs (plural), frog's (possessive, singular) frogs' (possessive, plural) – four written forms, but three of them are pronounced in the same way, so in speech there are only two distinct forms.

MAN – man (base form, singular), men (plural), man's (possessive, singular), men's (possessive, plural) – four forms

SEE – see (base form), sees (third person singular, present tense), saw (past tense), seen (past participle), seeing (progressive) – five forms.

6.12. Suffixes:

A number of thing + s (inflectional, plural) surprise me about the way that we categor + ise (derivational) words.

The child + ren (inflectional, plural) + 's (inflectional, possessive) shout + s (inflectional, plural) were becom + ing (inflectional, progressive) louder.

I hope you will be health + y (derivational), wealth + y (derivational) and happy.

The build + er (derivational, agentive) misled [N.B.: no suffix, but there is a prefix mis- followed by a past tense form of the root] me about the cost of the improve + ment (derivational) + s (inflectional, plural).

Exercises using clinical resources

6.13. ACE Syntactic Formulation subtest: 1 & 2, past tense; 3 & 4, past/passive participle. The other items target concepts that we consider elsewhere.

6.14. CAT, sections containing only morphologically complex items: 13, repetition of complex words; all 3 items have the structure prefix + root + suffix. 21, reading complex words: items 1 and 2 have the structure prefix + root +

suffix. It could be argued that item 3 has the form root + suffix, but no prefix.

6.15. ERB Sentence Scoresheet:
  a. Plural 1, 4, 6, 7, 9
  b. Progressive 2, 4, 10
  c. Past 2, 3, 10
  d. Third person singular, present tense 11

6.16. Suffixes are examined in the CELF-Preschool: Plural, possessive, third person singular, past tense, present progressive.

6.17. Syntax Summary of the Living Language programme. Irregular plurals – level V; third person singular present tense forms of verb – level III, apart from *is*; progressive forms of verbs – level II; irregular past tenses – level IV; irregular past participles – level VI.

6.18. PTT-2: drew/drawn, drove/driven, fell/fallen, flew/flown, rode/ridden, sat; VATT: made, gave/given, thought.

6.19. STASS:
  a. Plural 2, 3, 26, 29, 31
  b. Possessive 8
  c. Third person singular present tense 4
  d. Progressive 1, 2, 14, 20b, 25, 32
  e. Past tense 9
  f. Past participle 16, 19, 20b, 28, 30
  g. Comparative 27
  h. Superlative 28
  i. A derivational suffix 11, 20a

6.20. TALC compound words – level 4.

Chapter 7

General exercises

7.1.
  1. Yes. cf. <u>He</u> led the mission; The mission was led by <u>Neil Armstrong.</u>
  2. No
  3. No
  4. Yes. cf. <u>The Apollo 11 mission</u> was led by Neil Armstrong; <u>He</u> led it.
  5. Yes
  6. No
  7. Yes. cf. The mission was <u>dangerous</u>; <u>Funded by NASA</u> it was.
  8. No
  9. Yes. cf. <u>NASA</u> funded the mission; The mission was funded by <u>it/them.</u>

7.2.

Surprisingly	adverb
large	adjective
mice	noun
very	adverb (modifying *rapidly*)
rapidly	adverb
built	verb
an	determiner (indefinite article)
exceedingly	adverb (modifying *comfortable*)
comfortable	adjective
nest	noun
behind	preposition
the	determiner (definite article)
cupboards	noun
during	preposition
the	determiner (definite article)
winter	noun

7.3.

1	The new house	Noun Phrase
	very impressive	Adjective Phrase
2	Into the secret drawer	Prepositional Phrase
3	chewed the edge of the carpet	Verb Phrase
4	by the shredder	Prepositional Phrase
5	exceedingly expensive	Adjective Phrase
	worthy of the name	Adjective Phrase
6	New components	Noun Phrase
7	right across the street	Prepositional Phrase
8	Not surprisingly	Adverbial Phrase
9	very strong	Adjective Phrase
10	Which committee members	Noun Phrase

7.4.

1	Two	Linguistics is important + although it is sometimes complicated.
2	One	What is your name and age?
3	Two	What is your name + and + when were you born?
4	Three	Measure two ounces of butter, + melt it in a pan + and + add the onions.

7.5. The joke depends on the syntactic structure of *Eats shoots and leaves*. With the interpretation 'consumes certain vegetable matter' *eats* is a verb used transitively and *shoots and leaves* is a Noun Phrase, the direct object of *eats*. With the interpretation 'consumes a meal, fires a gun and goes away' all three major words are verbs used intransitively and the punctuation might be *Eats, shoots and leaves*. There is convention, known as the Oxford Comma that requires a comma after *shoots*: *eats, shoots, and leaves*. Students often protest about examples where punctuation is omitted, perhaps feeling that they have been tricked. All that we can say, having read an awful lot of student essays in our time, is that students are no more diligent about punctuating written text than most people!

7.6. Direct [DO] and indirect [IO] objects:
Direct [DO] and indirect [IO] objects:
1. Catriona lent Angus [IO] the car [DO]. → Catriona lent the car [DO] to Angus [IO] .
2. The chef made a special meal [DO] for his favourite client [IO]. → The chef made his favourite client [IO] a special meal [DO].
3. My mum bought me [IO] a bracelet [DO]. → My mum bought a bracelet [DO] for me [IO].
4. Don poured a drink [DO]. This example has no indirect object so cannot be re-ordered. An example with a direct object would be *Don poured a drink* [DO] *for Faye* [IO] → *Don poured Faye* [IO] *a drink* [DO].
5. Norman brought flowers [DO] for Rosie [IO]. → Norman brought Rosie [IO] flowers [DO].
6. Alison showed her holiday photos [DO] to her friends at work [IO]. → Alison showed her friends at work [IO] her holiday photos [DO].

7.7.
1. Jennifer was <u>enthusiastically</u> **adverbial** chopping <u>logs</u> **object**.
2. She was <u>amazed at his lack of concern</u>. **complement**
3. Susan was appointed <u>president of the golf club</u>. **(subject) complement**
4. <u>My aunt</u> **subject** left Louise <u>her entire fortune</u>. **object**
5. The lawyer sent <u>Louise</u> **object** a copy of the will.
6. Having forgotten to have lunch, she became <u>very irritable</u>. **complement**
7. We sent all the documents <u>to London</u>. **adverbial**
8. <u>Through the window</u> **adverbial** she could see people queuing.

Exercises using clinical resources

7.8. Phrase level sequences specified on the STASS and DASS that can function in particular ways at clause level (**note of course that there are other possible combinations that could appear** – see chapter).
a. Subject D N; Adj N; NN; D Adj N; Adj Adj N; Pron^P; Pron^O; NP Pr NP; XcX
b. Direct object as Subject
c. Indirect object as Subject, plus Pr N; Pr DN; Pr D Adj N
d. Complement as Indirect Object (remember that prepositional phrases can be complements if they do not refer to a physical location) plus Int X (as well as other structures not mentioned)

7.9. CELF-Preschool, items explicitly targeting structures a–d; look at the Sentence Structure Item Analysis on the record form:

    a. Verb phrase –1, 4, 5, 6, 16, 18

    b. Prepositional phrase – 2, 3

    c. Indirect object – 8, 21

    d. Passive – 19, 20

7.10. TROG-2 Section Q – complement.

7.11. CELF-4 Recalling Sentences, passives: 1, 5, 7, 11, 12, 18, 19, 32.

7.12. CELF-4 Sentence Structure:

    a. Indirect object – 6, 14

    b. Complement – 8, 10, 18,

    c. Adverbial – 3, 4, 5, 9, 16, 23, 24,

    d. Two conjoined clauses 7, 26

7.13. ACE elements of the clause: 1, 3, 9, 10 – SVA; 16, 17, 24, 26 – SVOiOd; 19, 21 – SVC (note that the S contains a PP; try the substitution test).

7.14. Cookie Theft Picture sentences:

    a. SVOdA

    b. SV

    c. SVC

    d. SVOiOd

    e. SVA

Chapter 8

General exercises

8.1.

    1. Declarative

    2. Interrogative

    3. Declarative

    4. Imperative

    5. Interrogative

8.2.

    1. You like oysters, don't you?

    2. Susan didn't leave a message, did she?

    3. We will go to the cinema, won't we?

    4. Your brother can read German, can't he?

8.3.

    1. *had been* delayed: passive

       got soaked by a lorry: passive

    2. *had driven his lorry*: active

    3. *will be stored*: passive

    4. *will store until the end of the year*: middle

       The Independent Magazine 20th Oct 2007 p. 99 Anna Pavord *Be Amazed.*

5. *tells very interesting stories*: active
6. *tell very well*: middle
7. *is always being interviewed*: passive
8. *interview for other jobs*: middle
9. actually pours without spilling: active
10. *to correct*: middle
11. *were blown off the roof by the storm*: passive
12. *has scratched our new door*: active
13. *scratches "excessively during normal usage"*: middle
14. *installs painlessly*: middle
15. *polishes up very nicely*: middle
16. *translate easily*: middle
17. *are being thoroughly cleansed and disinfected*: passive
18. *to be lubricated with special oil*: passive
19. *to cleanse and lubricate properly*: middle

Exercises using clinical resources

8.4. Complex Sentences section of the New RDLS, items with the passive structure: practice item xxii and items 54–56.

8.5. Recalling Sentences sub-test of the CELF-4:
   a. Passive interrogative – 5
   b. Active Interrogative – 2, 3, 6, 9.
   c. Negative – 6, 7, 10, 11, 17

8.6. VATT ditransitive construction: IH2, IH5

8.7. TAPS-R short passive: 5, 8, 9, 10, 12, 14, 15, 16, 18, 20, 21, 23, 29, 31, 32, 35, 36, 38, 39, 41, 43, 44, 45, 48

8.8. ERB Sentence Imitation Test:
   a. Negative – 1, 6
   b. Yes-no interrogative – 4, 8
   c. Imperative – 6
   d. Ditransitive – 10

8.9. CELF-Preschool:
   a. Imperative – 15
   b. Wh-interrogative – 11

Chapter 9

General exercises

9.1.
   1. *that Sabrina doesn't like camping*: complement clause
   2. *she took so long to write*: relative clause
   3. *Once they had a good night's sleep*: adverbial clause; *they liked our idea of going sailing*: complement clause
   4. *when they would arrive?*: complement clause

5. *my grandparents lived in*: relative clause
6. *as she explained the route*: adverbial clause
7. *when he heard that Alice was leaving*: adverbial clause; *that Alice was leaving*: complement clause
8. *as though she had tasted something sharp*: adverbial clause
9. *that our friends had to sell the house they'd just bought*: complement clause; *they'd just bought*: relative clause
10. *although his sister tried several times to talk to him about his decision*: adverbial clause

9.2.

1. *that she might borrow our flat*: complement clause
2. *that she describes in her book*: relative clause
3. *the theory that she has been working on*: relative clause
4. *that plants and animals evolved over millions of years*: complement clause

9.3.

1. *you bought the other day*: contact relative clause, restrictive
2. *who waved to us*: wh relative clause, restrictive
3. *that Jack built*: th relative clause, restrictive
4. *you found this example in*: contact relative clause, restrictive
5. *on which I keep the exam questions*: wh relative clause, restrictive
6. *which our son persuaded us to buy*: wh relative clause, non-restrictive
7. *many of which were not relevant*: wh relative clause, non-restrictive

9.4.

1. Compound
2. Compound
3. Complex
4. Complex
5. Complex
6. Compound
7. Compound
8. Complex
9. Simple
10. Complex

Exercises using clinical resources

9.5. CELF-Preschool, Sentence Structure subtest item 7: adverbial clause of reason.

9.6. Sentence Structure subtest of the CELF-4, subordinate clauses: 4, 5, 12 – relative clauses; 17 – adverbial clause of concession; 24 – adverbial clause of time.

9.7. ACE Narrative Syntax – adverbial clause of reason.

9.8. CELF-4 Recalling Sentences:
   a. relative clause – 15, 16, 20, 22, 23
   b. adverbial clause of condition – 19, 24, 29

    c. adverbial clause of reason – 13
    d. adverbial clause of concession – 14
    e. adverbial clause of time – 21, 27, 31

Chapter 10

General exercises

10.1.

    1. *Sailing in shark-infested waters*: Type 1 gerund
    2. *to lend her laptop to James*: infinitive
    3. *sitting up in the tree*: Type 2 gerund; *watching us*: free participle clause
    4. *lying on my desk*: reduced relative clause
    5. *Although not very tall*: reduced adverbial clause
    6. *when using electric carving knives*: reduced adverbial clause
    7. *spending hours sitting quietly and watching*: Type 1 gerund
    8. *sitting quietly and watching*: Type 2 gerund
    9. *Seeing that the youngster was in difficulty*: free participle clause
    10. *working on his memoirs*: Type 2 gerund
    11. *watching the team outplay their opponents*: Type 1 gerund
    12. *for us to win the competition*: infinitive

10.2. *Made in the classic Médocaine*: style free participle clause
    to marry the blend: infinitive clause
    and imbue the wine with subtle oak flavours: infinitive clause
    Though drinking well now: reduced adverbial clause
    cellaring for a year or two: Type 1 gerund
    drinking: Type 1 gerund

10.3. *to blow it up*: infinitive clause
    and then slowly let out the air: infinitive clause (*to* deleted) *to have to do this at least once or twice to get over the apparent humour involved in the chorus of a classroom of 40 students emptying balloons simultaneously*: infinitive clause

    to get over the apparent humour involved in the chorus of a classroom of 40 students emptying balloons simultaneously: infinitive clause

    emptying balloons simultaneously: reduced relative clause **OR** Type 2 gerund

10.4. *to hear the sound of heavy cartwheels rumbling over stones*: infinitive clause
    rumbling over stones: Type 2 gerund
    bouncing off the hills: reduced relative clause doing the night shift: reduced relative clause
    to be done at night: infinitive clause
    to be brought in from the cold: infinitive clause
    slithering and dripping from cell to synapse to neuro-transmitter until they arrived in the receptor marked 'suspicion': free participle clause
    feeling cheerful, and hopeful for the future: free participle clause

Exercises using clinical resources

10.5. LIST p. 5 reduced relative clauses: 3, 5, 6, 11, 12, 15, 19, 20.

10.6. Boston Diagnostic Aphasia Examination Auditory Comprehension block, section D3. Items 1, 4 and 5 contain a reduced relative clause.

10.7. CELF-4 Understanding Spoken Paragraphs: infinitive, gerund, free participle.
The Surprise: sentence 5, *coming* ... , Type 2 gerund.
Max and Lewis: sentence 1, *playing* ... Type 1 gerund; sentence 2, *to play* ... Infinitive; sentence 3, *to play* ... Infinitive; sentence 4, *coming* ... Infinitive; sentence 6, *chirping* ... , Type 2 gerund.
Marcus' Big Day: sentence 5, *To get ready for school*, Infinitive; sentence 5, *shopping* ... , Type 2 gerund; sentence 8, *to find* ... Infinitive.
Sports Day: sentence 5, *to wear* ... Infinitive
A Lucky Bear: sentence 1, *sniffing* ... Free participle; sentence 2, *eating* ... Type 1 gerund; sentence 4, *to escape* ... Infinitive.

10.8. Boston Diagnostic Aphasia Examination, Complex Ideational Material: Infinitive, Free participle, Reduced relative.
Mr Jones ... Infinitives in sentences 1 (*to go* ...), 2 (*to take* ...) and 4 (*for him to catch* ...)
A soldier ... Infinitive in sentences 1 (*to cash* ...) and 2 (*to have* ...).
A customer ... Free participle, sentence 1, *carrying* ... Reduced relative, sentence 4, *carrying their own* ...

Chapter 11

General exercises

11.1.

1	I	personal pronoun
	her	personal pronoun
	there	spatial deictic
	that	demonstrative
	I	personal pronoun
	That (that's)	demonstrative
2	there	spatial deictic
3	I	personal pronoun
	this	demonstrative
	we	personal pronoun
	He	personal pronoun
	this	demonstrative
	he	personal pronoun
	I (I'm)	personal pronoun
	him	personal pronoun
	that	demonstrative
	you	personal pronoun

11.2. Version A: The audience will see the interior of the staffroom with Leonardo sitting in a corner.
Version B: The audience will see the corridor outside the staffroom with the police preparing to kick open the door.

11.3. Discuss the targets of the underlined deictics in the following examples.

1. The policy may work in your country but I don't think it will work <u>here</u>.
   [Speaker and addressee are sitting in a pub in York.]
   England/UK
2. We really have quite dry weather <u>here</u> compared with Cumbria.
   [same speaker and location as for (1)]
   Yorkshire
3. The traffic police <u>here</u> are very polite compared with the French ones.
   [A Home Secretary talking on a discussion programme.]
   England/UK
4. The major sources of pollution are <u>here</u> and <u>here</u>.
   [Speaker draws imaginary circles on map.]
   Not the circles on the map but the areas of land that they represent.
5. <u>She</u> clearly understands the topic inside out.
   [Speaker taps assignment she is holding.]
   The student who wrote the essay
6. I remember the riots of 1968. We were on holiday in Paris <u>then</u>.
   The time of the riots.

11.4.

1. *They hunt in the Autumn*
   They hunt very specific creatures. Anyone with the frame 'hunting in the UK' knows what they are: foxes, pheasants, partridges.
2. *She's hunting upstairs* (= She's hunting for her driving licence.)
   Only possible if the driving licence has already been mentioned: *James is looking for Katarina's driving licence in the study and she is hunting upstairs.*
3. Barry washes, Jim dries and Dot puts away.
   The speaker assumes that the listener has a frame 'Washing up after a meal in the UK when there is no dishwasher'.
4. I'm cooking just now — I'll phone you back.
   Highly specific direct object: *a meal*. Needs frame 'domestic activities at certain times of the day'.
5. The accountant is cooking just now — he'll phone you back.
   (=The accountant is cooking the books.)
   Not acceptable, No conventionally accepted frame.
6. Jane buys for John Lewis.
   Requires a frame 'the running of large stores'.

11.5.

From a cardboard packet containing a bottle of cough linctus
Warnings
[the cough linctus] May cause drowsiness. If [you are] affected, do not drive or operate machinery. Avoid alcoholic drink.

Do not use if [the] bottle seal is broken when purchased. Keep bottle tightly closed.

Store [the bottle of cough linctus contained in the packet bearing the instructions that you are reading] below 30°C.

Keep [the bottle of cough linctus contained in the packet bearing the instructions that you are reading] out of the reach of children.

Require a frame containing information about the taking of medicine and another frame about instructions on medicine containers. They are written so as to address the person about to take the medicine. The noun phrases without articles are to be interpreted as referring to the things and people involved in a act of taking medicine that is about to be performed.

Exercises using clinical resources

11.6. Recalling Sentences in Context sub-test of the CELF-Preschool, items with direct speech that potentially involve 'shifting reference': this is potentially the case for any items that include deictic expressions within the inverted commas, e.g. p2, *we, our, then*; p3, *we*; p4, *we*; p5, *I*; p6, *this*; p7, *that*; p8, *I*; p9, *there*; p10, *I, myself*; p11, *those*; p12, *here, your*; p13, *you, this*; p14, *I, this*; p15, *I, these*; p16, *we, now*; p17, *I, myself*; p18, *I*; p19, *I, my*; p20, *you*; p21, *you*; p22, *tomorrow, we*; 23, *I, our, tomorrow*. (Note that this concept is not necessarily the aspect of processing that this subtest is trying to target.)

11.7. Questions that contain deictic expressions:
   a. Boston Diagnostic Aphasia Examination (p. 2, section A of the record booklet) – 1, *you, today*; 2, *you, here, before*; 3, *you, we*; 4, *you*; 5, *you, here*; 6, *your*; 7, *your*.
   b. Western Aphasia Battery (Part 1) – 1, *you, today*; 2, *you, here, before*; 3, *your*; 4, *your*; 5, *your*; 6, *you, here*.

11.8. Items that specifically target client's processing of deixis:
   a. CAPPA (Part A, section 1) – item 6
   b. CCC-2 – item 10 (item 1 mentions personal pronouns, but the focus is gender rather than deixis; similarly item 17 is about subjective and objective forms of pronouns).

(Note that other items do require incidental processing of deixis, as in question 2.)

Chapter 12

General exercises

12.1.
   a. Find an ATM. Stand well back from anyone already using it. When the ATM is free, step forward. Insert your card. Punch in your code. Read the menu. Guide the cursor to the arrow at the box you want, state how much

money you want to withdraw (if you are withdrawing money), take the money when it appears in the slot, take your card and take your receipt.

b. Stay in your seat until the seat belt sign goes out. Collect any hand baggage and any other belongings. (Depending on adrenalin and where you are seated) stand up and wait for the line of passengers to start moving OR stay seated and join the line of passengers once some space has appeared in the aisle. Leave the plane and EITHER walk through the bridge into the terminal building OR walk down the steps from the door of the plane to the ground and get on a bus. Once at passport control, join one of the queues. Once you get close to the passport officer's desk or booth, get out your passport and have it ready to hand over. Once the passport is returned, go to the baggage carousels, find which one your plane's baggage is going to arrive on, collect a trolley and wait. (If you have no baggage to be delivered to the carousel, pass through the baggage hall and out into the hall where people wait to meet friends and relatives who are arriving.)

12.2.

1. We're going to my parents for Christmas but I don't know how we'll get the Christmas tree into the car.
   Frame for Christmas includes Christmas tree, a conifer to be decorated. A central part of Christmas decorations.

2. A train drew into the station and the driver got down onto the platform. Most trains still have drivers. In train stations in the United Kingdom, trains stop alongside platforms which allow travellers easy access to the carriages.

3. We leave St Pancras at 11. The train arrives in Paris at 12.30.
   Frame: St Pancras is the train station from which the Eurostar trains leave for Paris. People book seats on specific trains.

12.3.

1. In her new school she blossomed.
   Source domain: Boys and girls learning and maturing at school.
   Target domain: Plants or trees being cultivated, growing and producing flowers.

2. The proposal turned out to be a lead balloon.
   Source domain: Putting forward a proposal for consideration by a committee or by friends, etc.
   Target domain: Balloons, made of a very light material, being inflated and rising into the air. Lead is a very heavy material. Balloons are not made of lead but any balloon that was made of lead would not rise off the ground at all. Proposals and ideas are often said to take off or fly, or to go down like a lead balloon.

3. In their anger they had a heated argument.
   Source domain: Anger
   Target domain: Heat (from a fire)

4. He can't get over the death of his wife.
   Source domain: Death and grief
   Target domain: Climbing over an obstacle.

12.4.

1. Vera <u>even</u> handed in her essay on time.
   There are many things that Vera does not do and handing in her essay on time is one that she usually never manages. This time she has accomplished a number of things, including the most unexpected one.
2. <u>Even</u> Vera managed to attend all the classes.
   Of all the students, Vera is the one who misses most classes and the one least likely to attend all of them in a given period of time.
3. Louise <u>almost</u> fell over the cliff.
   Louise was on the edge of the cliff, slipped or lost her balance, was beginning to fall and would have fallen if, e.g. somebody had not grabbed her.
4. Louise <u>almost</u> bought a ticket.
   Louise thought about buying a ticket (say, a lottery ticket), was tempted to do so but in the end decided not to. She didn't actually start the process of buying a ticket (whereas in (3) she did begin to fall).
5. Louise <u>almost</u> finished writing her bestseller.
   Louise began writing the book, kept at it and just had another chapter to write (when she fell ill/got fed up).
6. I <u>really</u> like your theory.
   Believe me, I'm very enthusiastic about your theory.
7. I don't <u>really</u> know him.
   I know who he is but I don't know anything about his character or interests.
8. I <u>really</u> don't know him.
   I know you think I know him but, believe me, I don't.
9. <u>Evidently</u> they are going to sell the estate.
   The speaker has heard from some source, possibly not reliable, that the estate is to be sold.
10. I haven't written that reference <u>yet</u>.
    The reference is not written but the speaker intends to write it (soon).

12.5.   1.   A: Have you sent Ken an e-mail?

B: I am.

B is engaged in composing an e-mail to send to Ken.

2.   A: Would you like me to deliver the computer to your house?

B: Could you?

Would A be able to deliver the computer to B's house?

Would A be willing to deliver the computer to B's house?

3.   I suggested he leave it till next week but he didn't agree.

The person the speaker asked to wait until next week before taking some action did not do what the speaker requested.

Exercises using clinical resources

12.6. TALC/frames and scripts: this resource has a variety of picture tasks that would draw on frames (to help with the processing of scenarios like a playground, a supermarket or a birthday party). There are also pictures that have to be sequenced; these would draw on scripts. Children are expected to be able to use this information from level 2, when they need it to be able to 'describe a simple picture', then on into level 3 (sequencing) and beyond.

12.7. CAPPA, item 21: Informativeness, which enjoins speakers and writers not to say more than is required.

12.8. Sheffield Screening Test for Acquired Language Disorders, scripts – item 8, sequencing.

12.9. MCLA/metaphor – Verbal Abstract Reasoning (quotations and multiple choice).

12.10. CCC-2:
   a. Jokes – 15
   b. Irony – 54
   c. Scripts – 40 (particularly if talking about stereotypical events)
   d. The I-Principle – 37, 42, 61

12.11. In the ASDS, identify items that focus particularly on
   a. Jokes and sarcasm – 4
   b. Levinson's principles – 1 (M); possibly also 2 (I)

Chapter 13

General exercises

13.1.

   1. I bet on the horses but only occasionally.
      Not performative. The speaker describes an act that he or she carries out from time to time.
   2. I bet you fifty quid her horse will win.
      Performative. The speaker makes a bet in uttering the words.
   3. A   What did Brian say just now?
      B   He bets you fifty quid that Alice's horse will win.
      Not performative. The speaker describes a bet that someone else has just made.
   4. Louise says she speaks French but I bet she's never been near the country.
      Not performative. The speaker is not actually making a bet. This is an extended use of *bet*.
   5. I'm asking you politely not drop your rubbish in my garden.
      Not performative. The speaker is describing the act. The most likely scenario is that the speaker is saying that they are not threatening the addressee but asking them politely.

6. I ask you: have you ever seen such a mess?
   Performative, but only used in situations when the speaker is taken aback or dismayed by some state of affairs.

7. I give you notice that you are no longer a member of the club.
   Performative. Very formal.

8. I'm giving you notice that you are no longer a member of the club.
   Not performative. The speaker describes the act they are about to carry out, perhaps handing over a written notice.

9. I apologise for any delay but air traffic control have just asked us to go into holding.
   Performative.

10. I'm apologising for the loss of your luggage but not for the delay in landing.
    Not performative. An explanation of an act just carried out.

13.2.

1. Have you received the cheque I posted to you last week?
   Preparatory conditions
   The speaker is entitled to ask the question.
   The addressee is in a position to answer the question.
   Sincerity conditions
   The speaker is being truthful with respect to the cheque.
   The speaker does not know the answer to the question.
   The speaker genuinely wants to know the answer.

2. Who helped Fiona to organise the party last Saturday?
   Preparatory conditions
   The speaker is entitled to ask the question.
   The addressee is in a position to answer the question.
   The speaker is correct in presupposing that a party took place.
   Sincerity conditions
   The speaker does not know the answer to the question.
   The speaker genuinely wants to know the answer.

3. Do you think we're made of money? (Parent to child)
   Preparatory conditions
   The speaker is entitled to ask the question.
   The addressee is in a position to answer the question.
   Sincerity conditions
   The speaker does not know the answer to the question.
   The speaker genuinely wants to know the answer.

4. Why can't we buy a Wii? Everybody else has one.
   (Child to parent for the nth time)
   Preparatory conditions
   The speaker is entitled to ask the question.
   The addressee is in a position to answer the question.
   Sincerity conditions
   The speaker does not know the answer to the question.
   The speaker genuinely wants to know the answer.

5. The car won't be ready till tomorrow, will it?
   Preparatory conditions
   The speaker is entitled to ask the question.
   The addressee is in a position to answer the question.
   Sincerity conditions
   The speaker is not completely confident of the answer to the question.
   The speaker thinks the answer is 'The car won't be ready till tomorrow'.
   The speaker genuinely wants to know the answer.
6. The car will be ready tomorrow, won't it?
   Preparatory conditions
   The speaker is entitled to ask the question.
   The addressee is in a position to answer the question.
   Sincerity conditions
   The speaker is not completely confident of the answer to the question.
   The speaker expects/would like the answer to be 'The car will be ready by tomorrow'.
   The speaker genuinely wants to know the answer.
7. Can you close the window?
   This is not a genuine question. The sincerity conditions are not met. It is an indirect request to the addressee to shut the window. This type of question is so frequent that analysts talk of the preparatory and sincerity conditions for questions being short-circuited. Addressees go straight to the conditions for commands and requests.

13.3.

1. From B3 to C13 the supertopic is 'School visit to outdoor activities centre'.
2. A1–B2 Initial subtopic: going to university
   B3–C13   events at the outdoor activities centre
      B3–C2   introduction
      C3–B6   canoeing
      C6–C13   camping
         C6   rucksacks
         B7–B9   hillwalking
         C9–C13   abseiling
   B13–B14   another school camp
   A12–C17   sixth-year students

3. Topic introductions
   Major introductions of new topics
      A1   What about eh what aspirations do you have you know for University? What kind of life do you think you'll have when you get there? You must have some views about it.
      A4   Are you interested in sport?
      B13   We're going on a school camp at the end of May which should be similar – the same type of thing.
      A12   What is your sixth year like? You know, what kind of personalities?
   Smooth shifts from one sub-topic to a related sub-topic.
      A4   Are you interested in sport?

B3   Well certain things. Like we were at an activities – an outdoor
       education centre
C3   Well the first day we went canoeing and
C5   and the next day we canoed round Loch Lomond which was a
       good day
C6   And they decided they would take us camping overnight
B7   except we had to hillwalk up a hill with the rucksacks on
C9   It was good at night. We went abseiling the next day
A6   Yeah. I've heard that word before. How do you spell that word?
       I've often wondered.
B12   Except I'm a bit of a coward and I didn't go down a big face
C12   I did.
A10   What was that like.
B15   And there's one girl — she's a real extrovert you know.
A13   There's only four boys?

4. Topic shifting: Major shifts of topic are done by A asking questions.
5. Repair: all self-initiated self-repair
    B3   Well certain things. Like we were at an activities – an outdoor
           education centre
    A8   Yeah. I've heard someone – my brother did it before.
    A12   What is your sixth year like? You know, what kind of personalities?
6. Joint narrative: C3–C13. Joint characteristics: C3-C6: the speakers take
    it in turn to produce main clauses. From B4, each main clause is linked
    by 'and' with the preceding one and adds another event to the narra-
    tive. C7 and C8 add bits of description to the events described in B7
    and B8.
7. Ellipsis
    B3   Well (**we're interested in**) certain things.
    B9   Yeah. It was. (**really bad**)
    A9   Is it? (**great**)
    C11   Oh yeah. (**It's**) Great.
    C12   I did. (**go down a big face**)

Exercises using clinical resources

13.4. Items in the CCC-2 that particularly refer to
    a. Conversational openings – 21, 31,
    b. Politeness – 59, 60
    c. Paralinguistic skills – 8, 14, 20, 39, 56, 57, 65, 70
    d. Topic management – 5, 26

13.5. CELF-4 Pragmatics Profile:
    a. Opening conversations – 1, 3, 16, 20
    b. Closing conversations – 2, 3, 16
    c. Turn-taking - 4, 21, 22
    d. Adjacency pairs and preference structure – 1, 2, 3, 11, 20
    e. Paralinguistic skills – 5
    f. Topic management – 6, 7, 8, 9, 10, 11, 12

13.6. Identify items in the ASDS that particularly refer to
   a. Opening conversations – Language subscale, 9
   b. Paralinguistic skills – Social subscale, 1, 2, 4, 9
   c. Turn-taking – Social subscale, 13

13.7. CAPPA:
   a. Opening conversations – 16
   b. Repair – 12-13
   c. Turn-taking – 17, 18, 19, 20
   d. Topic management – 23-26

13.8. MCLA: the following items are part of the Pragmatic Rating Scale
   a. Opening conversations – Initiation
   b. Turn-taking – Turn-taking
   c. Paralinguistic skills – Intonation, Facial expression, Eye contact, Gestures, Proxemics
   d. Topic management – Topic maintenance

13.9. 'Inconsistent Messages of Emotion' in the Understanding Ambiguity resource: paralanguage.

Chapter 14

General exercises

14.1. Cohesion
   I decided to try and write a popular book about space and time **after** I gave the Loed lecture at Harvard in 1982. There were **already** a considerable number of books about the early universe and black holes, ranging from the very good, **such as** Steven Weinberg's book, *The First Three Minutes*, **to** the very bad, **which** I will not identify. **However** I felt none of them really addressed **the** questions that had led me to do research in cosmology and quantum theory: **where** did the universe come from? **How** and **why** did it begin? Will it come to an end and if **so**, how? **These** are the questions that are of interest to us all.

Exercises using clinical resources

14.2. Written Narrative Rating Scale

14.3.
   a. Cohesion in the 'Renfrew Bus Story'
      1. Words, phrases and clauses marking the order of events.

      Paragraph 4:   As soon as he saw . . . he tried to stop
                          When the driver found . . . he telephoned

      Otherwise no items. The order of events is conveyed by one clause following another or connected by *and*. Compare the answer below for 'Peter and the Cat'.

2. **Words, phrases and clauses marking causal connections.**

Paragraph 2:   But
                    because

Paragraph 3:   But So
Paragraph 4   But So

3. **Full nouns and pronouns marking new items and given items.**

Paragraph 1:   bus his driver
Paragraph 2:   He (linking with *the bus* in paragraph 1)
                    a train they (they = the bus and the train)
                    the bus he he
                    a policeman his

Paragraph 3:   bus he he he
Paragraph 5:   bus he he he his he, driver he,
                    (found where the) bus (was) him him

4. **Ellipted subjects signalling same subject (i.e. same participant as in the situation described by the previous clause.**

Paragraph 1:   decided to run away
Paragraph 2:   made funny faces raced
Paragraph 3:   paid ran on
Paragraph 4:   tried to stop
                    didn't know how to put on
                    he fell and stuck
                    (a crane) to pull put him

Background events

Paragraph 1:   While his driver was trying... decided

b. **Cohesion in 'Peter and the Cat'**
   1. **Words, phrases and clauses marking the order of events.**
      Once there was, One day, At first, Then the cat meowed,
      When he got to the top, again and again, Finally + after a long time,
      When he saw, When Peter got home.
   2. **Words, phrases and clauses marking causal connections.**

      Maybe if I call + So Peter yelled
      scolded him + because
   3. **Full nouns and pronouns marking new items and given items.**

   p.3   Peter he him he
          the cat it (This sequence occurs twice.)

   p.7   Peter he he
   p.9   Peter wondered he thought
          Peter yelled he could He yelled again heard him

   p.11   Peter heard him
   p.13   he saw [*he* is an anaphor – it picks up the reference of *a man* on
   p.11   but is simultaneously a cataphor, pointing forward to *the man*
          in *the man* quickly got a ladder.

p.17   Peter his him
        his mother asked her
        his mother

4. Ellipted subjects signalling same subject (i.e. same participant as in the situation described by the previous clause.

p.5   decided + to climb + to rescue
p.7   He sat + hanging on
p.9   wondered what to do
p.13   got + and helped

5. Background events

p.3   was walking
p.11   watering (= 'who was watering')
p.15   shaking with fright

Chapter 15

General exercises

15.1. Given and new

Silk-Cotton Blouse	The caption above the description.
this rather light silk-cotton mix	given; already mentioned in the caption.
You	given; writer pretends they are addressing each reader individually.
all the style and breathability you demand	given; assumed to be known to the reader.
[It is] Exquisitely finished	given; subject noun is omitted because the blouse and the material it is made from, plus two other properties, have already been mentioned.
notch neck	new; first mention.
neat Mandarin collar	new; first mention.
gentle pleating from the shoulder	new; first mention.
the shoulder	given; frame containing information about garments for the upper body. They all have shoulders.
self covered buttons	new; first mention.
Stylish Silk Trousers	The caption above the description.
Pure Fuji silk trousers	new; the referent is treated as new for the reader because although stylish silk trousers have been mentioned, pure Fuji silk has not.
a matt sandwashed finish	new; first mention.
discreet back elastication	new; first mention.
smart flat front	new; first mention.
two side pockets	new; first mention.
this classic straight leg trouser	given; salient in the photograph. Readers have a frame for trousers containing the information that all trousers have legs.
your perfect summer outfitter	given; addressed to each reader individually and is in the summer catalogue.

15.2. Given and new

i. Three people:

the man referred to by the Bursar: *him [5]*, *He [6]*, *he's [7]*

the Bursar: *me, He [1], his [2], his [3], he [4], I* in *I've, I* in *I don't know, He [8], his [9]*.

the Librarian: *he [10], [He's] Not good*

ii. General convention that third person pronoun relates to the nearest full noun phrase: *He [1]* picks up the referent of *the Bursar* at the end of the immediately preceding sentence. By convention, any following third person pronouns of the same gender pick up the same referent., i.e. *He [1], his [2], his [3], he [4]*. The next sentence represents direct speech by the Bursar. *him [5]* and *He [6]* cannot therefore refer to the Bursar, nor to the Dean. The only other possible referent is 'that man'. The sentence *He [8] blew his [9] nose* is taken by convention as not seriously separated from the earlier sequence of *he* and *his* by the direct speech, so the third person pronouns are interpreted as referring to the Bursar. Out of context the referent of *he [10]* is mysterious. Anyone reading the book knows that the Bursar is inquiring after the Librarian, and two lines further down the page the phrase *The Librarian* occurs.

15.3. Theme

The theme phrases are shown in bold.

The Entrance Hall

Entering the room the visitor immediately notices the sturdy columns and rounded arches that divide the room into three. **The single column on the right** carries two arches, has an octagonal capital, in contrast to the two plainer columns on the left, which support three arches. **Above the fireplace** a decorative map shows the town as it was in the seventeenth century. **Unfortunately** the map suffered water damage in the flood of 1981.

Going through the door to the right of the fireplace the visitor enters the kitchen. **It** has a surprisingly wide stone fireplace. Inside the fireplace is a nineteenth-century kitchen range. **Beside the range** is an early eighteenth-century settle in elm. **The wall clock** is by a local clock maker. **Another item of note** is a Flemish iron-bound oak coffer with a domed lid.

Some phrases are in theme position because they have to do with the visitor moving around the building and with the visitor's gaze being directed to particular locations in each room: *Entering the room, Above the fireplace, Going through the door to the right of the fireplace, Beside the range*. These themes act as a bridge from one location to the next.

Note the theme phrase *The single column on the right*. At first glance it doesn't look like a location phrase but it contains the phrase *on the right*.

The wall clock is the subject noun phrase in a straightforward clause. The main participants in the narrative are the items in the rooms and the visitor. In addition *The wall clock* ties in with the last phrase of the previous sentence, *an early eighteenth-century settle in elm*. If the sentence had been *A local clock maker made the wall clock*, it would have made prominent a new participant and put the given participant, or given information, to the end of the sentence. Given information is usually mentioned first and new information is brought in at the end of a clause.

The theme *Another item of note* acts as a bridge from the previous sentence. It is part of a sequence going from the settle, to the wall clock, to 'another thing that the visitor should pay attention to'. It states what is important – you should look at what is about to be mentioned – and avoids a sequence of noun phrases: *the X, the Y, the Z*.

15.4. IT clefts
i) Jane Austen
    It was Jane Austen who wrote *Pride and Prejudice* . . .
    Jane Austen is treated as new information.
ii) *Pride and Prejudice*
    It was *Pride and Prejudice* that Jane Austen wrote in the sitting-room . . .
    Pride and Prejudice is treated as new information.
iii) in the sitting-room
    It was in the sitting-room of the parsonage at Chawton that Jane Austen wrote *Pride and Prejudice* round about 1805.

    in the sitting-room of the parsonage at Chawton is treated as new information.
iv) round about 1805
    It was round about 1805 that Jane Austen wrote *Pride and Prejudice* in the sitting-room of the parsonage at Chawton.
    round about 1805 is treated as new information.

And note the newer alternative construction for (iii) and (iv).
It was in the sitting-room of the parsonage at Chawton **where** Jane Austen wrote *Pride and Prejudice* round about 1805.
It was round about 1805 **when** Jane Austen wrote *Pride and Prejudice* in the sitting-room of the parsonage at Chawton.

To construct an IT cleft focusing on *at Chawton* you have to split up the phrase *in the sitting-room of the parsonage at Chawton*:
It was at Chawton, in the sitting-room of the parsonage, that Jane Austen wrote *Pride and Prejudice* round about 1805.

15.5. Focus constructions: use and misuse
Fiona Dalhousie wanted to enter the diplomatic service and at university she studied languages. Her father died before she completed her degree. Her mother was also dead, so she had to rely on her own efforts and earn her living. She was always keen on foreign travel and moved heaven and earth to get a job as a courier with a large travel firm. Her knowledge of several foreign languages was in her favour, plus her experience of several Alpine

ski resorts. She had also travelled to India. A vacancy that arose, she applied for the post, and was appointed.

15.6. Focus in a written narrative

A warm welcome to our summer silk collection!

This is a text sentence containing just a noun phrase. The first chunk is a fixed expression: *A warm welcome*. It requires little processing effort. The important phrase, *summer silk collection*, is at the end of the text sentence, a position in which words and phrases are relatively prominent.

Nothing beats the luxurious feel of natural fibres against your skin and summer is the perfect time to try our range of exquisite fabrics.

From cosy cotton nightwear to comfortable stylish daywear we have something for everyone.

The important phrase conveying the range of clothing on offer is right at the beginning of the sentence: *From cosy cotton nightwear to comfortable stylish daywear*. This is a position where words and phrases are also prominent, and it is an unusual position for this type of prepositional phrase, which also catches the reader's attention.

Travelling is made easy, silk tees pack away to nothing and keep you cool and fresh always.

Note the middle construction in *silk tees pack away to nothing*. The writer avoids a more complex piece of syntax such as *You can pack silk tees away to nothing*. By avoiding any mention of an agent the writer keeps the focus on the silk tees and by using the middle is also able to keep *silk tees* at the centre of the sentence by continuing to the next clause, which does not need an overt subject noun phrase: *and keep you cool and fresh always*. This clause also keeps the silk tees prominent by presenting them as agents, doing something for the wearer.

are so light, easy to wash and slow to crease that you can travel light and still have plenty of room for souvenirs.

Here again the use of the middle construction — *slow to crease* — keeps *silk tees* at the centre of the syntax and allows the writer to have three simple phrases resulting from chunks being ellipted from three clauses: *[silk tees] are so light, [silk tees are so] easy to wash and [silk tees are so] slow to crease...*

Crisp cottons and silk dresses see you through a casual day out or a special event.

A transitive clause with the items of clothing presented as agents doing something for the wearer and made prominent by being referred to by the subject noun phrase.

Exercises using clinical resources

15.7. The IT-Cleft

15.8. The FAST River Scene:
FM = first mention
D = deixis
FR = information from frame
P = perspective

The picture [Given FM] shows a landscape [new FM]. In the foreground [Given FR FM] is a river [new FM] and there are hills [new FM] in the background [Given FR FM]. Right in the front [Given FR FM D] of the picture [Given] there is a man [New]. He [Given] is walking his dog [given]. The dog [Given] is standing still looking at something out of the picture [given]. The man [given] is waving to another man [new] on a barge [new]. This man [given] is standing at the stern [given FR] holding the tiller [given FR]. Close to the bank [given] is a kayak [new FM] paddled by a boy [new FM]. Just beyond [D] the barge [given] there is a rowing boat [new FM]. The oars [given] are very long compared with the paddle [given FR] being used by the person [given] in the kayak [given]. This rowing boat [given] is going upstream [D] and is about to go under a bridge [new FM]. The bridge [given] is built of stones and has the shape [given FR] of an arch. On this side [given] of the bridge [given] there are steps [new FM] going up [D P] to a road or path [new FM] and there are two tall trees [new FM]. Between the rowing boat [given] and the barge [given] there is a duck [new FM] swimming and close to the spot [given] where the man [given] is walking there are two more ducks [new FM]. On the opposite [D] bank [given] from the man [given] is a warehouse [new FM], and beyond [D P] the bridge [given], partly hidden by a tree [new FM], is a house [new FM]. No smoke is coming [D P] out of the chimneys [given FR] and the trees [given] have all their leaves [given FR]. The man [given] walking his dog [given] is in his shirtsleeves [given FR], so it is probably a summer day [new FM].

Chapter 16

General exercises

16.1. End weight
Restructured examples
1. The principle of end weight is not relevant to this example because it contains no long or complex noun phrases.
2. Barnabas showed the new puppy they had just collected from the kennels to his friends.
Barnabas showed his friends the new puppy they had just collected from the kennels.

3. That the Government made a mistake in downgrading the level of threat to the embassy is now beyond doubt.
   It is now beyond doubt that the Government made a mistake in down-grading the level of threat to the embassy.
4. That this is a serious error has been agreed.
   It has been agreed that this is a serious error.
5. That the directors persuaded the CEO to make illegal payments has been discovered by the inquiry.
   It has been discovered by the inquiry that the directors persuaded the CEO to make illegal payments.
6. Whether the attacks will succeed in dislodging the guerrillas or merely turn out to be a huge waste of resources is difficult to predict.
   It is difficult to predict whether the attacks will succeed in dislodging the guerrillas or merely turn out to be a huge waste of resources.

Exercises using clinical resources

16.2. Boston Diagnostic Aphasia Examination, Cookie Theft Picture narrative.
Prog = Progressive
Sp = Simple Present
Perf = Perfect
Futbg = 'be going to' Future
FM = first mention
D = deixis
FR = information from frame
P = perspective
gen ref = generic reference
TH = clause theme (follows the theme phrase)

Almost in the middle [given FR] of the picture [given] TH you [given FR] can see a woman [new FM] in a kitchen [new FM]. Behind her [given] TH are two children, a girl [new FM] and a boy [new FM]. The woman [given] TH is standing [Prog] at the kitchen sink [given FR]. She [given] TH 's drying [Prog] a plate [new FM] and [given ellipsis] seems to be thinking [Prog] about something else [new FM] because she [given] TH has not noticed [Perf] that the water [given FR] TH is pouring [Prog] over the edge [given FR] of the sink [given] and on to the floor [given FR]. But she [given] TH will probably notice quite soon because a puddle of water [new FM] TH has appeared [Perf] round her feet [given FR] and [given ellipsis] is getting [Prog] bigger. On the countertop [given] beside the sink [given] TH are two small bowls [new FM] and a plate [new FM]. It TH looks as though the family [given] TH have just had [Perf] lunch. Along the end wall [given] of the kitchen [given] TH is a row of cupboards [new FM] and in one of them [given] TH, on the top shelf [given], is a jar of biscuits. The boy [given] TH has climbed [Perf] up on a three-legged stool so that he [given] TH can reach the jar. [given] He [given] TH has taken [Perf] one biscuit from the jar [given] and [given ellipsis] has been handing [Perf] it [given] to the girl [given]. Unfortunately three-legged stools [gen ref] are not very stable and the stool [given] has begun [Perf] to topple over. The girl [given] is reaching [Prog] out her hand [given] to take the biscuit [given] the boy [given] is holding [Prog] out to her [given] but there is going to [**Futbg**] be a nasty accident. The boy [given] TH is going to [**Futbg**] fall to the floor [given] and unless he [given] TH lets go, he TH 'll [**Fut**] pull the jar of biscuits [given] down with him [given].

16.3. Fish Story (Version 1)
Prog = Progressive
Sp = Simple Present
Perf = Perfect
TH = theme

The story begins [**Sp**] in the living room of a house. A boy is standing [**Prog**] beside a fish tank containing one fish. His mother comes [**Sp**] into the room and he asks [**Sp**] if he can have money to buy another fish to keep the first one company. He sets off [**Sp**] for the shops. In the third picture he is walking [**Prog**] along a path with grass on either side and is carrying [**Prog**] an orange bag. In the fourth picture he has reached [**Perf**] the town centre and is walking [**Prog**] along a street. A motorbike passes [**Sp**] him. In the following two pictures the boy has arrived [**Perf**] at the pet shop and is pointing [**Prog**] to the tanks containing fish. The shop assistant has taken [**Perf**] a bowl of water, put [**Perf**] a fish into it and is putting [**Prog**] the bowl into the bag. The boy is walking home [**Prog**] when he meets [**Sp**] two girls he knows, an older girl and a younger girl. One of the girls is carrying [**Prog**] a yellow bag. The boy and the older girl go to a kiosk to buy ice creams. They leave the younger girl sitting on a bench. She takes [**Sp**] a doll out of the yellow bag and the bowl out of the orange bag but puts [**Sp**] the doll back in the orange bag and the bowl in the yellow bag. When they have finished [**Perf**] eating their ice creams and chatting they set off [**Sp**] for home but are going [**Prog**] in opposite directions. The big girl is carrying [**Prog**] the yellow bag, which now contains [**Sp**] the fish bowl, and the boy is carrying [**Prog**] the orange bag, which now contains [**Sp**] the doll. In the next set of pictures the boy has arrived [**Perf**] at his house and is taking [**Prog**] the doll out of the bag. He realizes [**Sp**] what has happened [**Perf**] and tells [**Sp**] his mother. She phones [**Sp**] the big girl's mother. In the penultimate picture the boy's mother is talking [**Prog**] to the two girls, who have come [**Perf**] to the boy's house to give him his fish bowl and collect their doll. The final picture shows [**Sp**] the new fish swimming in the tank with the first fish. The boy is pointing [**Prog**] to the tank and saying [**Prog**] something to the girls, hopefully 'Thank you very much'.

Annotated Bibliography

Bauer, L. (1983) *English Word-Formation*. Cambridge University Press.
Clear and comprehensive coverage.
Bauer, L. (1998) *Vocabulary*. London: Routledge.
A concise and very readable account of this topic.
Bracken, B. & Panter, J. (2011) Using the Bracken Basic Concept Scale and Bracken Concept Development Program in the assessment and remediation of young children's concept development. *Psychology in the Schools*, 48(5), 464–475.
Brown, E.K. & Miller, J. (1991) *Syntax: A Linguistic Introduction to Sentence Structure*. London: Harper Collins.
An introductory text that discusses various aspects of sentence structure within a traditional framework.
Cheepen, C. (1988) *The Predictability of Informal Conversation*. Open Linguistics Series. London: Pinter.
A clearly written, straightforward and short introduction. In spite of its age, it is very worthwhile reading it.
Coates, R. (1999) *Word Structure*. London: Routledge.
A more concise introduction.
Collins, P. & Hollo, C. (2000) *English Grammar: An Introduction*. Macmillan.
Very clear. More detailed account of English grammar and narrative than in this book.
Cruse, A. (2004 and later edition) *Meaning in Language*. Oxford University Press.
An advanced textbook on semantics but clear and with excellent examples.
Crystal, D. (1992) *Profiling Linguistic Disability*. 2nd edition. London: Whurr.
This text provides frameworks for analysis of various aspects of language, including the LARSP.
Cummings, L. (2008) *Clinical Linguistics*. Edinburgh: Edinburgh University Press.
An introductory survey of work on various aspects of clinical linguistics.
Fernandez, E.M. & Cairns, H.S. (2011) *Fundamentals of Psycholinguistics*. Chichester, West Sussex: Wiley-Blackwell.
A recent introduction to psycholinguistics.
Fudge, E. (1984) *English Word Stress*. London: Allen & Unwin.
Useful lists of prefixes and suffixes.
Greenbaum, S. & Quirk, R. (1990) *A Student's Grammar of the English Language*. Harlow: Longman.

Introductory Linguistics for Speech and Language Therapy Practice, First Edition. Jan McAllister and Jim Miller.
© 2013 John Wiley & Sons, Ltd. Published 2013 by John Wiley & Sons, Ltd.

A comprehensive discussion of parts of speech and other linguistic concepts.

Harley, T. (2008) *The Psychology of Language: From Theory to Practice*. Hove: Psychology Press.

Clearly written and a good introduction to the area.

Hudson, R. (1995) *Word Meaning*. London: Routledge.

A concise introduction to key concepts in word meaning.

Hurford, J.R. (1994) *Grammar: A Student's Guide*. Cambridge University Press.

An encyclopaedia-dictionary. The entries are excellent and cover the central concepts used in this book. It focuses on English.

Hutchby, I. & Wooffitt, R. (2008) *Conversation Analysis*. Cambridge, UK and Boston, MA: Polity Press.

A clear introduction to the analysis of conversation with good examples.

Leech, G.N., Rayson, P. & Wilson, A. (2001) *Word frequencies in written and spoken English: based on the British National Corpus*. Harlow: Longman.

Frequency information about thousands of words, including lists organised according to parts of speech and other useful categories.

Löbner, S. (2002) *Understanding Semantics*. London: Arnold.

An introduction to various relevant concepts.

Lyons, J. (1995) *Linguistic Semantics*. Cambridge University Press.

A comprehensive discussion of semantics.

Marshall, J., Byng, S. & Black, M. (1999) *The Sentence Processing Resource Pack*. Bicester: Winslow.

A clinical resource with an introduction that provides useful linguistic background.

Miller, J. (2008) *An Introduction to English Syntax*. Edinburgh University Press.

Takes a different perspective from this book but assumes no knowledge on the part of the reader.

Snodgrass, J.G. & Vanderwart, M. (1980) A standardized set of 260 pictures: norms for name agreement, image agreement, familiarity, and visual complexity. *Journal of Experimental Psychology: Human Perception and Performance*, 6, 174–215.

Stackhouse, J. & Wells, B. (1997) *Children's Speech and Literacy Difficulties: A psycholinguistic framework*. San Diego, CA: Singular.

Wooffitt, R. (2005) *Conversation Analysis and Discourse Analysis: A Comparative and Critical Introduction*. London: Sage.

A sociological perspective, but very insightful.

Index

active, 44–9, 111–2, 115, 120, 123, 127, 129
actor, 45
acts of reference, 27
adjacency pairs, 234–5
adjective, 71–4
　attributive use, 72
　predicative use, 72
adjective phrase, 116
Advanced Syntactic Test of Pronominal Reference A-STOP-R, 84
adverb, 78–80, 256–7
　of degree, 79
adverbial, 129–31
adverbial clause of concession, 156
adverbial clause of condition, 156
adverbial clause of reason, 156
adverbial clause of time, 156
adverb phrase, 116–17
affix, 87–9, 94
agent, 45–9
age of acquisition, 21–2
allomorph, 90–92
allomorphy, 90
alternant, 91
ambiguity, 217–18
　lexical, 217–18
　syntactic, 217–18
anaphoric reference, 66, 257
animacy, 32
antecedent, 65-6
antonym, 36
ARC database, 23
aspect
　in narrative, 280–83
　use of progressive, 282–3

back-channel, 235
bare-verb clause, 175
base, 88
basic construction, 138–9
beneficiary, 46
binary semantic features, 30
Boehm Test of Basic Concepts, 32
Boston Diagnostic Aphasia Examination, 52, 134, 180, 203
bound form, 89–90
bound morpheme, 89
Bracken Basic Concept Scale, 32, 35, 40
bridge (reference), 201
Bristol Norms, 17
British National Corpus, 19

CAPPA (Conversation Analysis Profile for People with Aphasia), 203, 222, 224, 241, 242, 246, 247
CAPPCI (Conversation Analysis Profile for People with Cognitive Impairment), 211, 224, 241, 242, 246
CAT (Comprehensive Aphasia Test), 15, 24, 83, 105, 117
cataphora, 257
cataphoric, 66, 257
category, 27
CCC-2 (Children's Communication Checklist), 9, 203, 222, 241, 246
CDI (communicative development inventory), 21
CELF-4 (Clinical Evaluation of Language Fundamentals), 3, 14, 28, 35, 39, 44, 66, 68, 84, 86, 92, 96, 102

Introductory Linguistics for Speech and Language Therapy Practice, First Edition. Jan McAllister and Jim Miller.
© 2013 John Wiley & Sons, Ltd. Published 2013 by John Wiley & Sons, Ltd.